S0-BAD-367

ESSENTIAL OILS

Ancient Medicine

DR. JOSH AXE
JORDAN RUBIN
TY BOLLINGER

NOTICE TO READER

This book is not intended to provide medical advice or to take the place of medical advice and treatment from your personal physician. Readers are advised to consult their doctors or qualfied health professionals regarding specific health questions. Neither the publisher nor the author takes responsibility for possible health consequences of any person reading or following the information in this book. All readers, especially those taking prescription or over-the-counter medications, should consult their physicians before beginning any nutrition or supplement program.

† These statements have not been evaluated by the Food and Drug Administration. This product is not intended to diagnose, treat, cure or prevent any disease.

Published in 2016 by Axe Wellness LLC
Copyright © 2016 Dr. Josh Axe
All rights reserved

Unless otherwise identified, Scripture quotations are taken from THE Holy Bible, New International Version®, NIV®. Copyright ©1973, 1978, 1984, 2011 by Biblica, Inc.®. Used by permission. All rights reserved worldwide.

Scripture quotations marked AMP are taken from The Amplified Bible. Copyright © 1954, 1958, 1962, 1964, 1965, 1987 by The Lockman Foundation. Used by permission.

Scripture quotations marked NLT are taken from Holy Bible, New Living Translation. Copyright © 1996, 2004, 2015 by Tyndale House Foundation. Used by permission of Tyndale House Publishers Inc., Carol Stream, Illinois 60188. All rights reserved.

No part of this publication may be reproduced or distributed in any form of by any means, electronic or mechanical, or stored in a database or retrieval system, without prior written permission from the publisher. All inquiries should be addressed to Axe Wellness at help@draxe.com.

Visit our website at www.draxe.com.

ISBN-13 HC: 978-0-7684-1187-4
ISBN-13 TP: 978-0-7684-1786-9

Book design: Allison Brochey
Recipe photography: Ayla Sadler
Cover photography: David Molnar

Printed in the USA
6 / 22 21 20 19 18

CONTENTS

PART III: CONDITIONS

PART IV: SPECIAL AREAS OF ESSENTIAL OIL USE

PART V: ESSENTIAL OIL RECIPES

FOOD

Breakfast

Drinks

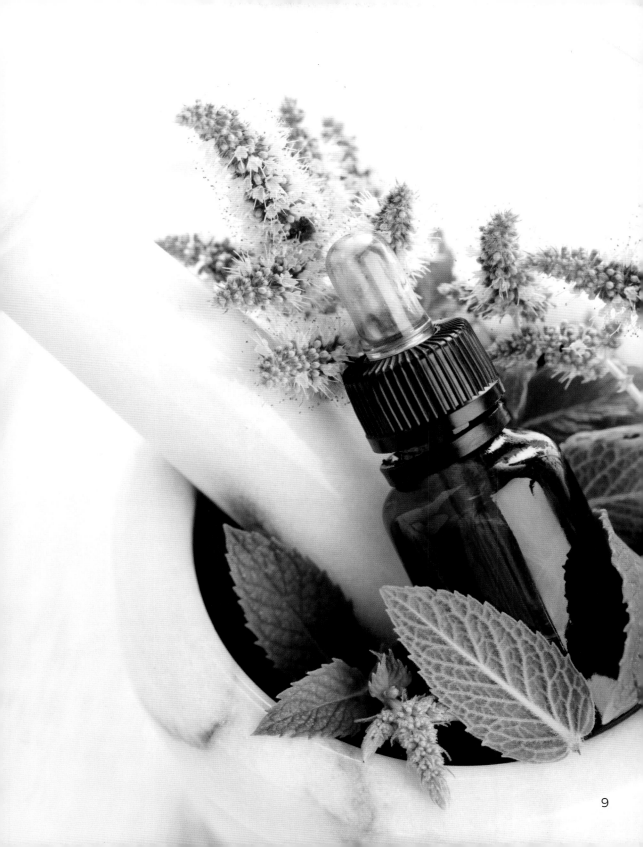

INTRODUCTION
Healing with Biblical Medicine

Let's travel back in time to over 3,000 years ago to visit the palace of King David in Israel's capital city, Jerusalem. You explore the immense castle until you stumble upon the private chambers of the king and discover a large cupboard. You've found King David's medicine cabinet! You swing open the heavy wooden doors, locate a treasure trove of healing balms, oils, spices and herbs inside, and you decide to take a closer look.

First, you find the woodsy and sweet-smelling sandalwood, which the king may use to clean wounds or as a natural aphrodisiac. Then you find some minty tasting hyssop that King David likely uses to soothe his aching muscles after battle and which acts as a powerful antiseptic. You smell the distinctive aroma of clean, energizing cypress, known for its ability to heal wounds and infections and serve as a powerful deodorant to keep the king smelling fresh in between his royal baths. You find smoky, bittersweet, sticky myrrh that the king and his royal family use to fight aging and help prevent gum disease. Then you pick up a vial of warm, spicy cassia, which boosts the body's immune system as it acts as a natural insect repellant to keep the king from being harassed by bugs during the hot Jerusalem summers. And finally, you find highly cherished and prized frankincense that King David uses in his and his wives' soaps and perfumes to hydrate and protect their bodies.

All of these oils and more are what the queens and kings of ancient days used as their medicine. There were no pharmacies on every corner; instead, there were simply herbs, spices and other plant parts known to promote health and healing.

Fast forward to today and step into our own personal homes. Inside, we invite you to look into our medicine cabinets. What you *won't* find is a single prescription medication. Instead, you will discover a cornucopia of ancient medicines and natural remedies based in nature, including herbs, spices, supplements and dozens of essential oils. Inside Dr. Josh's home, you'll always find frankincense; Jordan is never far away from a bottle of lavender; and Ty's office is drenched in the aromas of orange and peppermint.

We use essential oils in extensive ways in our lives; they wear many hats, if you will—as our medicines, our cleansing agents, our personal care products and countless other uses. Why do we rely on essential oils exactly, and why do we believe that everyone else should, too?

The reasons are simple: Instead of simply depending on prescription medications and synthetic drugs with a list of dangerous side effects, our families have opted for safer, natural remedies with thousands of years of history proving their benefits. Instead of using common household cleaners and personal care products that contain ingredients that cause toxicity, we have chosen superior alternatives that can achieve the same (or even better) results without the risk of damaging our bodies.

In the quest for health and vibrant living, the three of us have collaborated multiple times over the last several years in order to share important messages of health and hope. During this time, we have discovered that we all believe essential oils are one of the most powerful forms of plant-based medicine in the world. Now, we want to show you

We have seen essential oils benefit our families and our patients in some of the following ways:

- » Reduce toxicity
- » Balance hormones
- » Improve digestion
- » Boost energy
- » Improve brain function
- » Reduce emotional stress
- » Produce radiant skin
- » Boost immunity and fight infections
- » Alleviate aches and pains

And, a whole lot more!

how essential oils can transform the health of your entire family.

Essential oils can serve innumerable functions in your life—from fostering relaxation and caring for scrapes to helping fight disease and promoting healing.

Essential oils were placed on this Earth to benefit our health and provide rejuvenation. In fact, they have been a vital part of our individual journeys, both personally and in the pursuit of helping others find abundant health.

Allow us to share the roles essential oils play in our personal lives in order to equip and empower you to use them every day.

DR. JOSH'S STORY

I was 14 when my mother was diagnosed with breast cancer, and my family was blindsided by the diagnosis. The doctors recommended an aggressive chemotherapy treatment, and Mom consented to go this traditional route—which included a mastectomy—to eradicate the disease. I will never forget how sick my mom was from the chemo. I recall seeing her hair fall out in clumps and thinking she had aged 20 years in two weeks and praying for God to spare her life.

After her treatments, she was pronounced cancer-free, but she became sicker than ever. She struggled with leaky gut syndrome, hypothyroidism, weight gain, chronic constipation, candida yeast infections and depression, and she was on multiple medications and felt tired all the time.

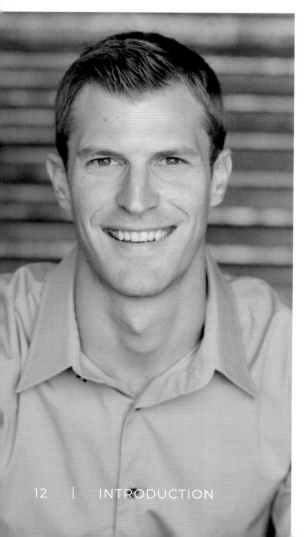

Ten years later, my mom was diagnosed with cancer yet again. I remember the phone call well. "Josh, I've got bad news. My cancer has recurred. What do I do?"

I immediately flew home; our family prayed together, and ultimately, we felt the Lord was leading us to take care of my mom naturally.

At this time, I had been training to become a doctor of natural medicine and a chiropractic physician and knew some of the top holistic doctors in the world. I started spending at least 12 hours each day researching natural remedies to fight cancer and talking to doctors who had experience in beating cancer naturally. Then, I put together an advanced health protocol for my mom.

The first thing we implemented was a massive change in Mom's diet. She started juicing vegetables and consuming homemade bone broth, antioxidant-rich blueberries, wild-caught salmon, probiotic-rich goat milk kefir and lots of organic green salads (yes, lots of kale!).

Amongst my thousands of hours studying the best natural cancer fighters, I discovered the power of essential oils.

I discovered essential oils such as frankincense, myrrh and oregano—which are some of the most effective agents to fight against unhealthy, irregular cells in the body—and started using these and other oils to support her health and to supplement the other natural cancer-fighting protocols we had implemented.

Today, my mother is cancer-free and thriving—and she uses essential oils now more than ever. I'm not claiming that essential oils alone are a treatment for cancer, but I absolutely do believe they can arm your body with powerful tools to win the battle against disease and regain your health when combined with key diet and lifestyle changes.

Inspired by these efforts to not only save Mom's life, but also *keep* her healthy, I have made essential oils a part of my daily regimen.

My wife and I use essential oils as a natural remedy for numerous health conditions, we use them for personal care and for cleaning, and I bring frankincense and lavender oils with me almost everywhere I go. I make my own homemade recipes with essential oils that have replaced so many of the products I used to buy, such as soap, shampoo, deodorant and toothpaste.

I have now recommended essential oils to thousands of my patients and to family members. In fact, I believe they are the most under-utilized form of plant-based medicine in the world today. One of my life's missions is to help transform the health of this world by teaching people how to implement essential oils into their daily lives.

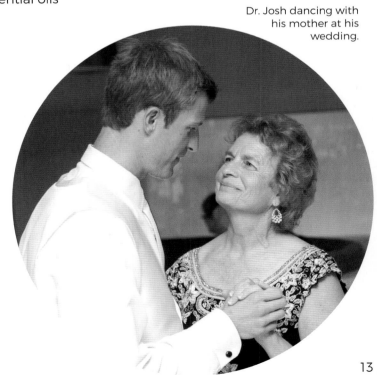

Dr. Josh dancing with his mother at his wedding.

JORDAN'S STORY

My journey with essential oils is equally personal and also involves a seemingly insurmountable battle with disease. My interest in essential oils initially was peaked after an intense study of the Bible in preparation for writing my book, *The Maker's Diet*, in 2003, a book that was inspired by my victory over Crohn's disease.

In an effort to follow what a California nutrition expert deemed as "God's Health Plan" in order to overcome severe Crohn's disease and more than a dozen health maladies, I had voraciously studied hundreds of books and thousands of Biblical references on health and wellness in body, mind and spirit, and I began a diet of strictly whole foods consumed in Biblical times: raw, organically grown, sprouted whole grains; organic fruits and vegetables; fermented dairy; grass-fed beef; and pastured eggs and poultry. I also added a daily regimen of probiotics teeming with beneficial bacteria called soil-based organisms. Thanks to these efforts, I beat the doctors' prognoses and was once again living a vibrant and healthy life free of the supposedly incurable Crohn's disease.

Through my studies, I was amazed to learn how valuable essential oils were in Biblical times—often cherished more than gold. I also began to understand their therapeutic value when used topically, through olfaction (inhalation) and oral consumption, and I began to comprehend the tremendous value and widespread application of essential oils for an extensive number of conditions and ailments.

Then came 2008—when I was diagnosed with an aggressive metastatic cancer. Essential oils became a critical tool in the fight and subsequent victory against catastrophic disease for the second time in my life, a triumph that came through natural and supernatural means and without the use of conventional treatments. During a 40-day period, I constructed a nutrition and detoxification program that involved the use of essential oils in multiple applications daily, including massaging my head and body with essential oils, diffusing oils 24 hours a day in my home, using them in hydrotherapy (shower, sauna and steam room) and consuming oils mixed in various nutritional beverages.

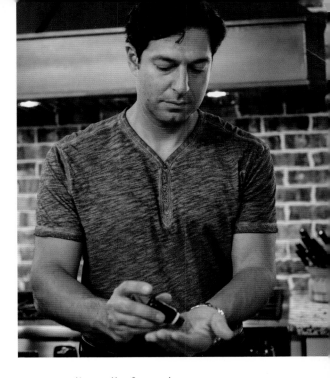

I have now used essential oils consistently for the past nine years, and they represent an indispensable tool in my family's health arsenal. My family of eight uses essential oils orally, topically, in our skin and body care regimen, in wound care and in recipes each and every day.

I also use essential oils daily during my meditation and quiet time with the Lord, and I anoint my wife and children daily with lavender oil while quoting parts of Psalm 23: "I anoint your head with oil. Your cup runs over. Surely goodness and mercy will follow you all the rest of your days and you will dwell in the house of the Lord forever."

I'm so thankful for essential oils and the protective measure they provide against the germs, toxins and stress surrounding all of us when we travel and interact with others, and even within our own homes. I have also recommended essential oils to many individuals whom I have helped coach back to health.

While essential oils have been such an important part of my daily life, I struggled to find a consistent source of practical information on the *how* and *why* of essential oils for the thousands of people who look to me for health coaching and guidance. That is why I teamed up with my good friends, Dr. Josh Axe and Ty Bollinger, to write *Essential Oils: Ancient Medicine*. We believe this book will demystify essential oils and provide you with the keys to unlock these powerful, hidden treasures inside the plants God created.

TY'S STORY

When I graduated from Baylor University with a Masters in Taxation in 1991, you could never have told me that one day I'd be a worldwide health freedom advocate, but life has a way of revealing its plans for you in unique ways. My career and life path change began when my father, Graham Bollinger, was diagnosed with cancer on July 1, 1996. Just 25 days after the diagnosis, he died.

My family and I were left in total shock after losing my father less than a month after discovering he had cancer, especially considering that at 52 years old, he was in excellent physical health at the time of his diagnosis. Dad had gone into the hospital with stomach pains, and we assumed the doctors would tell us it was gallstones. Instead, they informed us that he

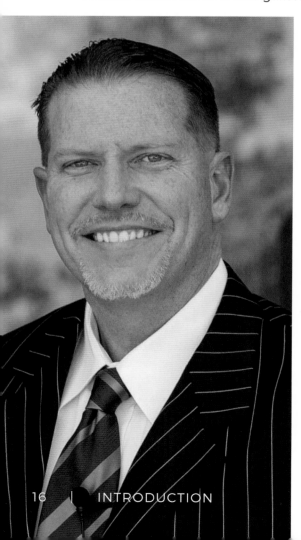

had numerous cancerous tumors in his stomach, and they were going to cut them out, which they proceeded to do.

He bled to death over the next three weeks after the surgery. His death certificate says he died from cancer, but in reality, he died from the surgery to remove the tumors in his stomach. What was even more troubling was the fact that his initial prognosis indicated he could have lived another year or two *without* treatment.

Over the course of the next seven years, both of my grandfathers, my grandmother, my dad's brother, a cousin and then finally my mother all died of cancer. Several of them died from the treatments for the cancer, not the cancer itself.

At the age of 41, I became the oldest person left in my family. The entire experience woke me up to the fact that we are clearly missing the mark when it comes to the methods we utilize to treat cancer today. With a medical system that is so advanced in many areas, like trauma medicine, why are we still in the dark ages when it comes to cancer treatments?

That is when my quest to learn all I possibly could about natural cancer treatments and the medical industry really began. In 2006, I wrote and published my first book, *Cancer: Step Outside the Box*. Before we knew it, the book was selling like crazy (it was #6 on Amazon at one point), and we had amassed a large following.

Since then, I've written multiple books before embarking on another unexpected journey— and that is filming, editing and producing documentary miniseries ("docu-series").

First, in the spring of 2014, we created a docu-series entitled *The Quest for the Cures*, which features my trek across the country interviewing patients, doctors, scientists and patients who all broke the code of silence to reveal some of the hidden truths about the cancer pandemic in our modern world.

After the immense popularity of this docu-series, in the fall of 2014, we released *The Quest for the Cures Continues*. Then, in 2015, I traveled the globe and interviewed over 130 cancer experts and patients, and we released The *Truth About Cancer: A Global Quest* to the entire world.

It is my mission to share the most remarkable discovery I made on my quests, which is that the vast majority of all diseases (including cancer) can be easily prevented and even cured without drugs or surgery.

During my search for living a healthier life free from disease, I discovered some of the many benefits of essential oils. My family and I now use essential oils in our daily lives. My wife uses frankincense and myrrh every day behind her ears and on her lymph nodes as a prophylactic, and we love to diffuse various oils throughout our home every day for everything from added mental clarity to extra immune support for our four children and ourselves.

During my research, I came to realize that essential oils are a largely overlooked piece of the health and disease treatment puzzle. As important and therapeutic as they are, they are still unknown and seem to be shrouded in mystery. Despite their enormous popularity, there are relatively few books that clearly explain the true benefits and uses of these gifts from God.

I believe books like *Essential Oils: Ancient Medicine* are going to change that. People are going to discover that they can use essential oils in place of so much of what is being used today in conventional medicine.

DESIGNED WITH YOU IN MIND

We hope this book will become the go-to guide for anyone who wants to protect and improve their health through the use of essential oils, but we also wrote it with a few specific groups in mind. First, we believe *Essential Oils: Ancient Medicine* can become a powerful resource for doctors and health practitioners seeking to provide their patients and clients with the best possible improvements in their health.

Second, the group of people who will benefit the most from reading this book will be moms. We know moms are dedicated warriors who are not only responsible for their own health but also charged with taking care of the health of their entire family. From children to pets to aging parents, they are constantly serving. If we could get a copy of this book into the hands of every mother in America, the health of our entire nation would radically change.

Essential oils are no fad—they are backed by thousands of years of history. They've been used in Biblical medicine, Egyptian medicine, Chinese medicine and Greek medicine—and they're still used throughout the world today. In fact, they're actually more popular in many other parts of the world than they are in the U.S.

Thankfully, America is now experiencing an essential oil revolution, and their use is growing in popularity every day. So, let's celebrate the fact that essential oils are becoming so popular! But it needs to stay that way—and in order for that to happen, you need to have easily accessible information that is simple to understand and implement.

We designed this book to give you clear, easy ways to use essential oils to benefit both your health and your family's health every single day. Our recommendations are supported by history and science. There are now thousands of research studies proving that essential oils are effective natural remedies and amazing ingredients for personal care and cleaning products—and we have utilized a great deal of this research in the writing of this book.

Ultimately, we want you to use this book to accomplish three things in your life:

1. To be **educated** about what essential oils are and why they are so powerful.

2. To feel **empowered** to use essential oils both safely and effectively to support your health and your family's health.

3. To be **equipped** with this trusted manual to turn to for utilizing essentials oils in your daily life—from boo-boos and stuffy noses to chemical-free personal care and household items and natural pet care.

So many of the diseases we see today are due to high levels of toxicity present within our bodies; chemical toxicants that have become *insidious invaders* in our daily lives through the foods we eat, the medicines we take, the products we use and even the water we drink.

Part of our collective mission is to teach people how to live free of toxins and medications. Essential oils can be used as a natural replacement for some medications, conventional personal care products, body products and home cleaning products. Essential oils can be used in so many ways that their only real limit is from a lack of knowledge of safe and proper use—and that is precisely what this book is designed to give you.

With the right tools in your arsenal, you and your family can experience a total medicine cabinet—and life—transformation.

If you are ready to experience more energy, better health, balanced hormones, improved digestion and an overall higher quality of life, then you have found the *right resource* at the *right time*. We want to provide you with everything you need to know about essential oils and everything you need to use them effectively, all in one place.

We hope this book provides you with the answers you've been looking for.

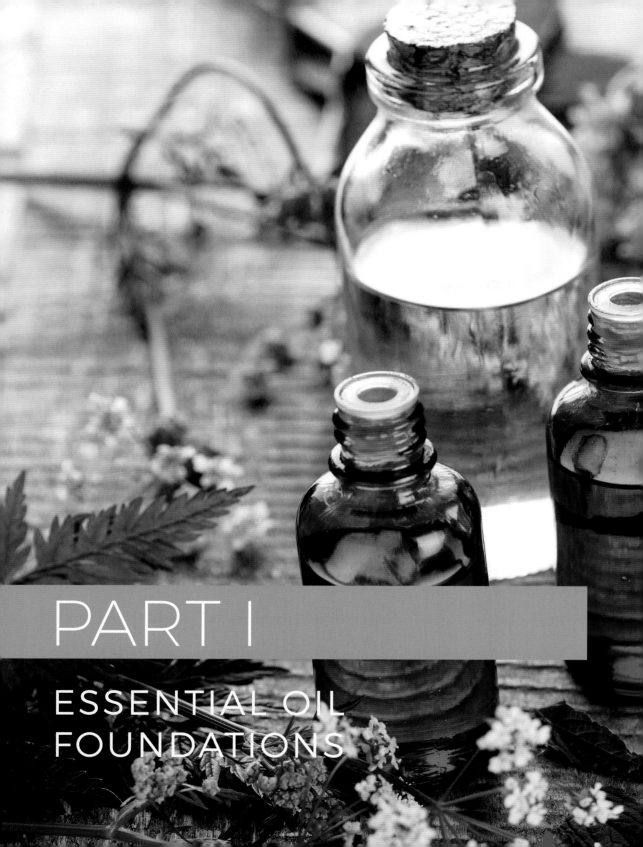

PART I

ESSENTIAL OIL FOUNDATIONS

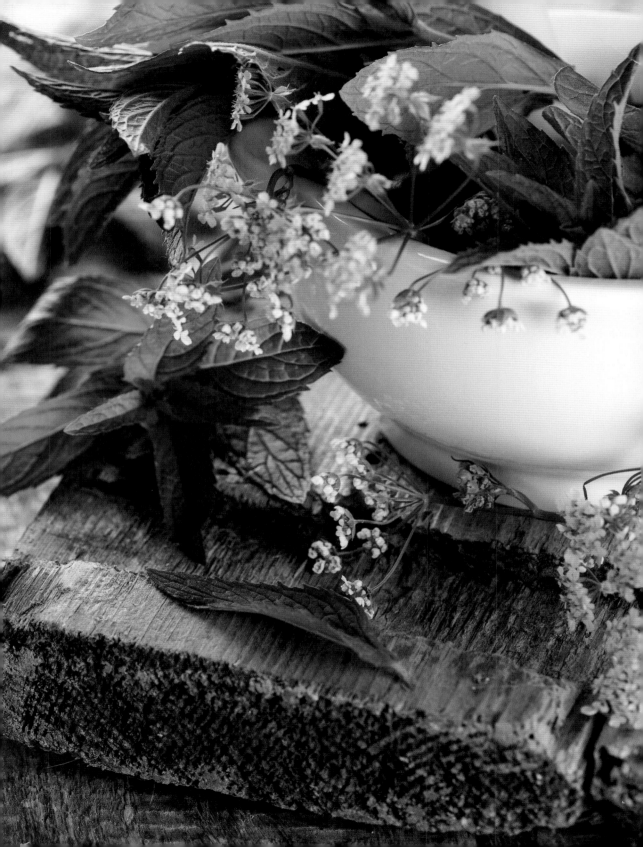

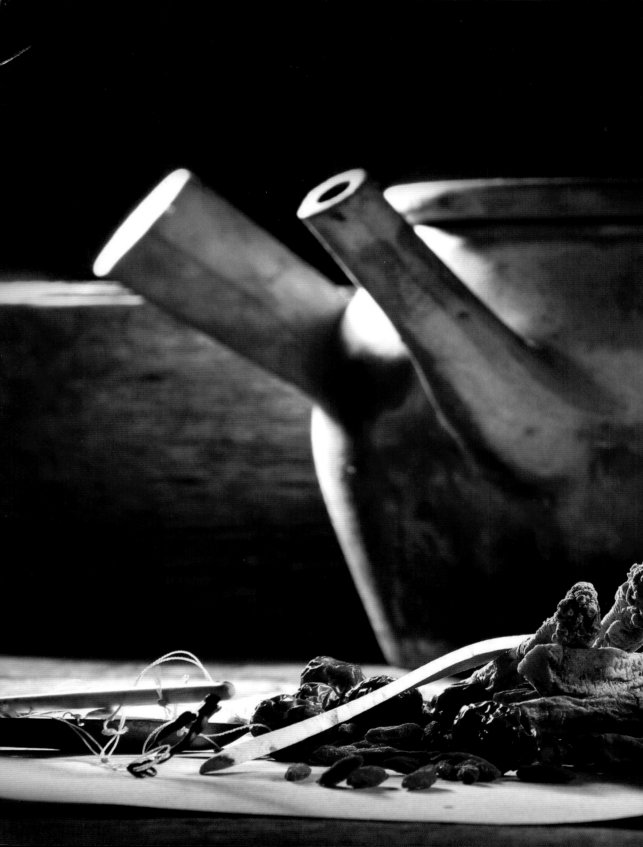

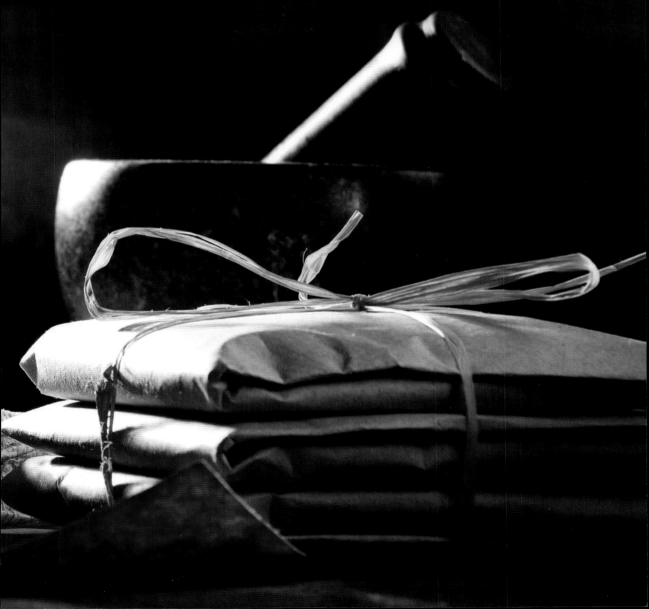

CHAPTER 1

FROM THE THIRD DAY TO THE MODERN DAY

After talking one day, the three of us discovered that our mornings start the same way—with praying, reading the Bible and meditating (oftentimes while applying or diffusing frankincense oil). In the course of our Bible studies of creation, it dawned on us that essential oils from plants have been available to mankind *since the very beginning*. More specifically, according to Genesis 1: 11-13:

> [11] *Then God said, "Let the land produce vegetation: seed-bearing plants and trees on the land that bear fruit with seed in it, according to their various kinds." And it was so.* [12] *The land produced vegetation: plants bearing seed according to their kinds and trees bearing fruit with seed in it according to their kinds. And God saw that it was good.* [13] *And there was evening, and there was morning—the third day.*

Because essential oils are derived from plants, we realized that on the third day of creation, even before God breathed life into Adam and well before sin, disease and death became reality, He created all the supportive tools and treatments everyone on this Earth would need for illnesses, ailments, aches and pains and placed them, quite literally, at our fingertips.

Now let's fast-forward to our use of these tools and treatments in the modern day. When Jordan was battling cancer in 2008, there was no shortage of people who believed his best chance of beating the disease was through one of conventional medicine's answers to cancer treatment. But he would not be deterred from his path to fight cancer naturally, and thanks to prayer, cleansing, a strict diet, a specific regimen of supplements and his use of essential oils, he beat the diagnosis—and he came out of cancer healthier than he was before.

Dr. Josh can relate to that victory. After his mother underwent chemotherapy for her first bout with breast cancer, she felt sicker after being pronounced "cancer-free" than she had felt while battling the disease. When the Axe family chose to fight her second cancer diagnosis through alternative treatments and lifestyle changes, his mother emerged healthier than she had ever been in her life. Sadly, Ty's mother and father never got that second chance.

We don't know a single person who has not lost a friend or loved one from cancer or some other form of disease. You may even be dealing with a diagnosis right now, and if you are, you are certainly not alone. According to the American Cancer Society, men have a 1 in 2 probability of developing cancer in their lifetimes, and 1 out of every 3 women will battle some form of cancer.

Whether you picked up this book looking for natural remedies for what ails you or as an overall reference, this is an exciting time. Essential oils *can* change your life, and together, we can prevent disease and change the way the world treats illness. Armed with the right information, we can spread the word and change the status quo.

We believe this is possible because the information in this book is backed by the latest scientific research, historical documentation and Biblical wisdom. It's time to change the way we view disease; it's time to change the products we are bringing into our homes and putting into our bodies.

This is a critical situation, and we are facing serious problems in the world today. Conventional treatments for both major *and* minor conditions are killing people. For example, diabetic drugs are causing vitamin B12 deficiency and permanent nerve damage. Drugs for depression are causing widespread dependencies, and the consequences of withdrawal include seizures and death. Drugs for high blood pressure are causing impotence among men and heart disease due to the vitamin and mineral deficiencies they cause. Drugs for lowering cholesterol are causing organ damage, memory loss and sexual dysfunction.

That's just a short list of the side effects of prescription drugs and doesn't include a discussion of the hundreds of drugs that have been overprescribed and resulted in a serious worldwide addiction epidemic. It also doesn't include the countless over-the-counter (OTC) drugs people use every day like acetaminophen, which has been linked to kidney disease and increased risk of heart attack and stroke.

According to an article published by the Harvard School of Public Health, there are nearly 2 million hospitalizations and 128,000 deaths every year from properly prescribed medications. This makes prescription drugs a major health risk, ranking it fourth among the leading causes of death.[1]

Conversely, how many reported deaths are from vitamins, supplements and essential oils each year? ZERO.

The solution for these serious and significant side effects is not more drugs. Modern medicine is designed to target the *symptoms* of disease and not the *source* of the problem. It's like getting a nail stuck in your car tire, and instead of removing the nail, you just keep filling up the tire with more air—without ever removing the nail. If you do not address the source of the issue (the nail), the air will continue to leak and eventually result in other problems, no matter how many times you patch it up and expect it to function properly.

The solution to this problem is found right in nature. We must remove as many of the toxins from our lives as possible (which come at us in our food, in our water, in our personal care and cleaning products, and in our air) and replace conventional medicines and products with innovations specifically designed by the Great Physician to heal, not to cause further harm.

There has never been a more critical time to act than now. Over 1,500 people a day are dying of cancer, and over 600,000 people will die of heart disease this year. And for the rest of us, quality of life is deteriorating thanks to poor diet and lifestyle choices, including our reliance on conventional drugs.

You don't have to wait for widespread mindset and policy changes to start acting. We believe you can start affecting change today—right now—through small, but specific actions.

For example, if you want to combat high blood pressure, start by using a combination of lavender, ylang ylang and frankincense. Diffuse cinnamon oil, grapefruit oil and ginger oil at your desk at work to support blood sugar balance. In clinical trials, essential oils have been proven to elevate moods, so start breathing in some bergamot, lavender and Roman chamomile to fight depression.[2,3,4]

The world of medicine offers many great wonders, and modern medicine and diagnostics are amazing on many levels. But the system is broken, largely due to the prevalence of pharmaceutical drugs being touted as cures.

Before the age of modern medicine, people did not rely on large drug companies for Band-Aid cures that often cause more problems than they treat. Instead, they relied on natural remedies made from plants to prevent and treat ailments. They relied on traditional herbal remedies like essential oils.

The funny thing about the word "traditional" is that people use it today to refer to medical practices that have only been around for 100 years or less. Medical professionals and others then lump essential oils into the "alternative" category, when in fact, nothing could be further from the truth. It is herbal remedies and essential oils that are "traditional," as they have been around since the third day of creation!

We believe in using the "traditional" treatments—in other words, those that come from the Earth. It's easy for people today to pass herbs, spices and essential oils off as "just plants," and that is because we've been conditioned to believe that "medicine" has to come from a lab.

But we believe that God's laboratory is far superior to the ones human beings have created, and that is precisely why you now hold this book in your hands.

When you use "God's Pharmacy" to treat your ailments and to provide preventative medicine, the options for treatment and healing are far more plentiful, the side effects are not so terrifying, and the results are longer lasting.

In order to more fully understand the inherent power and beautiful simplicity of God's Pharmacy, let's travel back in time to find out just how important essential oils once were before Earth was littered with pharmacies on every corner.

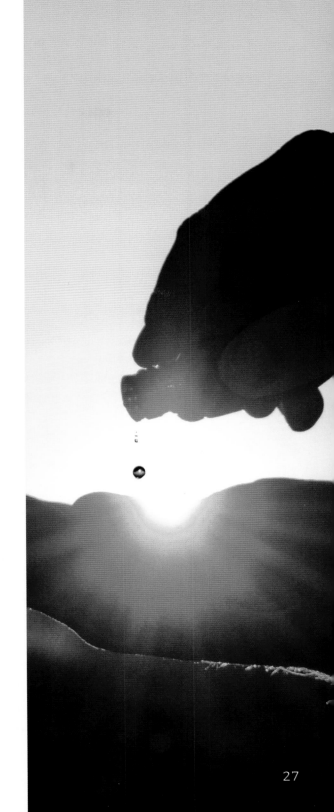

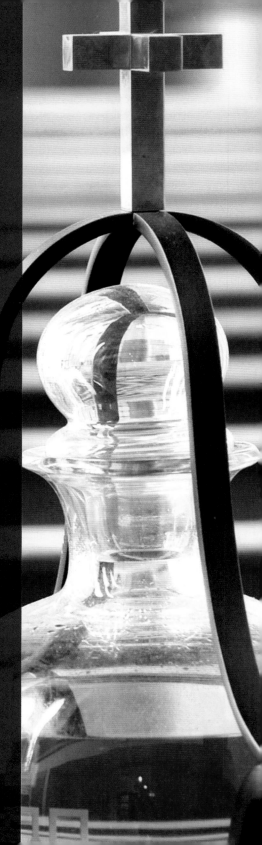

ESSENTIAL OIL'S BIBLICAL ROOTS

Essential oils have been an integral part of the daily lives of people for thousands of years. At least 33 specific essential oils and aromatic oil-producing plants are mentioned in the Bible, and the word "incense" is mentioned 68 times in Scripture. Psalm 45:7-8, Proverbs 27:9, Isaiah 61:3 and Hebrews 1:9 all reference oils in some way, as in "the oil of joy" and "the oil of gladness," and they speak of how oils "rejoice the heart."

Essential oils are also referred to in the Bible as fragrances, odors, ointments, aromas, perfumes and sweet savors.[5] In total, there are over 600 references to essential oils and/or the aromatic plants from which they were extracted in the Bible. For those of us who study the Bible, we know that the Holy Scripture is not filled with insignificant details. Therefore, there is obviously a tremendous importance surrounding oils and their many uses.

Oils such as frankincense, myrrh, rosemary, hyssop and spikenard were used for anointing and healing the sick. Moses and other Old Testament figures used essential oils to anoint kings and leaders; priests also used them for healing purposes. In fact, in Exodus 30:22-25, Moses was given a specific formula directly by God:

22 Then the Lord said to Moses, 23 "Take the following fine spices: 500 shekels [around 12 pounds] of liquid myrrh, half as much [around six pounds] of fragrant cinnamon, 250 shekels [around six pounds] of fragrant calamus, 24 500 shekels [around 12 pounds] of cassia—all according to the sanctuary shekel— and a hin [around a gallon] of olive oil. 25 Make these into a sacred anointing oil, a fragrant blend, the work of a perfumer. It will be the sacred anointing oil."

This formula was used to make a holy anointing oil that was poured onto the heads of those being appointed king or for those being prayed for by the priest. In other words, this anointing oil wasn't just used for rituals, but it was also known to have healing properties.

Another important reference to a holy anointing oil was when King David was anointed by Samuel in 1 Samuel 16: 12-13:

12 "So he sent for him and had him brought in. He was glowing with health and had a fine appearance and handsome features. Then the Lord said, 'Rise and anoint him; this is the one.' 13 So Samuel took the horn of oil and anointed him in the presence of his brothers, and from that day on the Spirit of the Lord came powerfully upon David."

When Jesus was born, the Bible tells us that three wise men from the far east gave the infant King gifts of gold to honor his royalty, frankincense as a perfume and myrrh for anointing oil. In those days, frankincense oil was often rubbed on children to reduce swelling because of its anti-inflammatory qualities as well as immune protection. Myrrh oil was known as a natural antiseptic and may have been put on the infant Jesus' umbilical cord area, as well as been applied to his mother, Mary, to help heal tissues and balance hormones.

There are also four different Gospel accounts of women honoring Jesus by anointing him with oil (also referred to as "expensive perfume" and "ointment"). John 12:3 tells of a particularly touching story in which Mary, the sister of Lazarus, performed this special action to pay tribute to Jesus:

12 "Then took Mary a pound of ointment of spikenard, very costly, and anointed the feet of Jesus, and wiped his feet with her hair: and the house was filled with the odor of the ointment."

In Esther's era, according to Esther 2:12, the future queen underwent "a six-month treatment with the oil of myrrh and six months with perfumes and other aloes." Queen Esther bathed in myrrh and olive oil for six months before her presentation to the king in order to purify her body.

Note that the essential oils referenced

in history and throughout the Bible were often herbs mixed with olive oil and not identical to what we think of as an essential oil today. (For more on how essential oils are made today as opposed to their production in Biblical times, see Chapter 3).

God created these wonderful resources for mankind's use—and undoubtedly for the eventual use of every subsequent generation. He gave us everything we need to support ourselves on an emotional, physical, mental and spiritual level, including wonderful aromatic plants and essential oils.

THE 12 OILS OF THE BIBLE

Here are 12 of the most revered oils of the Bible and their historic uses:

1. Frankincense. Frankincense is the king of the oils. It was used as a primary component of the holy incense, a medicine and a currency—and of course, it was a gift from the wise men to baby Jesus. In fact, at the time of Jesus' birth, both frankincense and myrrh may have been worth more than their weight in the third gift: gold.

2. Myrrh. Quoted in Scripture 156 times as having a variety of uses, including as an ointment, an incense, an embalming ingredient and used as a skin beauty treatment by Queen Esther in Esther 2:12. By far, myrrh's most common usage in the Bible is as a part of holy anointing oil.

3. Cinnamon. Like myrrh, cinnamon oil was a chief ingredient in holy anointing oil and used to cleanse the air, kill mold and act as a natural medicine. In Proverbs 7:17, Solomon uses this aromatic oil in the bedroom and as a natural perfume or cologne.

4. Cedarwood. King Solomon used cedarwood in building God's temple and Jesus was crucified on a cross made of cedarwood or cypress. It was thought to bring wisdom, was used for ritual cleansing and served as medicine in treating skin conditions and leprosy.

5. Spikenard. In Biblical times, "nard" was not only a very expensive perfume but also a precious ointment that was used as medicine. Interestingly, the "spikenard" used in the Bible may have in fact been lavender oil. In John 12:3, the Bible tells how spikenard was used to anoint Jesus just days before His death and resurrection.

6. Hyssop. In the Old Testament, God commanded His people to use hyssop in the ceremonial cleansing of people and houses. Hyssop appears at Jesus' crucifixion, when the Roman soldiers offered Jesus a drink of wine vinegar on a sponge at the end of a stalk of hyssop.

7. Cassia. An herb very similar to cinnamon, cassia is the fourth ingredient listed in the holy anointing oil detailed in Exodus 30:24. It may have been brought out of Egypt when the Israelites fled Pharaoh and was commonly used with myrrh and aloes to scent garments.

8. Sandalwood (aloes). In Scripture, sandalwood is referred to as "aloes" and is called one of the oils of joy and gladness along with frankincense, myrrh and cedarwood. Nicodemus and Joseph of Arimathea brought sandalwood (aloes) and myrrh to bury Jesus, and in today's market, the amount of oils used would be worth an estimated $200,000!

9. Cypress. Cypress is celebrated in Scripture as a symbol of strength, security and prosperity. The Bible mentions cypress as the choice wood for building, trading and even weaponry. In Genesis 6:14, God commanded Noah to "make yourself an ark of gopher wood," which in modern English is in fact "cypress."

10. Galbanum. Galbanum is a main ingredient of the holy incense used in the heart of the temple in Exodus 30:34. Interestingly, although galbanum itself has a somewhat foul odor, when burned with other sweet smelling oils in holy incense, it has the most beautiful scent and was thought to balance the emotions.

11. Rose of Sharon. Mentioned in the Song of Solomon, the rose of Sharon is not really a "rose" but instead similar to the hibiscus or tulip (which is also a source of saffron). Some Bible expositors see the rose of Sharon as Christ and the lily as the church, His bride.

12. Calamus. Also known as "sweet cane," calamus is an ancient herb that is perhaps what we now know as lemongrass. In Biblical times, calamus was used in perfumes, incense and as an ingredient in the special holy anointing oil used by the priests in the temple.

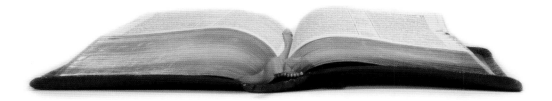

THE EGYPTIANS
EXTREME OIL LOVERS

In the days of Pharaoh, Egyptians made extensive use of essential oils in medicine and burial practices. The process of embalming and mummification was developed at this time, as the Egyptians searched for immortality. Frankincense, myrrh, galbanum, cinnamon, cedarwood, juniper berry and spikenard were used to preserve the bodies of their royalty in preparation for the afterlife; in fact, when King Tut's tomb was opened in 1923, archaeologists discovered 50 alabaster jars that contained essential oils, several of them completely full!

Aromatherapy (also known as essential oil therapy) was used in combination with their religious practices and mysticism. The Egyptians burned incense made from aromatic wood, herbs and spices in honor of their gods; they believed that as the smoke rose up to the heavens, it carried their prayers and wishes to the gods. Entire Egyptian temples were dedicated to the production and blending of oils, where oil recipes were written on the walls in hieroglyphics.

The Egyptians also used essential oils as part of their daily lives. The women of Egypt would use fragranced oils after bathing to rejuvenate their skin and protect them from the sun. Cleopatra, once considered the most beautiful woman in the world, was known to use essential oils. She used oils like rose, frankincense, cypress, neroli and myrrh for her personal beauty treatments. The queen was often described as "clouded in a scent of mystery." (We're not entirely sure if a "scent of mystery" is a good thing or a bad thing, but it certainly speaks to her love of essential oils.)

Today, we are finally beginning to embrace the wisdom of the Jews and Egyptians by using essential oils to combat the detrimental effects of stress and simultaneously restore beauty, peace and harmony into our daily lives.

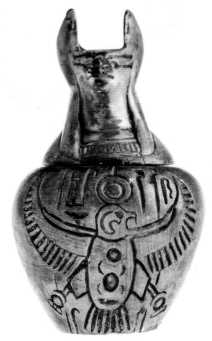

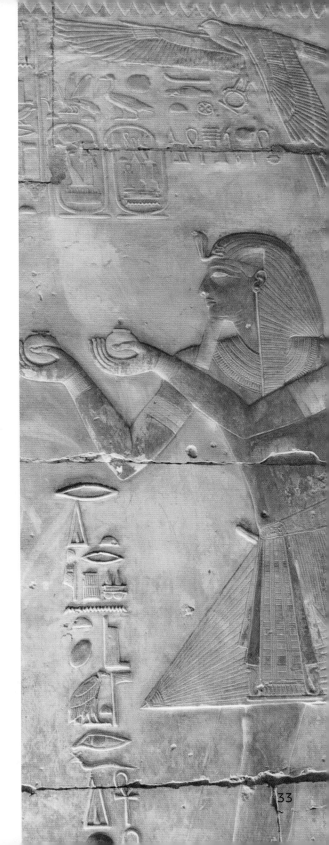

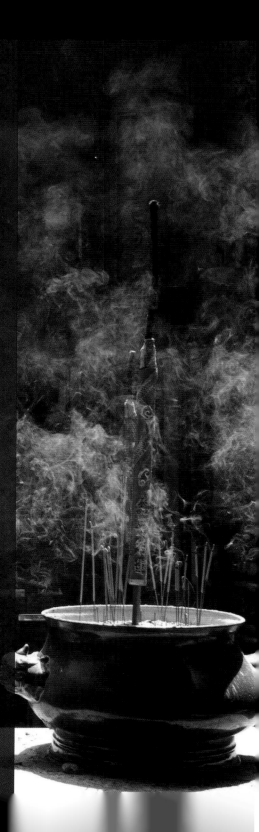

THE CHINESE
PIONEERING THE USE OF OILS AS MEDICINE

The ancient Chinese also believed in the power of essential oils. Some speculate that the Chinese may have begun studying aromatics at the same time as the Egyptians, or even before. The oldest surviving medical text is *Shennong's Herbal*, dated around 2700 B.C. Shennong was a mythical sage ruler of prehistoric China who reportedly consumed hundreds of herbs and tested their medicinal value. The upper class citizens in China also used plant oils frequently during the T'ang dynasties to scent their homes, clothing, temples, ink, paper and cosmetics.

In ancient Chinese medicine, it is understood that herbs have specific actions and properties. Some herbs are cooling, while others are warming; some herbs invigorate and others sedate. Each herb is explained through its energetics as well as its actions and effects. It is believed that the concepts of "Qi" (your life energy) and "Yin and Yang" (or Yin-Yang) form the base of this medical system.

For example, low Qi can be detected by feeling a weak pulse, low energy levels, hypothyroidism or depression. Having a Yin deficiency often presents as dry skin, food cravings and trouble sleeping. A Yang deficiency is often correlated with low libido, physical weakness and poor self-esteem.

In Chinese medicine, a practitioner may use a Yang essential oil such as ginger, which has warming properties to aid in digestion and help clear dampness (candida and colds) from the body. Then, they may use a Yin strengthening essential oil such as geranium to treat infertility and improve skin health. And then, to boost the body's Qi, thyme oil can effectively treat conditions such as low energy and weakness.

This method of diagnosis and treatment was a fascinating and forward-thinking early application of "holistic medicine," which is a form of medicine that emphasizes the need to look at the whole person (including analysis of all physical, emotional or spiritual imbalances) in the quest for optimal health and wellness.

As you can see, ancient Chinese medicine is an advanced form of holistic healing that has harnessed the benefits of essential oils for thousands of years.

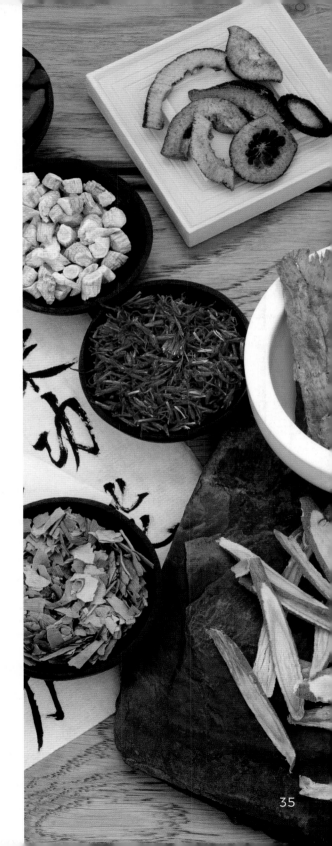

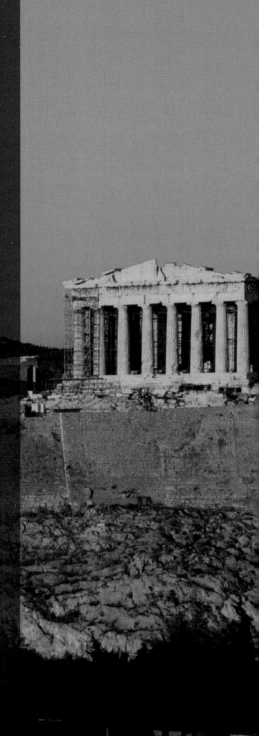

THE GREEKS
BOTANY
TRAILBLAZERS

Botany, also known as plant science, is the science of plant life and a branch of biology. The term "botany" comes from an Ancient Greek word meaning "pasture" or "grass." Historically, all living things were classified as either animals or plants, and botany covered the study of all organisms not considered animals. Therefore, the study of essential oils falls under the *botany* umbrella—and there are several men who are credited with creating and describing many of the fundamental principles of the science:

Hippocrates. Hippocrates is referred to as the "Father of Western Medicine," even though much of what he did would today be considered holistic. Hippocrates documented over 200 different herbs during his lifetime; he believed that plant-based medicine could save lives and surgery should only be used as a last resort. He was also one of the first to believe that diseases were caused naturally rather than view them as punishments by the gods.

Theophrastus. Known as the "Founder of Botany," Theophrastus wrote several botanical works. *The History of Plants* became one of the most valued botanical science references for centuries to come. Theophrastus investigated everything about plants and even how specific scents and different flowers' aromatic properties affected people's emotions.

Pedanius Dioscorides. Pedanius Dioscorides was a Greek military physician, pharmacologist and botanist. Between 50 and 70 A.D., Dioscorides wrote a five-volume book entitled *De Materia Medica* (meaning "On Medical Material"), which became the precursor to all modern pharmacopeias. In it, Dioscorides discussed 600 plants in total—detailing their descriptions, habitats, proper preparation, storage and healing properties.

Claudius Galen. Claudius Galen was a prominent Greek physician, surgeon and philosopher in the Roman Empire. Galen began his medical career working with gladiators by treating their wounds with medicinal herbs. He is often credited with helping to spread the doctrine of Humorism, which is a system of medicine detailing the makeup and workings of the human body, and it suggests that the human body is filled with four basic substances, called humors, which are in balance when a person is healthy.

Galen's system and the pioneering efforts of these men allowed physicians to formulate and prescribe medicines more accurately. In short, Greek Medicine became a system for healing that treats the person, not the symptoms of disease.

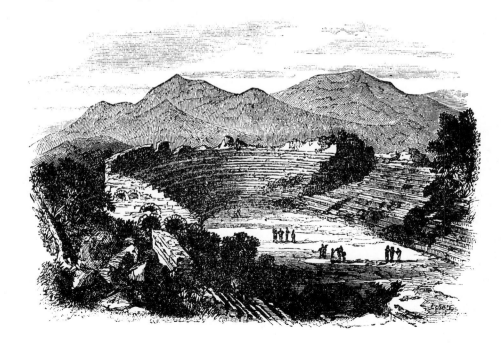

OILS CRUSADE INTO EUROPE

As civilizations transferred world power, the essential oil techniques from Greece traveled to Rome and favored aromatherapy and fragrances. After the fall of the Roman Empire, Persia picked up these healing techniques and perfected the essential oil distillation process that is still used today.

During the Crusades, the Knights and their armies were responsible for passing on knowledge of herbal medicines that they learned in the Middle East throughout Western Europe. The knights acquired knowledge of distillation and carried perfumes with them. (For more on the distillation process, see Chapter 3.)

This holistic approach to treating health conditions was largely rejected during the Dark Ages. During this era, it is believed that monks continued the healing tradition of essential oils and secretly kept herbal medicine alive in the halls of the monasteries. Because the Catholic Church viewed bathing as inappropriate during this time, the citizens favored aromatics to keep foul odors at bay. What they didn't realize is that many of these oils where also anti-bacterial, which meant that their perfume was also helping them to stave off sickness and disease.

After the invention of the modern distillation process, the popularity of essential oils spread through Europe. When the Great Plague became widespread, fumigations were conducted using aromatics to drive out sickness from the cities. In London, houses and workplaces were fumigated on a daily basis, and this reportedly protected the citizens from the plague. The oils were valued because of their anti-microbial properties, especially lavender and frankincense.

History tells us that there are several variations of a protective blend that were used to guard citizens from the plague. One such blend was called "Four Thieves," and the legend states that it was a powerful blend of vinegar, herbs and oils. While the legend changes as much as the precise formula for this blend, the gist of the story is this:

During the plagues (the Black Plague is the most common one cited), a group of four brothers began robbing the dead. At first, their crimes were largely ignored, because everyone knew they would eventually pay the price by catching the plague themselves. To everyone's surprise, they managed to avoid catching the plague and continued robbing graves, amassing a great deal of wealth. They became legendary, and everyone wanted to know how they managed to escape what seemed like inevitable death.

When they were finally captured, it was discovered that these men were the sons of a perfumer and herbalist, and they had learned about essential oils from their parents during childhood. Thanks to their parents' knowledge, the brothers knew a certain combination of oils would protect them, so they rubbed this concoction on their bodies and used the blend to clean anything they brought back from infected homes and gravesites. The powerful, legendary blend typically contains some combination of eucalyptus, clove, rosemary, thyme and sage.

Although the details of this story may never be fully verified, one thing is certain. The oils in that blend were once widely known to fight disease and protect the body, and a whole host of other oils continued to be used in perfumes, medicine and other uses for many centuries.

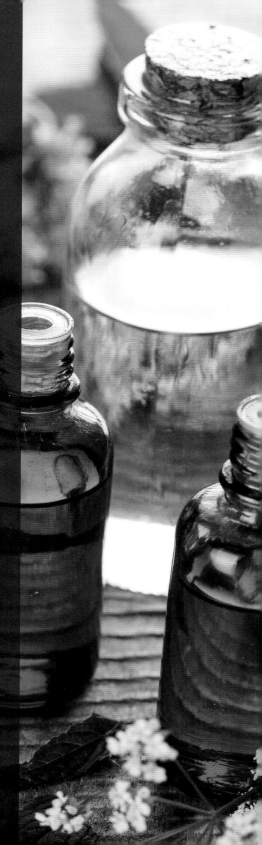

MODERN MEDICINE EMERGES

By the 1800s, pharmaceutical companies emerged, including Abbott, Parke-Davis and Squibb. Eventually, pioneering drug companies like Pfizer, Bayer, Merck and Johnson & Johnson became mainstream, and although these companies were still using plant-based medicines, synthetic drugs were gaining momentum. By the 20th century, many people stopped using whole-plant remedies and essential oils; instead, drug manufacturers offered convenient and effective medications, including penicillin and insulin.

These modern and life-saving discoveries left the idea of plants as medicine in the dust—and there essential oils sat for many years, joining the realm of seemingly obsolete folk medicine.

In 1928, essential oil use began to reemerge when French chemist René-Maurice Gattefossé used lavender oil to heal a burn on his hand. He then decided to further analyze the properties of lavender oil and how it could be used to treat other types of skin infections, wounds or burns. With this, the term "aromatherapy" was officially born.

Gattefossé and a colleague conducted further research on the healing properties of lavender and introduced it to many of the hospitals in France. During the outbreak of Spanish influenza, there were no reported deaths of hospital personnel, which was credited to the use of lavender.

The use of these oils continued to spread once again throughout Europe, especially with practitioners of alternative medicine, such as massage therapists and beauticians. Aromatherapy did not become popular in the U.S. until the 1980s, when product makers began to add essential oils to various lotions, candles and perfumes.

Today, there are trained professionals such as aromatherapists, herbalists, massage therapists, nutritionists and doctors of natural medicine who use aromatherapy in their practices and are trained in specific uses for essential oils.

Even so, their use as medicine is so highly contested and has undergone such harsh scrutiny in recent years that it has caused many people to wonder, "Are essential oils the real deal?"

The answer is a resounding YES, essential oils are "real" and, when used properly, are effective without side effects, unlike their synthetic drug counterparts. By incorporating essential oils into your daily life, you can make over your health, home and body and create a medicine and personal care cabinet fit for a king or queen.

According to the NIH (National Institute of Health) PubMed database, **there are currently 17,277 medical studies on essential oils**, many proving their therapeutic benefits. Essential oils have been used to support the body, mind and spirit since before the time of recordkeeping. They were long looked upon as sources of healing, and they were highly prized and valued. In fact, Proverbs 21:20 says: "There is treasure to be desired and oil in the dwelling of the wise."

The possession of oil in one's house was once a sign of wisdom—and we believe it can be that way again.

Medicine doesn't have to be so complicated. Health and healing don't have to be so elusive. You simply have to unlock the power of the plants that God made on the third day of creation in order to both simplify your life and enjoy a happier, healthier existence for you and your family.

CHAPTER 2

CONTROVERSY, CURES AND HEALING COMPOUNDS

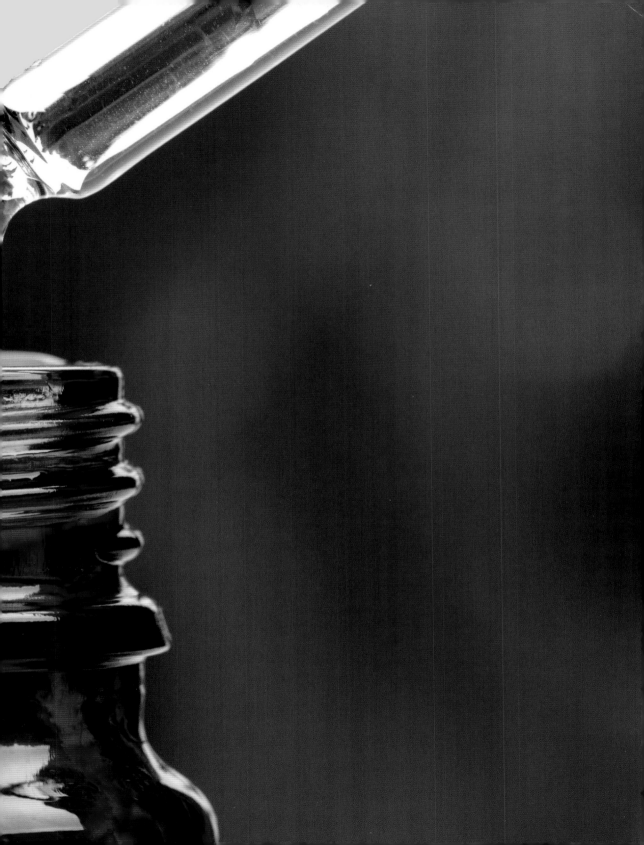

In the search for healthy alternatives to prescription drugs, chemical household cleaners and toxic personal care products, essential oils were the natural answer for the three of us.

When Jordan became a father, he knew he wanted to use only the safest products and natural medicines for his children. With six kids at home, Jordan and his wife Nicki feel good about the fact that they use oils of frankincense, lemon and thyme to support their children's immune systems during cold and flu season. They also exclusively use shampoos and cleansers made with botanicals and essential oils such as rosemary and clove, which contain free radical-fighting antioxidants.

Dr. Josh and his wife Chelsea appreciate that when you walk in their door, it smells great inside—and not because of chemically laden air fresheners, but because of the essential oils they diffuse. Their soap is filled with lemongrass, Roman chamomile and aloe vera that work to naturally clean. After a workout, they like to rub on an essential oil blend that contains turmeric, peppermint and rosemary for relief from sore and tired muscles.

Ty also diffuses oils in his home to purify the air and to enhance his and his family's natural immune response. He and his wife Charlene use oils like ginger to ease an upset stomach when one of their three children feels unwell, since studies have shown that when ginger oil is inhaled or consumed, it is effective in reducing nausea.[6,7] They also use lavender, with its highly known anti-microbial properties, to speed the healing of their kids' cuts and scrapes.

Essential oils have become so common in our households that we could not imagine our daily lives without them. But you may wonder, what exactly are essential oils? How are they different from other oils? Why are they so powerful?

There have also been a lot of questions concerning proper usage and safety of essential oils.

In the next few chapters, we will answer your questions by first explaining what essential oils really are and how they are made today and then providing the most critical information every essential oil user needs to know to use them safely and effectively.

In this chapter, we will start with the most basic fundamentals for those who are new to essential oils, or for those want to know more about their derivation and properties. The sections in Chapters 2 and 3 each begin with a question, and you can use the headings as an educational resource or a quick reference guide for answers to some of the most frequent questions we receive about essential oils.

We believe the reason some people don't understand the power of essential oils is because they don't have the right information. This is your opportunity to gain the best knowledge and empower your health and well-being.

WHAT ARE ESSENTIAL OILS?

Essential oils certainly don't seem like "oil" in the most widely recognized sense. To understand essential oils a little better, let's first examine the other more common family of oils called "fixed oils." Fixed oils are non-volatile (which means they don't evaporate into the air) oils of animal or plant origin; they are the ones we all know the best and often use in the kitchen (such as olive, grapeseed and coconut).

Essential oils, which are known as "volatile oils," function very differently from these oils because they evaporate readily and will pass more easily and more quickly into the body through the skin. The oil's volatility is what makes it aromatic and useful in aromatherapy—the molecules released as vapor into the air carry the essential oil's scent.

For instance, if you put coconut oil on your skin, it will still look "oily" or "greasy" two minutes later; but if you put frankincense oil on your skin, two minutes later there will be no remnant of it because some has evaporated and the rest penetrated your skin and is being passed deeply into the cells, tissues, organs and bloodstream.

Essential oils are obtained from plants—including flowers, leaves, roots, barks and peels—using a steam-distillation, cold pressing or CO_2 extraction process. Some companies sell plant extracts that they call essential oils, but to be a true essential oil, an extract must be obtained without the use of chemical solvents.

We will discuss how to ascertain the quality of essential oils in the next chapter.

WHY ARE THEY CALLED "ESSENTIAL" OILS?

When something is described as "essential," it is only natural to think of the item as a necessary thing since that is often what the word "essential" means. For instance, some vitamins and minerals are described as being essential because the body can't produce them and requires them to remain healthy.

Essential amino acids are those that the body needs but cannot produce on its own. These amino acids must be derived from the foods we eat. Given the use of the word "essential" to describe nutrients that our bodies need, it is no wonder that there is some confusion as to what essential oils are and why we call them essential.

However, when used to describe essential oils, the word "essential" is a different word altogether. It is a shortened version of the word "quintessential." In modern times, the word "quintessential" means "embodying or possessing the essence of something." This essence is the term that describes essential oils; these natural liquids are drawn from the very essence of the plant.

The word "quintessential" has a history that dates back to the discovery of essential oils, and the two have been interlinked since that time. "Quintessential" can be literally translated to mean "the fifth essence." This quinta essentia was thought to be the fifth and highest element, and it was believed that when the quinta essentia combined with earth, air, fire and water, it made up the whole of a being.

The quintessence was the life force or spirit of the being or plant. A similar comparison in humans would be the word "pneuma" (also spelled numa or nooma), which means the spirit or "breath of life" in the Bible.

While essential oils aren't really comprised of the spirit of the plant, they are the plant's essence. That essence is made up of beneficial compounds that can support our health in numerous ways.

HOW DO ESSENTIAL OILS WORK?

Plants are more complex than many imagine; they are the only living things that can produce their own energy using the light of the sun. The rest of us, human and animal alike, are dependent on plants at some level to provide us with the energy and nutrients we need for survival.

Plants, though not sentient, have an "intelligence" of their own. More than just roots, stems and leaves, plants have a complicated system of communication, both within each individual plant and also with the surrounding environment. These communications are made by means of chemical messengers.[8]

These natural plant chemicals are created with unique tastes, aromas and colors to protect the plant from predators, sweet smells to attract pollinators and coatings to keep bacteria and fungi at bay. Some plants even release a chemical that prevents competing plant species from growing in the first plant's territory!

This is fundamentally why essential oils are so powerful as natural remedies. We are capturing the healing properties of the plant and using them to support our own bodies. For instance, most flowers give off scents that are attractive in nature to bees. Similarly, throughout history, women have used floral oils such as rose, jasmine and lavender to attract men.

The plants of oregano and thyme naturally repel pathogenic bacteria, viruses and parasites in nature, actions that protect the plant itself. When we use their oils, they can benefit our bodies in the same way if we suffer with infections from candida, the flu or the common cold.

As you can see, essential oils are complex and life-giving compounds that benefit the plant as well as humans.

As it says in Genesis 1:12, "The land produced vegetation, all sorts of seed-bearing plants and trees with seed bearing fruit. Their seeds produced plants and trees of the same kind. And God saw that it was good." You can harness more of the goodness that God gave us by using essential oils.

ARE ESSENTIAL OILS SAFE?

When trying any new product, it is important to remember that everybody is different. "Natural" is not a synonym for "safe." Essential oils are highly concentrated compounds. Whether inhaled, applied to the skin or consumed, using this level of concentration means that any sensitivity or allergy to the source plant will be magnified. Strong fragrances may trigger respiratory reactions in people with asthma or similar conditions, and applying the oil directly to your skin may cause a skin reaction.

Additionally, some plants have natural medicinal qualities that can react with your prescribed medications or exacerbate a medical condition. So, to be safe, always start slowly when using a new essential oil. Dilute the oil before using it on your skin. Check with your physician if you are taking medication or suffer from allergies. Furthermore, some essential oils should be avoided if you are pregnant. It is always a good idea to research the specific risks associated with the essential oil you are considering.

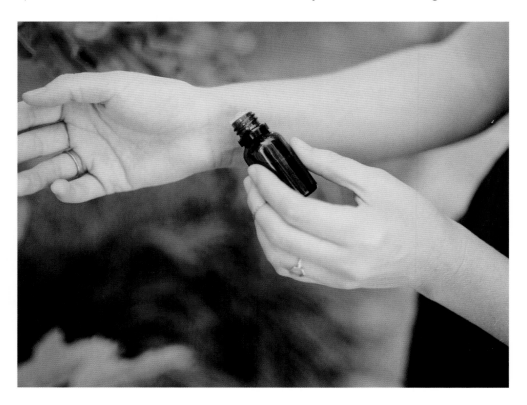

ESSENTIAL OIL SAFETY FACTORS

According to the National Association for Holistic Aromatherapy, factors that influence the safety of essential oils include:

1. **Quality of the essential oil being utilized:** Adulterated essential oils increase the likelihood of an adverse response. Therefore, the need for pure, authentic and genuine essential oils is of the utmost importance (see the oil quality guidelines under "How Can I Tell I'm Getting the Best Oils?" in Chapter 3).

2. **Chemical composition of the oil:** Essential oils rich in aldehydes (like cinnamon) and phenols (like clove and oregano) may cause skin reactions. The oils rich in these constituents should always be diluted prior to application to the skin (see safety precautions in Chapter 5).

3. **Method of application:** Essential oils may be applied on the skin (dermal application), inhaled, diffused or taken internally. Each of these methods has safety considerations (see safety precautions in regard to method of application in Chapter 5).

4. **Dosage/dilution applied:** Essential oils are highly concentrated, and a little bit goes a long way. When using topically, a carrier oil may be used. Any excessive usage of essential oils may cause irritation or other undesired effects due to their lipophilic (fat-liking) nature (for more on proper application and dilution, see Chapter 5).

5. **Integrity of skin:** Damaged, diseased or inflamed skin is often more penetrable and may be more sensitive to dermal reactions. It is potentially dangerous to put undiluted essential oils onto damaged, diseased or inflamed skin.

6. **Age of user:** Infants, toddlers and young children are more sensitive to essential oils. Also, some essential oils should simply be avoided for children, pregnant and breastfeeding women and the elderly.

For a more complete list of safety information and precautions for using essential oils, refer to the safety guidelines in Chapter 5 and throughout this book.

CAN ESSENTIAL OILS CURE DISEASE?

Many modern medicines include plant-derived compounds, and as we discussed in Chapter 1, ancient remedies were based on natural ingredients. Herbalists and natural healers have known about the benefits of botanicals for generations. Yet widespread information about essential oils remains limited until recently, when the number of published articles and research studies available on the effectiveness of essential oils has skyrocketed.

In many instances, studies have shown a correlation between a specific essential oil and a health benefit, and we will share this information throughout the book.

The use of essential oils in the U.S. for therapeutic purposes is still limited, but medical aromatherapy is common in Europe, where essential oils are most often used as part of a comprehensive treatment plan. Approximately 100 varieties of essential oils are used in Austria and Europe for aromatherapeutic purposes.

The benefits of essential oils are probably best realized when they are used as a supplement or adjunct to other treatment protocols, along with a healthy diet of real food that comes from nature and is free from chemicals, pesticides, antibiotics and added hormones.

The use of essential oils can enhance your life in many ways, but they are not cure-alls. If you are dealing with a serious disease, their use should be a part of a supervised treatment plan.

Now that you know the basic *what* and *why* of essentials oils, in the next chapter, you will discover more about how they are farmed and then extracted.

What is amazing is that each and every plant has unique properties that make it ideal for unique, specific uses. God put such thought and meticulous design into each plant from which we extract these amazing oils.

He really is the ultimate scientist.

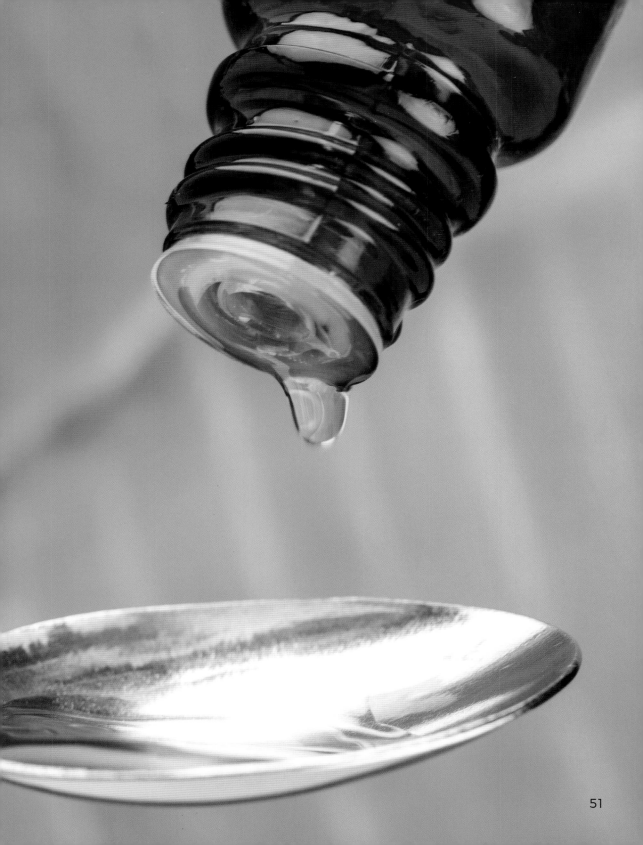

CHAPTER 3

GO ORGANIC AND GET WILD

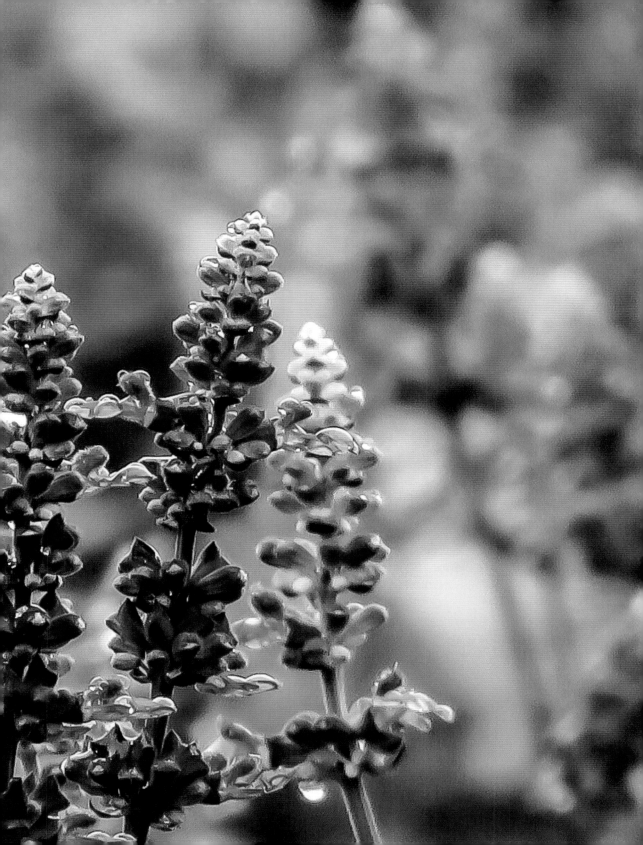

In today's toxic world, going organic and following a holistic approach to health is more important than ever. We know that many health conditions—from autism to cancer and autoimmune disease to eczema—have been linked to toxicity. And if you're like us, you want to keep your home and family toxic-free by only purchasing the highest quality foods, supplements and essential oils. One action the three of us all believe in very strongly is supporting organic farming methods that are free of pesticides and allowing plants to grow to their peak ripeness before being harvested and extracted without the use of chemicals.

We've all been exposed to the ugly side of modern-day agriculture and the heavy toll our planet is paying—all in the name of greed and profit. Sourcing exclusively from organic, non-GMO growers is a great first step, but Jordan wanted to do more. That is why he started the Beyond Organic Ranch and Heal the Planet Farm in southern Missouri.

What you will find there is nothing short of amazing when you consider how most of our food is raised. The livestock on Jordan's farm, including cows, sheep, goats and chickens, are "pasture raised," which means their food comes from grazing in open pastures, the water they drink is from a deep aquifer and they are some of the best cared for animals in the world. Likewise, all of the crops grown on Heal the Planet Farm are organic and grown without the use of chemicals.

Pierre Chardin, a French philosopher and Jesuit priest, bestowed this wisdom upon the world: *The future belongs to those who give the next generation hope*. That is why Jordan likes to say, "We are farming for our future."

Since essential oils are derived from plants, this is a relevant discussion because an essential oil is only as good as the plant from which it originated. This chapter will educate you on the proper making of essential oils, what to look for in terms of quality and some critical issues when it comes to safety.

If you are like us, you are willing to do whatever it takes to ensure a healthy future for your family. Those actions should include using only the highest quality essential oils that are properly farmed, harvested and extracted for maximum therapeutic benefit.

HOW ARE ESSENTIAL OIL PLANTS FARMED?

The farming of essential oil plants is a highly specialized process. It is also extremely important, because just as the type of food and water given to a cow affects the toxicity level of the dairy or meat it produces, the terrain and soil used to grow the plants directly correlates to the purity of the oils.

Plants must be both grown and harvested by knowledgeable farmers who will allow the plant time to mature properly and without the use of harsh chemicals or pesticides. If a field is sprayed with toxic chemicals, this affects the chemistry of the plants and, ultimately, their therapeutic quality.

For instance, a recent study done on blueberries found that wild Alaskan blueberries contain 3 to 5 times more antioxidants than conventional blueberries grown in North America.[9] This demonstrates the difference the proper soil, climate and harvesting method make in creating an exceptional food, supplement or essential oil.

Most essential oil crops do well in temperate, Mediterranean and subtropical regions. For example, lavender is a Mediterranean plant, and it requires a similar climate to thrive. The Provence region of France is where most lavender is commercially grown, as the climate, with mild winters and warm, sunny summers, is ideal for lavender production.

Because of environmental toxicity and soil depletion, crops grown just decades ago were much richer in vitamins and minerals than are the varieties most of us get today—and with the growing popularity of essential oils, essential oil crops are in danger of being grown in over-farmed, depleted soil, which would in turn lessen their therapeutic benefit.

Just like the animals and crops on Jordan's farm, essential oil plants do best when they are allowed to grow and thrive in an environment that most closely resembles the wild—given no chemicals, situated in their ideal climate, allowed to grow to maturity in nutrient-rich soil and fed with natural sunlight and the purest water available.

HOW ARE ESSENTIAL OILS MADE?

Essential oils are present inside the plants because God created the oils for highly specific purposes within their living hosts. In fact, they serve four distinct purposes in nature:

1. Essential oil constituents **protect plants** by attacking organisms that threaten the survival of the species.

2. Essential oils **defend plants** by preventing animals or insects from eating them. The oil constituents are able to repel these pests because the scent is noxious or irritating to many animals.

3. The unique fragrance of essential oils is thought to be inviting for a pollinating insect, even more so than color; therefore, essential oils are able to **increase pollination**.

4. Essential oils **prevent other plants from growing too close** to the plant. This biological phenomenon is called allelopathy, which happens when plants produce biochemicals that influence the growth, survival and reproduction of organisms.

Regardless of the amazing and varied functions they serve in a plant, essential oils must be extracted if we wish to use them. The methods of extraction depend on the plant material, the type of product to be liberated and the availability of equipment. The three basic methods of essential oil production are steam distillation, expression and extraction.

Steam distillation. Steam distillation is the most common method for producing essential oils today. The method for extracting essential oils was invented when Avicenna, an Arabian physician, added water to rose petals and distilled the mixture in the 10th century. The rose water he collected is considered to be the first modern perfume.

Although Avicenna is credited with the invention, evidence of distillation occurring thousands of years earlier was found in Tape Gowra, Mesopotamia. It consisted of a pot, which held almost 40 liters, and a collecting ring that had a capacity of about 2 liters. This apparatus dates back to 3600 B.C.

In steam distillation, plant material is exposed to steam, whose heat causes the essential oil to evaporate. Subsequent cooling of the hot vapors causes condensation of both water vapor and oil. Because the oil and water will not mix, they are easy to separate at that stage.

Although the water is always separated from the essential oil during a steam distillation, it is often reserved (called a *hydrosol*) and used to add a pleasant fragrance to linen sprays, perfumes, moisturizers and hair and body products. See Figure 3.1 for an illustrated guide to steam distillation.

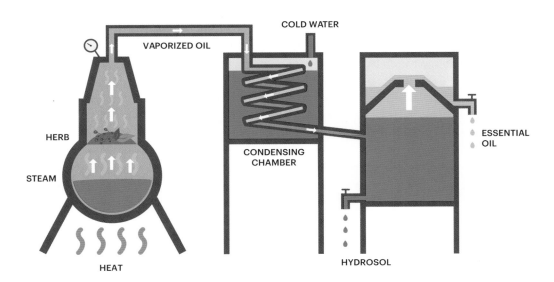

Figure 3.1. The Steam Distillation Process. The most common method for extracting essential oils, steam distillation also produces hydrosol (a scented water also known as "flower water").

Expression. The expression process is used to obtain oils from citrus fruit, because the heat of distilling essential oils easily damages citrus oils. This technique is sometimes called *cold-pressing* because the oils are literally pressed out of the peel by hand or machine at ambient temperatures.

A more modern method of cold-pressing extraction, which is less labor-intensive, has been termed the "ecuelle a piquer process," where the fruit is placed in a device and rotated with spikes on the side puncturing the oil cells in the skin of the fruit. The puncturing of the rind will release the essential oil to be collected in a small area below the container.

Carbon dioxide (CO_2) extraction. Oils extracted by the CO_2 (carbon dioxide) method are commonly called *CO_2 extracts* or *supercritical fluid extractions*. This method uses carbon dioxide to carry the essential oil away from the raw plant material. CO_2 extracts are removed by pressurizing carbon dioxide until it becomes a liquid. The liquid carbon dioxide then acts as a solvent on the natural plant matter, and the essential oil content then dissolves into the liquid CO_2. Before being pressed through the plant, the carbon dioxide is then chilled, which causes the CO_2 to evaporate back into its gaseous state—and what is left is the resulting oil.

Supercritical fluid extraction produces a pure and unaltered essential oil. Spicy-smelling oils like ginger and clove can be produced with carbon dioxide. Other oils produced via CO_2 extraction include turmeric, frankincense and myrrh. The CO_2 supercritical extraction process eliminates the need for potentially harmful solvents like hexane that is often used in the manufacturing process of absolute oils, avoiding unnecessary environmental pollution and potential human bodily harm. It is a process that is growing in popularity as more and more essential oil companies embrace the concept of using CO_2 extracts.

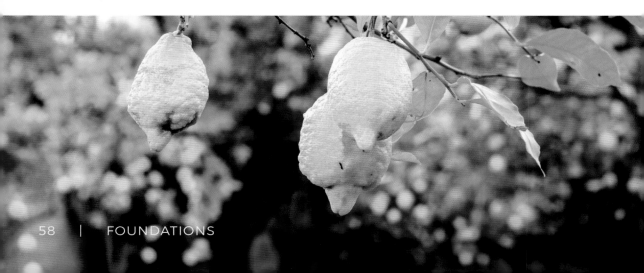

IS THERE A DIFFERENCE IN THE QUALITY OF OILS?

The answer to that is absolutely! You've heard the popular saying, "Quality over quantity." This holds especially true when it comes to essential oils. Many people think that when they buy oil that is labeled "100% pure," they are getting good oils. This is often far from true. Pure, unadulterated essential oil is more difficult to come by than many imagine, and it can be expensive. One reason for this is because it can take as many as 500 to 2,000 pounds or more of raw plant material to produce just a pound of essential oil. For example:

» It takes 27 square feet of lavender plants to make one 15 mL bottle of lavender oil.
» It takes 256 pounds of peppermint leaves to make 1 pound of peppermint oil.
» It takes 75 lemons to make one 15 mL bottle of lemon oil.
» It takes 60 roses to make a single drop of rose oil.

No wonder quality oils are costly!

Remember, in the Bible, it was said that a jar of nard (lavender) was worth a year's wages, and frankincense and myrrh were valued alongside gold.

To be truly therapeutic, an essential oil must be free of chemicals and slowly and carefully extracted through methods that keep the original compounds in their natural state. The oils should also be bottled in dark glass containers to protect them from oxidation and sunlight, identified with their Latin name (to avoid confusion between the identification of some essential oils and their uses for therapeutic purposes), and tested to meet the standard of the species.

When purchasing essential oils, you should always buy essential oils produced from organic ingredients whenever possible. Don't be afraid to ask questions about the origins, extraction process and quality of any essential oil you purchase. The only way to get a pure and high-quality essential oil is from oils that are unprocessed and sourced directly from nature, with nothing added. This allows the oils to remain rich and complex—just as God created them.

HOW CAN I TELL I'M GETTING THE BEST OILS?

One of the most vital rules you must remember about essential oils is this: *Not all essential oils are created equally.* In fact, many are worthless to your health and can even be potentially toxic due to synthetic chemicals and other additives. Here is a quick guide to the four grades of essential oils available:

Synthetic and altered oils. These oils are created in laboratories and are considered the lowest grade of oil. Although chemists have successfully recreated multiple chemical constituents of plants, those man-made constituents do not have the same healing properties as essential oils.

Natural and "pure" oils. Although of better quality, these oils are overly processed, so they lose healing compounds. Natural oils are the most commonly sold type of essential oils. Just like the use of the word "natural," there are many loopholes involved with the use of the word "pure." It is possible for essential oils to be labeled as "100% Pure" or "100% Natural," but not be the highest quality as one would hope or expect. For example, lavender oil is often cut with lavandin, which has very little therapeutic quality.

Pure also does not mean it has no additional ingredients added to it. It could be 75 percent vegetable oil and 25 percent essential oil and still be labeled "100% Pure." In the U.S., you are only required to have 5 percent essential oil in the bottle to label it "Pure."

Therapeutic-grade essential oils. These oils are said to have been steam-distilled and unadulterated, containing an array of beneficial compounds. However, therapeutic-grade is an unregulated term and is really defined by the company that produced them with no outside third-party validation. The only negative associated with therapeutic-grade essential oils is that they may come from plants and herbs that may have been grown with the use of chemical fertilizers and sprayed with pesticides.

Certified organic essential oils. These are the highest grade of essential oils with the greatest healing properties. You can smell, feel and taste the difference between certified organic oils and those produced from conventionally grown plants. Organic essential oils can cost between 2 to 4 times the price of their conventional counterparts, and some organic oils are in very short supply, which are the only real reasons an essential oil manufacturer would choose not to use organic oils.

It is important to note that although "therapeutic-grade" essential oils are generally considered the safest oils, currently there is no regulatory standard for the descriptive use of the term "therapeutic-grade," which means anyone can claim something is therapeutic-grade since there is no quality standard for authentication.

Two organizations, the International Organization for Standardization (ISO) and the Association French Normalization Organization Regulation (AFNOR), provide specifications as a guide to essential oil compositions. However, there is also no company or agency that officially certifies essential oils or their quality.

Ethical companies who are committed to quality will use certain guidelines like those set by ISO and AFNOR as well as their own internal standards to make sure the oils they are creating will preserve the properties and integrity of the plant.

In the labeling of essential oils, what you have are instances of ethical questions rather than legal ones, which may make it seem difficult to find the best oil. However, if you want to ensure the quality of the oil you use, there are several ways to assess an essential oil's potency and therapeutic quality:

1. Check to see if certain testing has been performed. It is ideal to purchase essential oils from a company or manufacturer who performs gas chromatography and mass spectrometry (GC/MS) testing. These testing techniques can analyze the constituents in oils. Gas chromatography (GC) is a technique that provides a fingerprint of the oil and can reveal additives. A mass spectrometer (MS) can measure the presence and quantity of chemical constituents that give essential oils their therapeutic benefits.

GC/MS testing can detect if two or more oils with similar chemical composition have been mixed together, if an oil has had certain chemical constituents removed or if an oil has been rectified (made with lower quality plant parts). It will also reveal traces of solvents or mineral oils.

2. Know your Latin names. One of the simplest things you can do to be certain you are purchasing the right essential oil is to read the label. Many

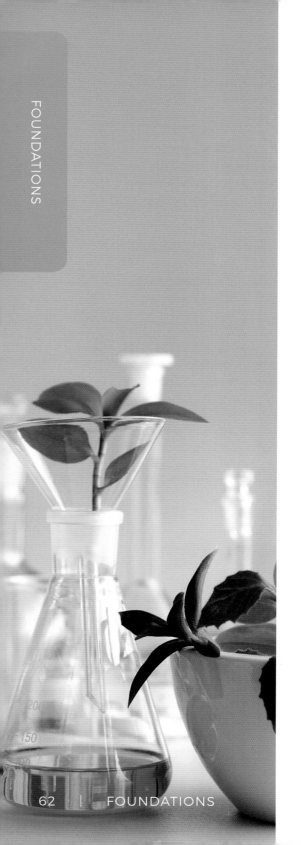

plant names around the world also have similar common names but come in different varieties that can produce different results. If purchasing an unknown brand of essential oil, purchase by the Latin name, and always check for the correct botanical name.

Lavender is a good example of the importance of Latin names. *L. angustifolia*, also referred to as "true lavender," is the preferred lavender for clinical aromatherapy—not lavandin (*L. intermedia*). True lavender has almost no camphor, whereas lavandin can have up to 40 percent.

This matters because camphor is known to have a stimulating effect. Since lavender's reputation is primarily that of a sedative, if you purchase lavender using just the common name, you could end up with an oil that will keep you alert rather than relaxed.

3. Check the price tag. There is an awareness that a price that is very low comparatively may indicate that an oil is not sourced from the correct plant or part of the plant, or that it is diluted in a base oil or is otherwise adulterated.

Generally, higher, premium priced oils designate superior quality.

4. Trust your nose. The smell, taste, feel and look of essential oils can provide important information about its quality and whether or not it should be used. In short, the more potent the fragrance, typically the more pure and powerful the oil.

TIPS FOR PURCHASING HIGH-QUALITY OILS

When purchasing essential oils, keep these questions in mind to ensure you are getting the best quality:

» Is it from a reputable company that is known for its quality products?

» Has the essential oil been tested or verified by a third party?

» Is the essential oil certified organic or at the very least wild crafted?

» Is the price of the oil in line with similar companies? If the price is significantly cheaper than oils from similar companies, it may not be a high-quality oil.

» Does the label provide legitimate information, such as the plant's Latin name and common name?

If you are new to the world of essential oils, it can seem overwhelming. Ask around and find the most trusted brands from friends and family who are seasoned essential oil users. A well-known reputation for producing high-quality oils will go far in the industry, but oils made by smaller distillers who use the proper techniques and test their oils for quality are excellent choices as well.

Always remember to trust your instincts—and your nose!

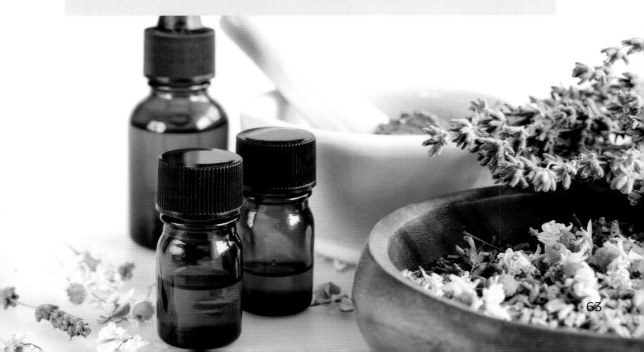

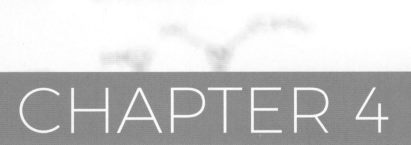

CHAPTER 4

ESSENTIAL OILS
CHEMISTRY 101

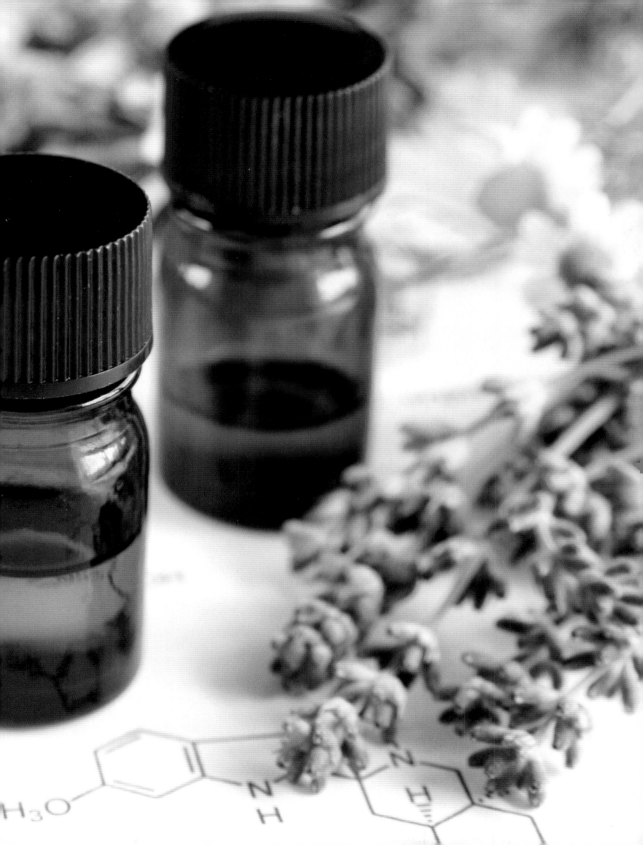

H_3O NH N NH

Many of today's synthetic drugs carry potentially serious side effects. The Nutrition Institute of America funded an independent review of "government-approved medicine" that was published in 2006. Professors Gary Null and Dorothy Smith, along with doctors Carolyn Dean, Martin Feldman and Debora Rasio titled the report, "Death by Medicine."[10]

The researchers found that America's leading cause of death isn't heart disease or cancer: it's conventional medicine. Over the course of a decade, the scientists predict that iatrogenic deaths will total about 7.8 million, "more than all the casualties from all the wars fought by the U.S. throughout its entire history," a death rate equivalent to that caused by six jumbo jets falling out of the sky every day.

What that means is we are spending billions of dollars every year on conventional treatments that are killing us at a faster rate than the ailments for which we are being treated.

Essential oils, on the other hand, represent a gentle, supportive approach to healing. Because of their chemical structure, they're metabolized in the cells like other nutrients. Essential oils are volatile and therefore evaporate quickly. So, unlike many synthetic drugs, they don't accumulate in the body. The remarkable qualities of essential oil chemistry make using oils a safe and natural alternative for healing the body.

When Dr. Josh's mom was diagnosed with cancer for the second time, frightening statistics about iatrogenic death rates were not widely available; yet his family felt strongly that she would soon become a statistic if they followed the conventional path to cancer treatment again.

That is when she started following an all-natural plan that included vegetable juicing, probiotic foods, immune-boosting supplements, stress-reducing techniques, prayer and essential oils.

After only four months, the tumors on her lungs had shrunk significantly and one year after that, she was again diagnosed as being "cancer-free" and healthy. Ten years later, she is in her mid-60s and in the best shape of her life, regularly water skiing, running and still going strong.

We want to be clear—we are not claiming that what Dr. Josh's mother did is a proven cancer treatment. We're also not attributing her results solely to the use of essential oils, as they played a supportive role in her recovery. But we believe natural therapies, either used by themselves or in conjunction

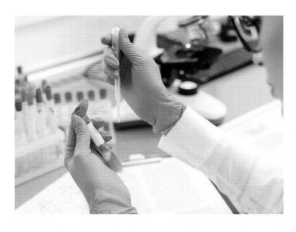

with conventional medical treatments, may support the body in the healing process.

Dr. Josh is often asked, "What exactly did your mom do?" Among other regimented therapy plans, one of the things she used was essential oils, such as *frankincense, myrrh, lavender and oregano oil*. Frankincense essential oil is one of the most effective natural cancer fighters and is now the subject of numerous research trials. Specifically, Indian Frankincense (*Boswellia serrata*) has been shown clinically to be an adjunctive remedy for various forms of cancer. [11,12,13,14,15]

According to researchers out of Baylor University Medical Center in Dallas, the potential cancer-fighting effects of frankincense are due to its chemistry—components in frankincense give it the ability to influence your genes to promote healing.

In each of our families, essential oils are a natural, first choice for supplementation. The reason for our confidence in them is based on their rich history of use, the thousands of articles and studies proving their effectiveness and, ultimately, the chemistry of essential oils, from which their distinct abilities are derived.

Essential oil chemistry reveals an elegance that is nothing short of astounding. Learning about their complex nature provides greater insight into how essential oils can affect your health.

CHEMISTRY DEMYSTIFIED

Essential oils have been called the "lifeblood" of a plant. They circulate through plant tissues and pass through cell walls, carrying nutrition into cells and carrying waste products out. Because the chemistry of pure essential oils retains the healing intent of the plants from which they originated, they manifest an ability to organize and balance our energies as well. If our bodies are out of balance and experiencing illness or dysfunction, the oils serve to restore order and balance (or homeostasis) to our various systems.

Research has found that people who consistently use essential oils have a higher level of resistance to illnesses, colds, flus and diseases than the average person. Further indications show that after contracting a cold, flu or other illness, these individuals will recover 60 to 70 percent faster than those who do not use essential oils.

There are two main groups of essential oil constituents that define the chemistry of essential oils: 1) hydrocarbons and 2) oxygenated compounds, and both types are further divided into subgroups. Oils contain multiple constituents, which is why they have so many varied properties and uses.

For example, a major component of frankincense oil (40 percent of its composition) is alpha-pinene, which is a monoterpene hydrocarbon. That enables frankincense to take on the therapeutic qualities of monoterpenes. Frankincense also contains 98 other constituents—and the end result is an essential oil that has innumerable value and uses.

In the remainder of the chapter, we will briefly look at each chemical compound subgroup in order to highlight each constituent's therapeutic benefits, as well as which oils contain large percentages of each.

Hydrocarbons

Monoterpenes is a chemical family made up of components that are considered "top notes," as they are the first aromas to hit your nose in a blend. Monoterpenes are found in almost all essential oils in some percentage. Essential oils with more than 60 percent monoterpenes include frankincense, grapefruit, cypress, lemon, juniper berry and sweet orange. Here are some of the therapeutic qualities of monoterpenes:

> » Analgesic
> » Anti-bacterial
> » Antiseptic
> » Decongestant
> » Excellent for diffusing since they kill airborne germs
> » Expectorant
> » Great for getting deep into sore muscles, tendons and ligaments
> » Rubifacient (increases circulation)

Sesquiterpenes are present in almost all essential oils. Research from the Universities of Berlin and Vienna show increased oxygenation around the pineal and pituitary glands with the introduction of sesquiterpenes. Further research has shown that sesquiterpenes have the ability to surpass the blood-brain barrier and enter the brain tissue.[16,17] Although they are difficult to generalize, here are some therapeutic qualities and examples of sesquiterpene-containing oils:

» Analgesic
» Anti-fungal
» Anti-inflammatory
» Anti-spasmodic
» Antiseptic
» Sedative

Oxygenated Compounds

Phenols have excellent therapeutic properties because they are stimulating to the nervous and immune systems. They are an excellent choice for combating an aggressive infection. Examples of oils containing high amounts of phenols are wintergreen, oregano, clove and tea tree. Here are some of the therapeutic qualities of phenols:

» Anti-bacterial
» Antiseptic
» Disinfectant
» Stimulant

Alcohols are divided into monoterpene and sesquiterpene alcohols. Sesquiterpene alcohols are not commonly found in large quantities in essential oils, but when found (like bisabolol in German chamomile), they have great properties, which include liver and glandular stimulant, anti-allergen and anti-inflammatory. Other oils that contain sesquiterpene alcohols are sandalwood, ginger, patchouli, vetiver, carrot seed and valerian. Monoterpene alcohols have very few known side effects and have an uplifting, energizing effect. High levels of monoterpenes alcohols are found in lavender, rose, geranium, juniper and tea tree oil. They also have the following properties:

» Anti-fungal
» Anti-viral
» Antiseptic

» Bactericidal
» Germicidal

Esters are the most relaxing, calming and balancing of all the essential oil constituents. They regulate the nervous system and are anti-spasmodic. Some of the essential oils with the highest percentages of esters are Roman chamomile, jasmine absolute and helichrysum. Here are some of the other therapeutic qualities of esters:

» Analgesic
» Anti-inflammatory
» Sedative
» Soothing
» Stress-reducing

Aldehydes are calming to the nervous system. They are best known to relieve stress and promote relaxation. Aldehydes can be quite irritating when applied topically, but may have a profound calming effect when inhaled. Cinnamon bark and lemongrass contain high amounts of aldehydes, which have the following therapeutic properties:

» Anti-bacterial
» Anti-fungal
» Anti-inflammatory
» Anti-spasmodic
» Fever reducer
» Sedative

Ketones have distinctive fragrances and are calming and sedative. They also stimulate cell regeneration, promote new tissue growth and liquefy mucus, making them ideal for respiratory issues. Peppermint has more ketones than most other essential oils, although rosemary, vetiver and spike lavender have effective amounts as well. Ketones also generally provide the following benefits:

» Analgesic
» Anti-spasmodic
» Cicatrisant (scar healing)
» Rubifacient
» Wound healing

Oxides are expectorants that can be mildly stimulating. 1,8-cineole or eucalyptol is the most prevalent member of the oxide family, and it is wonderful for respiratory issues. Eucalyptus, ravensara and rosemary contain high amounts of oxides. Other therapeutic properties of oxides include:

» Anti-bacterial
» Anti-fungal
» Anti-viral
» Can stimulate blood flow to the brain when inhaled

THE CHEMISTRY OF ESSENTIAL OILS

If you're interested in the therapeutic use of essential oils, some knowledge of their chemistry can be highly useful. Not only will you better understand how and why essential oils work, but the great importance of using natural, high-quality oils will also be made clear. Essential oils have different chemical make-ups than other oils, and the differences can significantly affect the healing potency of topical, inhaled and oral applications for you and your family. In the next chapter, you will learn more about the potency of oils and how to use them safely and effectively in a variety of applications.

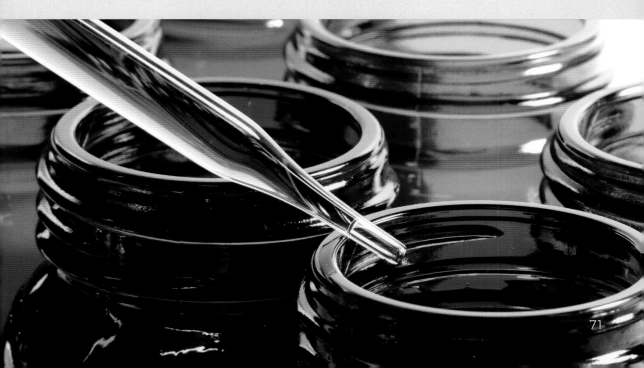

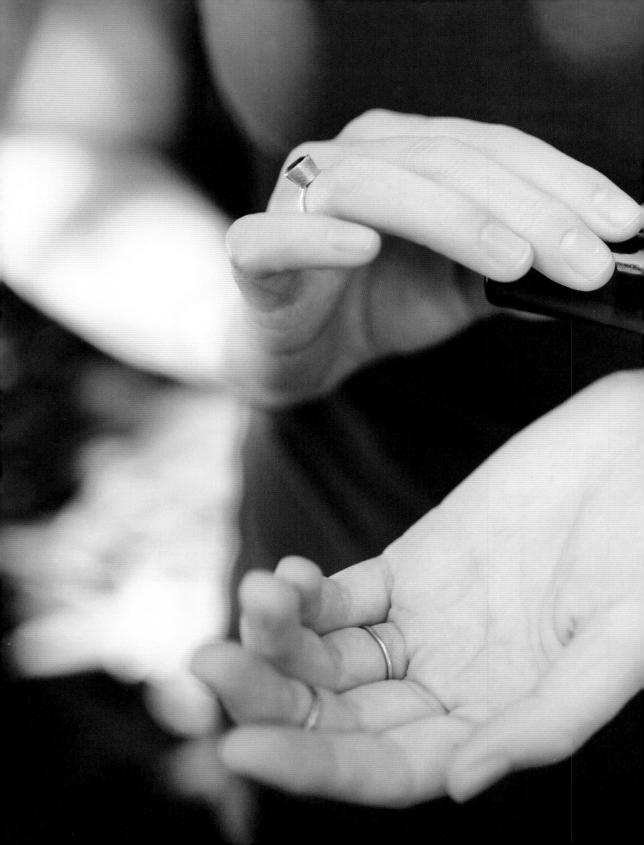

CHAPTER 5

USING ESSENTIAL OILS SAFELY AND EFFECTIVELY

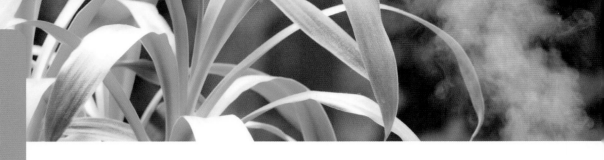

Everyone has a different "essential oil style." Some people use essential oils as natural remedies while others use them to fragrance the air. Some use them to replace toxic personal care products. Finally, other people use essential oils for everything—it becomes part of their cleaning products, shampoo, toothpaste, detergent, deodorant and used as first aid remedies.

The three of us have our own essential own styles that are unique to our families.

Jordan has seen his life transformed by the use of essential oils every day. His essential oil style might be called "ancient healing." As he anoints his family with oils each morning, he is reminded of the wondrous power within the oils as he thanks the Great Physician who created them.

Ty's essential oil style is one of "soothing air." He prefers to diffuse his oils because he believes that is the best way for his entire family to experience the immune boosting, restorative, energizing abilities of essential oils each and every day.

Dr. Josh enjoys finding new ways to use essential oils. His essential oil style is "infinite possibilities" because he and his wife use it to clean their air, care for their dogs, improve their sleep, stop headaches, improve concentration and countless other uses.

What's your essential oil style? Everybody has one—even those who are just beginning to explore the world of essential oils. The good news is that there are so many oils and so many ways to use them that the options for use are virtually limitless.

There are, however, a finite number of ways essential oils may be used when it comes to our bodies. The ways in which they are used are dependent upon the needs or desired outcome of the individual using the oil. This chapter will describe the three main methods of essential oil use: 1) aromatherapy applications (direct inhalation and diffusing), 2) topical use and 3) internal use.

THE FRAGRANT WORLD OF AROMATHERAPY

The aromatic nature of essential oils stimulates powerful mental, emotional and physiologic responses. Not only does the aroma of the natural essential oil stimulate the brain to trigger a reaction, but also when inhaled into the lungs, the naturally occurring chemicals can supply therapeutic benefits. For example, diffusing eucalyptus essential oil is an effective way to help ease congestion.

When a person simply breathes in the aroma of an essential oil, this is called direct inhalation. Here are some methods of **direct inhalation**:

» Open an essential oil bottle and breathe in the aroma.
» Place a drop or two of oil or a blend of oils in the hands, rub them together, make a cup around the nose and mouth and breathe in. (Note: Use caution when practicing this method. Some essential oils require prior mixing with a carrier oil, such as coconut oil, to dilute the concentration and prevent skin irritation.)
» Place a drop or two of oil or a blend of oils on a piece of cloth or tissue, hold it close to the face and inhale.

Another popular method of aromatherapy is **diffusing essential oils** into a room. When using a diffuser, the essential oil is evaporated into the surrounding environment. Diffusing essential oils can alter your mood by relaxing or stimulating the mind. It can also kill airborne pathogens and treat a respiratory condition. Here are some ways to diffuse essential oils:

» To clean the air, add a blend of lemon, clove, orange, cinnamon, eucalyptus and rosemary oils to a diffuser.
» To improve energy, add peppermint to a diffuser.
» To reduce stress or combat a headache, or just to relax, add lavender to a diffuser.

There are four main types of diffusers:

1. **Atomizing:** No water is involved when using atomizing diffusers—the essential oil bottle is connected to the diffuser to create a pure vapor that is extremely powerful and therapeutic.

2. **Vaporizing:** These diffusers use water with the essential oil; ultrasonic waves are used to emit the oil and water particles into the air. Vaporizing diffusers are very quiet, so they are popular with therapists, yoga instructors and other professionals who are looking to achieve a peaceful environment.

3. **Fan or evaporative:** Evaporative diffusers are usually lower in cost and used in a smaller area. A fan blows air from the room through a pad or filter that has essential oils on it. The air blowing through the pad causes the oils to evaporate more quickly than with other diffusers, and the air with the evaporated oil is blown into the room.

4. **Heat:** Like evaporative diffusers, heat diffusers also cause the essential oils to evaporate quickly; these diffusers use heat instead of blowing air to accomplish diffusion.

Another way to diffuse a room with essential oils is by using a **spray bottle**. Oils can be mixed with water or alcohol and then sprayed in the air, on surfaces or on the body. This will create a refreshing and energizing environment.

LET'S GET TOPICAL

When essential oils are **applied directly to the skin**, they are absorbed and enter the bloodstream (this is because the oils are fat-soluble). When an oil is applied to the skin with no carrier oil, this is called a "neat" application. The soles of the feet is one area of the body that is sometimes exposed to a neat application. It is also one of the most popular places to apply oils. There are several reasons for this:

Less irritation. When oils are administered on the soles of the feet, there is a lower risk of skin irritation. The skin there is less sensitive than the skin on the rest of the body.

No sebum. The soles of the feet and the palms of the hands are the only sites on our body without sebaceous glands. Sebum is an oily substance that helps lubricate and waterproof the skin. Since the palms and the soles do not secrete sebum, they are more ready to absorb oil.

Bypass the liver. When you apply oils to the soles of the feet, the oils bypass the liver and will not accumulate there. Instead of being processed by the liver, the oils reach the lower bronchial capillaries via the circulatory system and the entire organism unprocessed.

Other key points of application on the body include behind the ears, neck, abdomen, upper back, temples and along the spine. When applying essential oils, sensitive skin areas should be avoided, such as the eyes, inner ears, genitals and open skin.

Essential oils are commonly **combined with a carrier oil**, which not only dilutes the essential oil but also prevents easy evaporation. Because using a carrier oil dilutes the potency of the essential oil being used, the chances of experiencing an irritation or skin reaction are reduced. Some of the best carrier oils include coconut oil, jojoba oil, grapeseed oil, olive oil, almond oil, pomegranate seed oil and avocado oil:

- *Coconut oil*—The best all-purpose oil to use in personal care products, from making homemade body care products like lotion, deodorant and toothpaste to diluting for topical use. When used topically, *fractionated coconut oil* works best due to its liquid state at room temperature.

- *Jojoba oil*—Ideal for both very dry and oily skin to help bring balance back. Use it with geranium, lavender and tea tree for tough skin conditions.

- *Magnesium oil*—Known as the ultimate relaxer. Blend it with Roman chamomile and lavender to reduce stress and improve sleep.

- *Arnica oil*—Best for treating bruises, pain and skin inflammation.

- *Shea butter*—The best carrier oil for moisturizing very dry and aged skin. It's also great for making a homemade body butter recipe.

- *Argan oil*—Known to firm and tighten skin, which is great for anti-aging effects. Mix it with frankincense, myrrh and geranium to improve skin tone. It's also packed with vitamin E.

- *Evening primrose oil*—Great for hormone balance because it contains high levels of GLA (gamma linoleic acid), which produces hormone-regulating prostaglandin. Mix it with clary sage, thyme and ylang ylang to support healthy hormones.

There are many other beneficial carrier oils such as olive, rosehip, hemp, sea buckthorn, black cumin, almond, apricot and pomegranate. For a more complete list of carrier oils, including their key benefits, please refer to Part II, which details individual essential and carrier oils.

Topical Use Recommendations
The appropriate dosage for topical use of essential oils is different for each oil and individual—taking into consideration the individual's personal circumstances and health conditions.

When determining an appropriate topical dose, age and size are the biggest factors. The younger and smaller the person, the less essential oil is needed. It is safest to start with a small amount and repeat the application 20 minutes later if necessary. *In most cases, essential oils should be diluted with a carrier oil for use on the skin.*

A generalized suggested ratio for dilution with a carrier oil is as follows:

FOR INFANTS

1 drop of essential oil to
1 tablespoon carrier oil

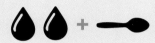

FOR CHILDREN

1 to 2 drops of essential oil
to 1 teaspoon carrier oil

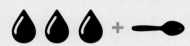

FOR ADULTS

3 to 6 drops of essential oil
to 1 teaspoon carrier oil

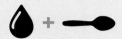

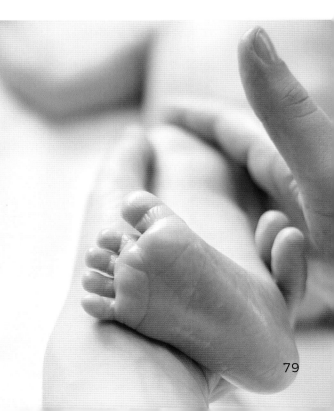

Once the essential oils are mixed with the carrier oil, rub the oils together in the palm with your fingers and apply the mixture to the specific area in circular, light massage movements.

Here are some other ways to use essential oils topically:

Baths. Adding oils to bath water is a mix of aromatic and topical applications. In order to disperse the oil throughout the bath water, add 5 to 15 drops of essential oils to bath salts or Epsom salts, which will dissolve in the water. This can help improve circulation, relieve sore muscles, soothe skin, open airways, relax the body and improve sleep. Soothing oils like eucalyptus and lavender are especially beneficial when added to an aromatherapy bath.

Compresses. Using a warm compress will increase the absorption of essential oils. Add 10 drops of oil per 4 ounces of water. Soak the cloth with the oil and water mixture and apply it to bruises, infections, aches and pains. (Peppermint is one of the best oils for muscle aches, while lavender is great for treating infections.)

Salves. A salve is an ointment that is used to soothe the surface of the body. You can make salves by adding 15 drops of essential oils to 1 ounce of a carrier oil (2.5 percent dilution). Salves can be stored in a metal or glass container and used on cuts, scrapes and sore muscles.

Personal Care. Essential oils can be used in common home remedies like homemade toothpaste, deodorant, shampoo, conditioner, body wash, face wash, perfume, cologne, lip balm and body lotion. To make homemade teeth- and gum-supporting toothpaste, mix ¼ cup coconut oil, 3 tablespoons bentonite clay and 10 drops of peppermint or clove essential oil together and put the mixture into a rubber tube or sealed glass container.

TAKING ESSENTIAL OILS INTERNALLY

Essential oils are more potent than whole plant material. Remember that a single drop of rose oil contains the chemical constituents present in 60 roses. That is why when essential oils are used internally, it should be in small amounts only. However, research does show that many oils can be safe and effective when taken orally, so it may be worth the necessary preparation and caution for certain conditions and for short periods of time.

When an essential oil is consumed in high doses, it can result in overuse or toxicity. That is because essential oils are fat-soluble, meaning they are not easily eliminated from the body and must travel through the liver and then the gut. To avoid ingesting toxic concentrations of essential oils, labels should be read carefully and professional guidelines should be followed.

When we get the question, *"Are essential oils safe to use internally?"* our answer is always, "It depends upon which oil and the person taking the oil."

There is a sub-population of therapists who believe that essential oils should not be taken internally unless recommended by a physician. They recommend only topical or aromatic use. It's important to remember that a large amount of published articles and studies have demonstrated that many essential oils provide tremendous benefits when used internally, and traditional practitioners of Chinese and Ayurvedic medicine have used essential oils therapeutically for thousands of years.

It's all about using wisdom, applying common sense and remembering that following product usage directions is key in all supplement use—and when in doubt, use the oil topically. The three of us have personally used essential oils for ourselves and our families, clients and patients.

Some oils, like peppermint and lemon oil, can be consumed in small doses at 1 to 2 drops, two to three times a day. Other oils like oregano should only be consumed for a maximum of 10 days and under the guidance of a health care professional. Wintergreen should only be used topically or aromatically (diffused) and should never be used internally. People with liver disease and those who have higher levels of sensitivities need to be cautious. All essential oils should be taken with food or a beverage and not on an empty stomach.

Suggested internal use methods for adults include:

Add 1 to 2 drops to a glass of water, almond milk or coconut milk

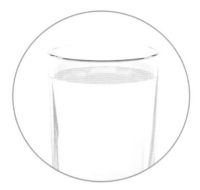

Put several drops of oil into an empty capsule and swallow with water

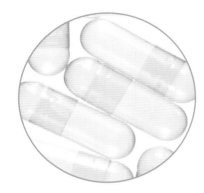

Add 1 to 2 drops to 1 teaspoon of raw honey and then consume

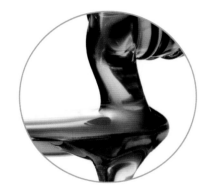

Add 1 to 2 drops to 1 teaspoon of coconut oil and then consume

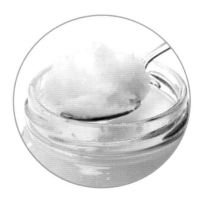

Drop certain oils directly under the tongue

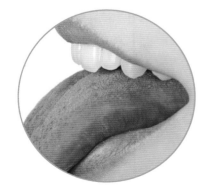

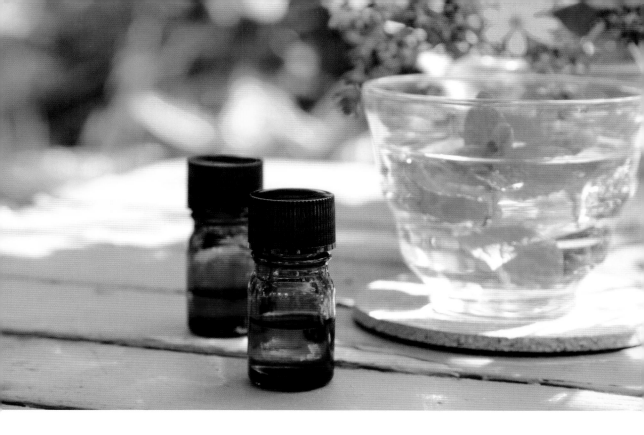

If you're someone who purchases and consumes organic foods, you should do your best to consume essential oil products that are certified organic.

When it comes to using oils on your body (topically) or taking them internally, safety is based on the properties of the oil itself, not the "quality" of the brand. *Some oils are simply not safe to take internally.* It is not wise to believe a company statement that asserts, "All of our oils are safe for internal use."

A bottle label may say "safe for supplemental use," but even then that doesn't necessarily mean it is safe when taken internally. *Some oils that are not safe for ingestion* include oils from the needles of trees such as pine essential oil and some bark oils such as cypress. Some essential oils are only suitable for external use because they have been linked to liver toxicity. These oils include aniseed, bay and tarragon.

Always consult with a doctor or healthcare practitioner before using essential oils internally. When in doubt, remember that with most essential oils, benefits can be found from topical and aromatherapy use.

RESPECT THEIR POWER: OIL SIDE EFFECTS AND INTERACTIONS

A scientific review published by the *U.S National Library of Medicine* in 2014 states that safety testing on essential oils shows very few negative side effects or risks when they are used as directed. Some essential oils have been approved as ingredients in food and are classified as GRAS (generally recognized as safe) by the U.S. Food and Drug Administration, within specific limits.

However, like all medicine, they are not without their risks and possible complications.

It takes a small amount of essential oils to prompt a powerful therapeutic benefit. Because essential oils are so concentrated, they must be used with care. Labels should be read carefully and guidelines followed vigilantly. *Essential oils should never be applied to the eyes or ear canals.* After handling essential oils, avoid accidental eye contact by washing your hands. If essential oils get into the eye, place a few drops of a carrier oil in the eye and blink until the oil clears out.

If you are taking prescription or over-the-counter (OTC) medications, be aware that using an essential oil along with a drug can increase the drug's side effects. The chemical constituents of the essential oil could inhibit the drug's metabolizing enzymes, rendering the drug unable to be excreted or metabolized properly. Grapefruit essential oil specifically has been shown to interfere with medications.

Before using essential oils, research the oil's drug interactions or speak to a health care provider about possible outcomes. For example, people who are taking heart medications, such as blood thinners, should avoid using clary sage, cypress, eucalyptus, ginger, rosemary, sage and thyme oils.

The International Fragrance Association has banned several essential oils because they are toxic when ingested or applied topically. These oils include cade oil crude, costus root, elecampane, fig leaf absolute, horseradish, nightshade, pennyroyal, rue, sassafras, savin, southernwood, stinging nettle, stryax gum, tea absolute, wormseed and wormwood.

Allergic reactions and skin irritation may occur, especially when essential oils are in contact with the skin for long periods of time. In fact, sun sensitivity may develop when citrus or other oils are applied to the skin before sun exposure.

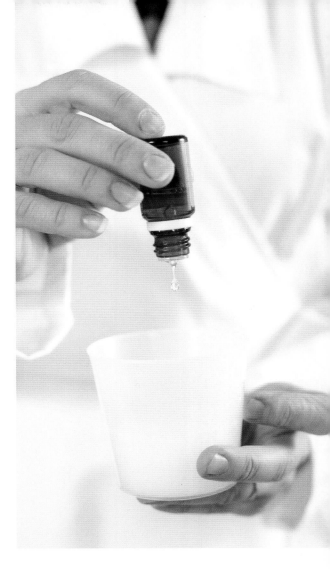

Finally, lavender and tea tree oils have been found to have hormone-like effects similar to estrogen. On the other hand, many studies, including one published in *Evidence Based Complementary Alternative Medicine* concludes that lavender oil effectively relieves stress, anxiety, depression, neurological conditions and cognitive conditions.[18] Lavender oil and tea tree oil are known to reduce pain and work as antioxidants and anti-inflammatory agents. Some essential oils that are better for regulating hormone levels include Roman chamomile, sandalwood and clary sage.

Keep in mind that **essential oils are highly concentrated substances**. One drop is powerful enough to soothe sore muscles, relieve an itchy bug bite or stop a cold in its tracks. Don't be fooled by their "natural" origin. Their power must be respected—they have the potential to cause minor reactions, such as skin irritation, or more serious consequences like respiratory failure, when not used appropriately.

Before experimenting with an oil, become familiar with its properties, dosage instructions and precautions. When in doubt about a condition or an oil, consult a qualified medical specialist. There is no regulated standard, which means it is up to users to educate themselves on the proper use of each essential oil before using them.

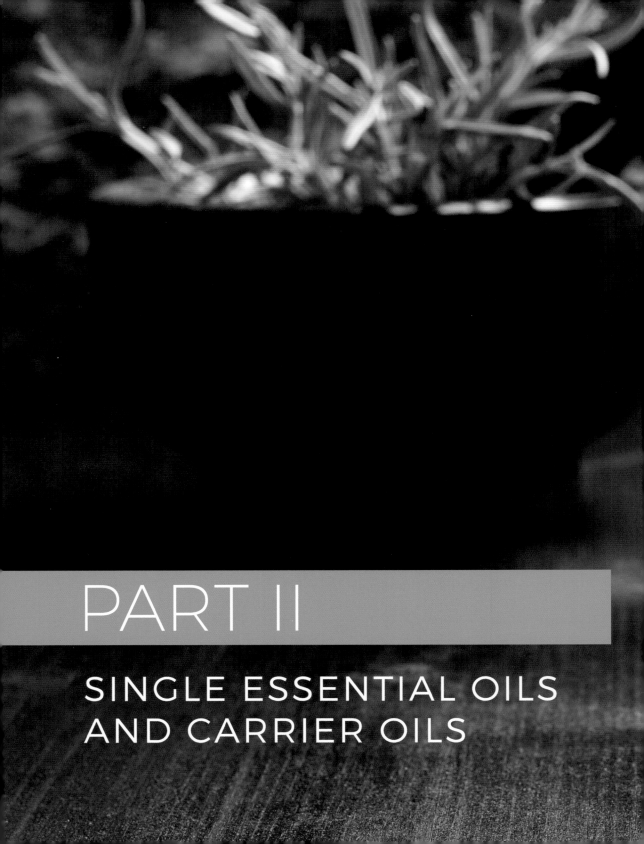

PART II

SINGLE ESSENTIAL OILS AND CARRIER OILS

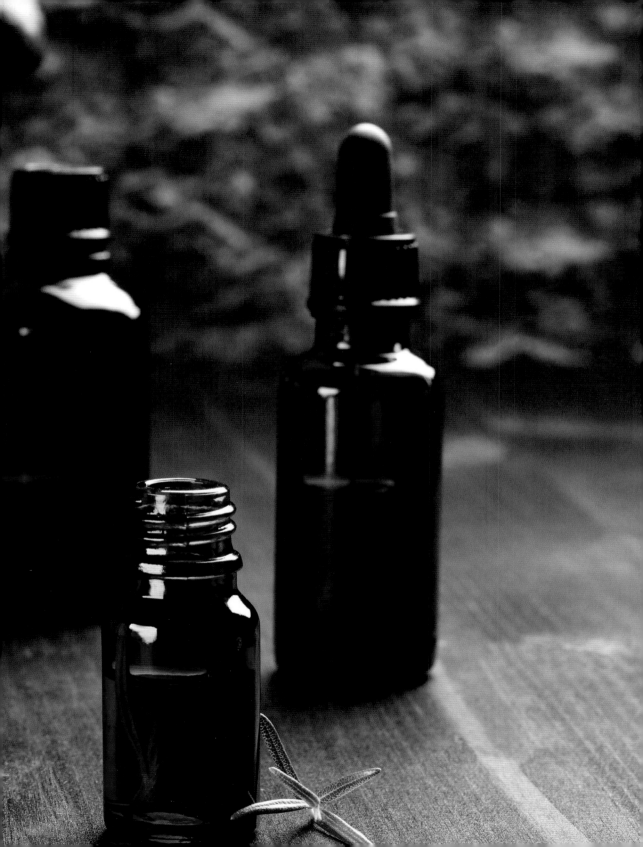

Essential oils are so much more than just extraordinary aromas—each one features a vast array of uses and benefits. Every essential oil contains compounds that possess unique therapeutic benefits. In the pages that follow, we will explore the rich history of many different oils, while examining their aromas and most prevalent therapeutic qualities.

EACH OIL PROFILE CONTAINS:

 Description: A brief account of the oil's history and its most common uses from antiquity to modern times

 Research: A summary of research studies demonstrating the therapeutic properties of its primary chemical constituents

 Key Benefits: A list of the major benefits associated with the oil's chemistry

 Therapeutic Compounds: Highlights of the oil's important nutrients and beneficial compounds

 Safety: Unique safety considerations for the oil

 Super 7 Rx Uses: Seven uses and practical applications for the oil

NOTE: Throughout this section, we have provided you with suggested uses for each oil. Here are the guidelines for use:

Aromatherapy Use. Place 5 to 7 drops of the desired oil in a diffuser with fresh, filtered water.

Topical Use. Apply 2 to 4 drops to the affected area. Refer to cautions about which oils are "hot" oils. For sensitive skin, always mix the essential oil with a carrier oil.

Internal Use. Place 1 to 3 drops in a beverage, on a spoonful of honey or coconut oil or under the tongue. See the specific guidelines for each oil for more information.

We have also included our own personal favorite uses for particular oils to provide even more examples of how they can be used. For example, Dr. Josh relates how he and his wife use myrrh, Ty talks about how he uses lemon oil and Jordan discusses his use of frankincense oil.

You can use each essential oil by itself and/or gain enhanced therapeutic benefits by blending oils together. One option is to combine essential oils with a carrier oil and use this mixture in the place of potentially toxic personal care products (see The Role of Carrier Oils). In some cases, simply adding a few drops of essential oil to an existing product will greatly enrich its benefits. (For more on the art of blending oils, refer to the introduction in Part V: Essential Oil Recipes.)

Our hope is that you feel inspired to utilize essential oils in new and unexpected ways to provide healthy alternatives to many chemically-created products available today.

The Role of Carrier Oils

Carrier oils serve a key role in delivering essential oils both topically and internally. The most common carrier oil for everyday use is coconut oil, which is often fractionated (meaning it's liquid at room temperature), but there are other options that can provide you with additional advantages. For more carrier oil options, as well as information on their key benefits, see the list of carrier oils at the end of Part II.

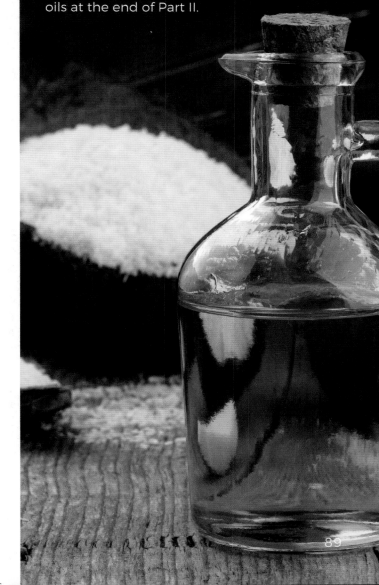

GENERAL SAFETY AND COMMON SENSE GUIDELINES

Here are some important safety recommendations that apply to the use of all essential oils. Read this list carefully—and then go enjoy your oils!

» When it comes to essential oils, a little goes a long way. Start with one to two drops and assess your tolerance and desired results before increasing amount.

» Many oils can be applied NEAT (undiluted, or without a carrier oil), but check each oil first to ensure it is safe to do so. When in doubt, dilute.

» Stop use immediately if irritation occurs.

» **Some oils are not safe to take internally.** Check the warnings for each oil before ingesting and only consume essential oils that are certified organic and labeled as dietary supplements.

» **Some essential oils are not safe to use while pregnant.** Check the warnings for each oil before use during pregnancy.

» If you are prone to mouth or throat irritation, put essential oils into a capsule or dilute it with a carrier oil or food (honey, applesauce, etc.) before swallowing.

» When adding essential oils to food or liquid, start with one drop and taste before adding more.

» Most essential oils should be taken with food and not on an empty stomach.

» Talk to your healthcare practitioner before using essential oils if you are taking any prescription medications, as some oils may have interactions when taken along with certain drugs.

» Do not use essential oils in the eyes or in the ear canals.

» Only use certified organic oils to ensure highest quality and purity—and to ensure safety for use on or in your body.

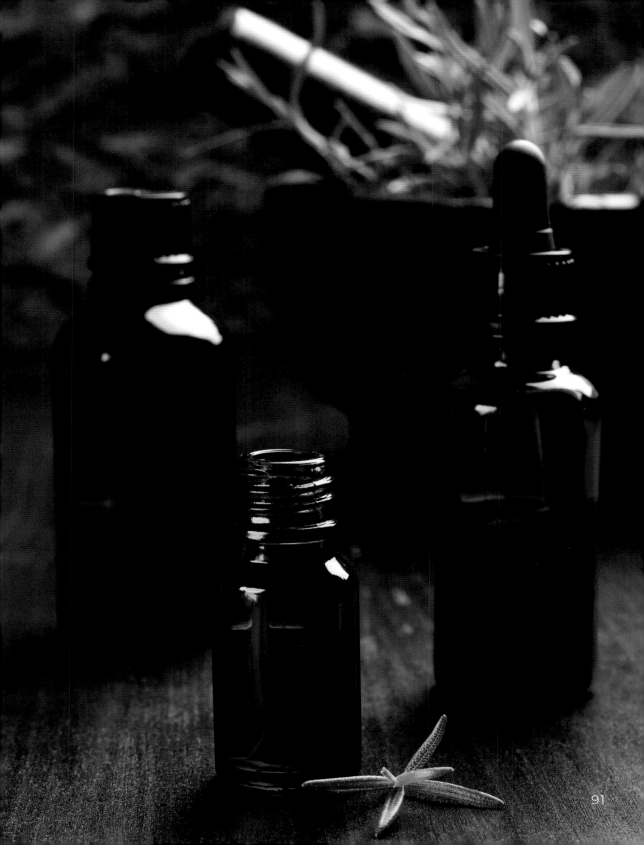

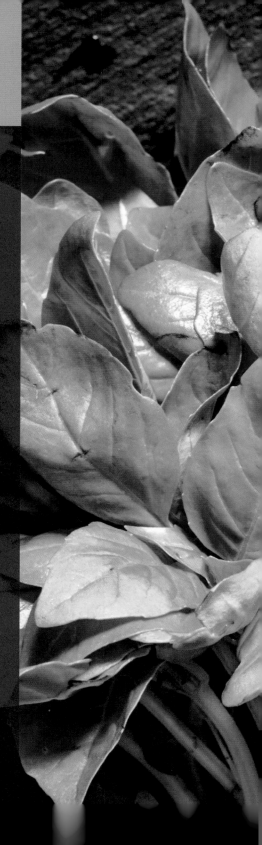

BASIL

OCIMUM BASILICUM

An ancient herb found in Egyptian pyramids, the kings of old were often anointed with basil in special ceremonies. In Asia, basil is commonly used to counter venomous poisons from snakes and insects. In India, basil is sacred; it is planted around temples and graves. It is also used in Ayurvedic and Chinese medicine to treat colds, flu, fever, muscle aches and earaches. Centuries ago, basil was considered to have an alluring scent; Italian women wore the oil and even set pots of basil outside their windows to attract possible suitors.

Basil essential oil, sometimes called "sweet basil oil," has a naturally sweet, warm, spicy and herbal smell and is derived from the *Ocimum basilicum* plant through steam distillation. You probably know basil to be an herb that is used to enhance the flavor of many recipes. However, its uses today extend far beyond the culinary world. Basil essential oil is used to treat various wounds and infections, and it often serves as a calming agent to combat inflammation, help reduce adrenal fatigue and treat nerve and muscle conditions.

RESEARCH STUDIES

A study found that basil oil, along with other plant oils, including fennel, demonstrates inhibitory properties against powerful strains of bacteria, including Listeria monocytogenes and Salmonella enteriditis.[1]

According to a 2014 review, basil oil has been effectively used as a traditional medicinal plant for the treatment of headaches, coughs, diarrhea, constipation, warts, worms, kidney malfunctions and more.[2]

KEY BENEFITS

- Contains anti-bacterial properties
- Reduces inflammation
- Combats free radical damage
- Helps relieve congestion
- May increase urine output
- Stimulates the nervous system
- May balance adrenal hormones
- Serves as an aid for ear infections

SAFETY

Do not use during pregnancy. Basil is also not appropriate for those with epilepsy. Dilution is recommended for topical use.

THERAPEUTIC COMPOUNDS

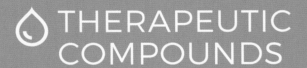

Eugenol Linalool

Methylchavicol

SUPER 7 RX BASIL USES

1. Acts as an Anti-bacterial and Anti-fungal Agent

To combat bacteria and fungus in and around the home, diffuse or vaporize basil oil, or combine it with a natural cleaner in a spray bottle to rub down surfaces and help remove bacteria from kitchens and bathrooms.

2. Relieves Cold and Flu Symptoms

Diffuse basil throughout the home to fight common cold and flu symptoms such as congestion. Add 2 to 3 drops to a steam bath, or combine 2 drops of basil oil with 2 drops of eucalyptus oil and a carrier oil to help open up the nasal passages.

3. Freshens the Air

Aid in eliminating odor-causing bacteria and mold by diffusing basil oil, combining 4 to 6 drops with baking soda to clean kitchen appliances or spraying a mixture of water or natural cleaner and a few drops of basil oil in the toilet, shower and garbage can.

4. Aids in the Treatment of Urinary Tract Infections

Add 1 to 2 drops of basil oil to food, or dilute 1 to 2 drops with a carrier oil and take it internally to assist in detoxifying the urinary and digestive tracts.

5. Relaxes Muscles

Rub 3 drops of basil oil into painful, swollen muscles or joints to help relax them. To lessen tense areas and feel immediate relief, add Epsom salts, lavender oil and basil oil to warm bath water.

6. Reduces Ear Infection Discomfort

Rub equal parts basil and frankincense oil diluted with coconut oil behind the ears to help reduce swelling from an ear infection and encourage healing.[3]

7. Promotes Oral Health

Add a few drops of pure basil oil to your mouthwash or toothpaste. This will also help protect your teeth and gums from toothaches, ulcers, sores and viral blisters.

BERGAMOT

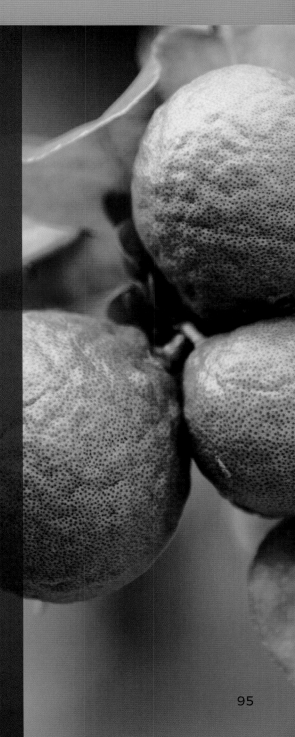

CITRUS BERGAMIA

Native to Southeast Asia, Bergamot is cold-pressed and then distilled from an evergreen citrus tree. The fragrant trees also line the Ivory Coast, Morocco, Tunisia and Algeria. Bergamot is defined as a hybrid between a sour orange and lemon—and it's the oil commonly used in black tea. In fact, just add a drop of bergamot oil to a cup of regular tea to make Earl Grey!

Bergamot is unique among citrus oils due to its ability to be both uplifting and calming, making it ideal to help with anxious and sad feelings. It is also purifying and cleansing for the skin while having a calming effect. Additionally, bergamot oil has been used to fight bacteria, help heal scars and reduce painful headaches and muscle tension, as well as stimulate hormonal and digestive juices.

RESEARCH STUDIES

In a 2011 study, applying a blend of lavender and bergamot oil to participants helped in treating depression or anxiety. Compared with the placebo, the essential oil blend caused significant decreases of pulse rate and blood pressure.[4]

Other research suggests that bergamot oil is able to minimize tension in the body.[5]

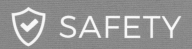 ## KEY BENEFITS

- Helps release emotional pain
- Contains anti-depressant qualities
- Helps reduce stress
- Soothes skin irritations
- Acts as a natural deodorant

- Helps relieve joint and muscle pain
- Aids the digestive system
- Has anti-bacterial and disinfectant properties

SAFETY

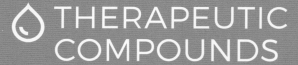 THERAPEUTIC COMPOUNDS

Avoid direct sunlight for up to 12 hours after external application. If you use bergamot oil and have diabetes, monitor your blood sugar levels regularly, as it may affect blood sugar control.

Limonene

Linalool

Linalyl formate

SUPER 7 RX BERGAMOT USES

1. Improves Mood and Serves as a Natural Anti-depressant

Bergamot can create feelings of joy, refreshment and energy by supporting healthy circulation. Rub 2 to 3 drops onto your hands and cup your mouth and nose. Breathe in slowly. Also apply it to your feet and the back of your neck.[6]

2. Encourages Lymphatic Drainage

Apply 2 to 3 drops to your feet before bedtime or combine 3 to 5 drops with a carrier oil for a calming and relaxing massage and to encourage lymphatic drainage.

3. Helps Digestive System

To support digestion and regulate appetite, rub 3 to 5 drops of bergamot oil onto your stomach. This may stimulate muscle contractions in your intestines and the production of digestive juices.

4. Acts as a Natural Deodorant

Add bergamot oil to deodorant or apply it directly to your armpits to help prevent the growth of germs that cause body odor. Combine bergamot oil with lemon, cedarwood or sandalwood oils to make a personalized fragrance.[7]

5. Aids in Reducing Stress

Relieve stress and anxiety by using bergamot oil in a diffuser. It can also be applied topically to help with stress by rubbing 1 to 2 drops onto your temples and wrists.

6. Manages Food Cravings

Diffuse in the classroom, at work or at home in between meals to help control hunger pangs.

7. Supports Immunity

To fight harmful bacteria and stress that can lead to illness, take bergamot oil internally, diffuse it, inhale it directly or add a few drops to a warm-water bath.

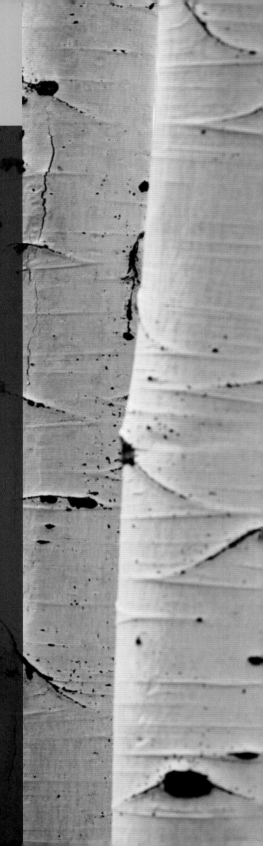

BIRCH

BETULA LENTA

Birch essential oil, also known as sweet birch oil, is rich in methyl salicylates and has a long history of use for sore and fatigued muscles. Birch essential oil is identical in chemical constituents to wintergreen essential oil, which is why the American Indians and early European settlers added both birch bark and wintergreen to tea in order to benefit from their warming and stimulating properties. The Native Americans took birch for various health conditions associated with the stomach, including dysentery, diarrhea and indigestion.

Birch oil has a minty and earthy aroma that relieves muscle pain and increases awareness in the sensory system. The wood of the birch tree is steam-distilled to extract the essential oils. Its active ingredients (salicylic acid and methyl salicylate) make this minty, versatile oil an excellent choice for supporting skin health. Consider adding it in very small concentrations to some of your favorite skin care routines.

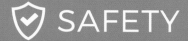 RESEARCH STUDIES

A 2006 study found that birch oil possesses anti-bacterial activity, and its vapors inhibit bacterial growth on tested organisms.[8]

A 1994 study found that chemicals in white birch bark slowed the growth of HIV. Researchers also found that the betulinic acid present in birch oil killed melanoma cells in laboratory animals. In addition, results indicated that birch may be an effective treatment for a precancerous skin condition.[9]

⊘ KEY BENEFITS

- Soothes achy muscles and joints
- Supports respiratory function
- Provides emotional balance
- Stimulates the senses
- Boosts skin health
- Helps relieve cramps
- Contains anti-inflammatory properties
- May ease symptoms of arthritis and tendonitis

🛡 SAFETY

Birch oil is not recommended for internal use. Avoid use if pregnant or breastfeeding. Dilute for topical use. Use the minimal amounts required to achieve benefits. Avoid if you're on blood thinners, are having surgery or suffer from bleeding disorders, salicylate deficiency, seizure disorder or ADD/ADHD.

◊ THERAPEUTIC COMPOUNDS

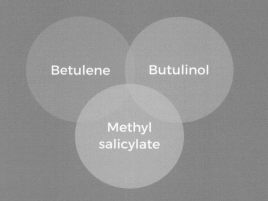

Betulene

Butulinol

Methyl salicylate

SUPER 7 RX BIRCH USES

1. Soothes Muscle Pain and Spasms

Birch oil has analgesic properties—it may help relieve muscle and joint pain and aid in alleviating spasms, headaches and toothaches. Apply it topically to the area of concern. For toothaches, apply 1 to 2 drops to the outside of your mouth.

2. Relieves Arthritis Symptoms

Birch essential oil may improve circulation and has detoxifying agents that aid in reducing swelling, rheumatism and arthritis. Apply it topically to the area of concern.[10]

3. Helps Reduce Chronic Inflammation Associated with Gout

Because birch oil helps alleviate inflammation, it may be useful to those suffering from gout. Apply 3 to 4 drops to the affected areas to help ease some of the pain associated with gout.

4. May Relieve Pain from Ulcers and Cramps

Due to its anti-spasmodic properties, birch oil assists in relieving pain from ulcers and cramps throughout the body. Apply 2 to 3 drops with a carrier oil to the abdomen, or add 3 to 5 drops to a warm-water bath.

5. Can Improve Mood and Self-Esteem

Birch oil stimulates the nervous, sensory and circulatory systems. It is warming and can provide a sense of peace, confidence and awareness. Diffuse birch oil or apply it topically to your wrists, the back of your neck and the soles of your feet.

6. Encourages Improved Circulation

Birch oil stimulates the circulatory system and can improve circulation. To encourage blood flow, apply to areas of poor circulation.

7. Supports Kidney Detox

Because birch oil is both diuretic and stimulant in nature, it aids in the removal of toxins through increased urination and perspiration. Dilute birch with a carrier oil and massage it into your skin to support kidney detox.

BLACK PEPPER

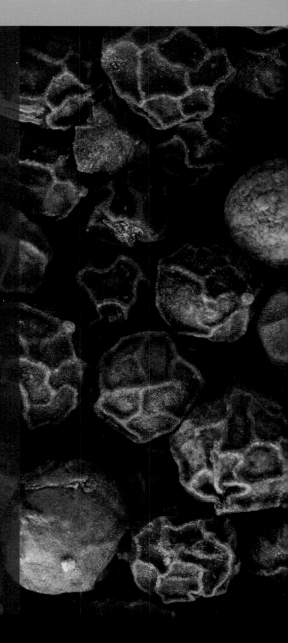

PIPER NIGRUM

Archaeological evidence of pepper use goes back to at least 2000 B.C. in India. References to pepper appear in Greek and Roman texts, suggesting an ancient trade between India and the West. The Romans loved adding pepper to their food; in fact, in the oldest known cookbook in existence, 80 percent of the recipes contain the spice. Signs of an ancient pepper trade from India to Egypt have also been found, including peppercorns that had been stuffed into the nostrils of Ramses the Great when he was mummified.

Derived from the fruit, black pepper essential oil is extracted through steam distillation. The essential oil has a spicy, warm, peppery and musky aroma. It is commonly used to aid the digestive and nervous systems—stimulating circulation and promoting emotional balance. Black pepper possesses a unique versatility that is both energizing and warming. In addition to invigorating the senses, black pepper can be used to enhance mental clarity. It is a favorite among athletes and those with an active lifestyle.

RESEARCH STUDIES

A 1994 study found that black pepper oil can suppress certain smoking withdrawal symptoms, including cravings for cigarettes. Cigarette smokers reported that cigarette cravings were significantly reduced and feelings of anxiety were alleviated.[11]

When patients applied a cream composed of black pepper, marjoram, lavender and peppermint essential oils to the neck daily for a four-week period, the group reported improved pain tolerance and significant improvement of neck pain.[12]

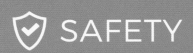 ## KEY BENEFITS

- May help relieve cramps and spasms
- Helps relieve respiratory conditions
- Helps soothe feelings of anxiety
- Contains anti-inflammatory and anti-spasmodic properties

- Enhances food flavor
- May aid digestion
- Encourages circulation
- Helps increase energy

SAFETY

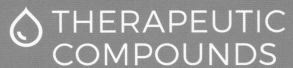 ## THERAPEUTIC COMPOUNDS

Dilution is recommend for topical use. Black pepper can be a strong irritant in high doses.

Carene

Limonene

Caryophyllene

SUPER 7 RX BLACK PEPPER USES

1. Aids Circulation

To increase circulation and blood flow to the muscles and nerves, add 3 to 5 drops of black pepper oil to a warm compress and apply to your abdomen or area of concern.

2. Improves Digestion

Black pepper may help ease the discomfort of constipation, diarrhea and gas. Take 1 to 2 drops of black pepper oil internally by adding it to a smoothie, soup or savory dish. It can also be applied topically to your abdomen.[13]

3. Helps Soothe Sprains and Tendonitis

Because of its warming, anti-inflammatory and anti-spasmodic properties, black pepper oil works to reduce muscle injuries and tendonitis. Apply topically to the area of concern.

4. Aids Respiratory Conditions

Black pepper oil supports the draining and cleansing of your respiratory and lymphatic systems. You can either take it internally or inhale the oil. To relieve congested airways, apply 2 to 3 drops topically to your chest.

5. Helps Reduce Cigarette Cravings

Black pepper oil may help reduce cravings for cigarettes and symptoms of anxiety in smokers deprived from smoking. Inhale or diffuse the oil to help with cravings.

6. Relieves Symptoms of Arthritis and Rheumatism

Due to its warming, anti-inflammatory and circulating properties, black pepper oil helps relieve symptoms of arthritis and rheumatism. Apply topically to the area of concern.

7. Helps to Detoxify the Body

Black pepper oil increases sweating and urination—helping to remove bodily toxins and excess water. This reduces swelling and inflammation and can lower blood pressure. Take internally or apply 2 to 3 drops topically to the soles of your feet.

CARDAMOM

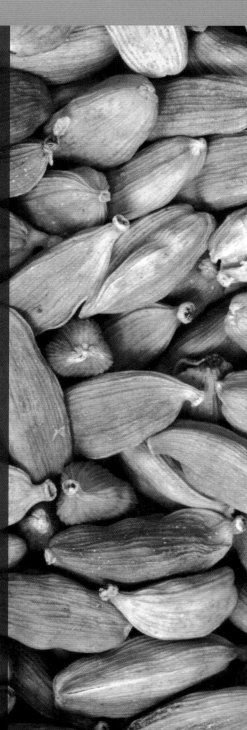

ELETTARIA CARDAMOMUM

Cardamom essential oil was one of the most prized spices in ancient Greece and Rome and is mentioned in one of the oldest known medical documents dating from 16th century B.C. Egyptians used it for medicines, embalming and other ritualistic practices. They also chewed the pods to clean their teeth and freshen their breath. It has been used medicinally to assist in treating colds, colic, diarrhea, nausea, gas and kidney and reproductive complaints.

Cardamom essential oil is steam-distilled from the seeds after they have dried for more than three months. The oil has a sweet, spicy and balsamic aroma. Today, cardamom is widely used and admired as a versatile spice around the world, thanks to its cool, minty aroma and flavor. Its woody aroma is both soothing and emotionally uplifting, and it assists mental function and may reduce drowsiness, all while improving concentration.

RESEARCH STUDIES

Cardamom essential oil has anti-inflammatory properties and proved to be an effective treatment for inflammation in laboratory animals. The oil has also shown analgesic activity, protecting mice against pain.[14]

Research states that cardamom essential oil can kill bacteria that produce bad breath and infections. It also has anti-microbial effects when used to fight oral bacteria and is effective against pathogenic organisms such as Streptococcus mutans and Candida albicans.[15]

KEY BENEFITS

- Supports digestion
- Soothes sore throat
- May ease muscle pain
- Eases mental fatigue

- Promotes relaxation
- May reduce menopause symptoms
- May alleviate cramps and spasms
- Improves respiratory conditions

SAFETY

Dilution is recommended, as cardamom can cause allergic reactions for those with sensitive skin. Do not apply on or near the face of infants or young children.

THERAPEUTIC COMPOUNDS

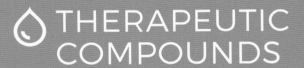

1,8-cineole
Linalool
Terpinyl acetate

SUPER 7 RX CARDAMOM USES

1. Helps Ease Digestive Concerns

Cardamom oil calms and promotes digestion, assists in alleviating discomfort from intestinal illnesses and helps reduce symptoms of vomiting, nausea and diarrhea. It may also help with loss of appetite. Take 1 to 3 drops internally, or apply it topically to your abdomen.

2. Diminishes Menstrual and PMS Symptoms

Apply 3 to 4 drops topically to your abdomen to help relieve some of the discomfort associated with menstruation and PMS.

3. Improves Sore Throat

Apply cardamom oil to your chest to soothe a sore throat. The oil's warming properties heat up the body, promote sweating and help clear congestion and coughs that may lead to a sore throat.

4. Serves as a Natural Aphrodisiac

Diffusing cardamom oil or applying 1 to 2 drops topically can have an arousing effect, making it helpful for impotence, erectile dysfunction, loss of libido and frigidity. It stimulates and invigorates the senses while working as a relaxing and warming agent.

5. Lessens Muscle Pain and Cramps

Because of cardamom's anti-spasmodic and anti-inflammatory properties, it helps relieve muscle and joint pain, which could alleviate some of the symptoms of arthritis, menopause and menstruation. Apply it topically to the area of concern.

6. Decreases Mental Fatigue and Brain Fog

Cardamom can clear the mind and ease mental fatigue because of its stimulating and invigorating properties. Apply 1 to 2 drops topically under your nose and the back of your neck.

7. Freshens Breath

Because of cardamom's antiseptic and anti-microbial properties, it can be used as a mouthwash to eliminate bad breath and reduce oral cavities. Add a few drops to water and swish in your mouth.

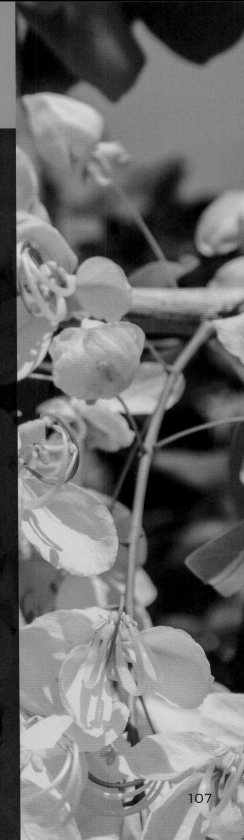

CASSIA

CINNAMOMUM CASSIA

Cassia is considered one of the 50 fundamental herbs in Traditional Chinese Medicine. Egyptians imported cassia from China and used it in the embalming process. In the ancient Middle East, people so valued cassia that it was worth its weight in gold or ivory.

Cassia is mentioned in the Bible several times and was often used in anointing oils. The root word, *kiddah*, in both Hebrew and Arabic, signifies a "strip" and refers to the strips of bark from which the spice is made. In the spiritual sense, cassia speaks of devotion (being stripped of pride) and consecration (set apart) with a servant's heart. The Israelites may have brought it with them when they left Egypt for the Promised Land. As the Israelites traveled throughout the Sinai Peninsula, they may have purchased cassia from traders who crossed the Peninsula from Arabia to Egypt.

Cassia essential oil is derived by steam distillation of the plant's bark, leaves and twigs. It has a spicy, warm aroma—similar to cinnamon but sweeter. It has been traditionally used in the treatment of leprosy, erysipelas, ulcer symptoms, cough, flatulence, dyspepsia, menstrual problems and tuberculosis. Cassia oil is often used as a supportive aid for bronchitis, anemia and constipation.

RESEARCH STUDIES

A 2016 study found that a chemical constituent present in cassia showed a preventive effect for the formation of atherosclerotic plaque (the plaque that builds up in your arteries).[16]

A study found that both cassia oil and pure cinnamaldehyde (the organic compound that gives cassia its flavor and odor) were equally effective in inhibiting the growth of various isolates of bacteria, including four species of candida, and molds.[17]

⊘ KEY BENEFITS

- Can improve circulation
- Alleviates menstrual symptoms
- Works as an anti-depressant
- Supports the immune system

- Inhibits the growth of bacteria
- Works as an astringent
- Serves as a natural bug repellant
- Balances blood sugar

🛡 SAFETY

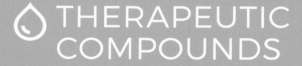 ## ◊ THERAPEUTIC COMPOUNDS

Use it internally in small doses only (1 to 2 drops). Cassia oil may reduce milk supply in lactating women.

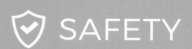

Cinnamaldehyde

Cinnamyl acetate

SUPER 7 RX CASSIA USES

1. Promotes Healthy Blood Sugar Levels

Studies suggest that cassia oil has the ability to naturally improve diabetes by helping to lower blood sugar levels. To support healthy blood sugar levels, take 1 drop of cassia oil internally with tea, coffee, oatmeal or any dish that has a warm and spicy flavor.

2. Boosts Metabolism

Cassia oil can act as a stimulant. Rub 2 to 4 drops of cassia oil onto the soles of your feet or abdomen in order to give your metabolism a boost.

3. Warms Cold Extremities

Rub a few drops of cassia oil on your legs and the soles of your feet or add 5 to 7 drops to a warm-water bath to encourage warmth and stimulate cold extremities.

4. Boosts Libido

Diffuse or put 2 drops of cassia oil on a handkerchief and inhale the scent to give your libido a boost.

5. Encourages Lung Detoxification

Diffuse or put cassia oil in a handkerchief and inhale to promote lung detoxification.

6. Reduces Food Cravings

Combine 1 drop along with a drop of lemon oil in a glass of water and consume to aid digestion and ward off hunger cravings.

7. Acts as a Natural Anti-depressant

To fight harmful bacteria and Cassia contains cinnamaldehyde, a component that has been studied and is known to alleviate stress-induced behaviors and conditions. Diffuse cassia oil or add it to a warm-water bath.[18]

CEDARWOOD

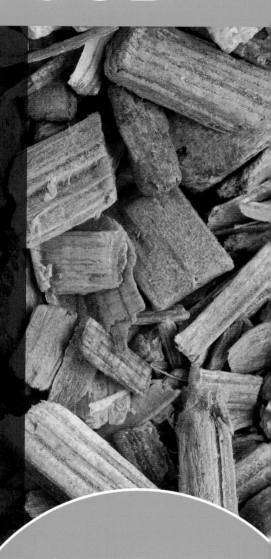

CEDRUS ATLANTICA

Cedarwood has been used medicinally since ancient times. The wood and its oil were used in embalming by the Ancient Egyptians. *Cedrus atlantica* is closely related to the Biblical Cedar of Lebanon. An enormous grove of cedars of Lebanon—from which King Solomon is said to have built his temple—exists still on the slopes of Mount Lebanon.

Cedarwood essential oil is comforting, reassuring and possesses a woodsy, pleasant scent. The oil is extracted through the process of steam distillation from wood pieces of the cedar wood tree, and it adds a warm tone to any blend of perfumes, colognes or oil mixtures. Cedarwood has the power to improve the look of your skin, help with organ function, tighten muscles, support metabolism and benefit your digestive system. It's no wonder why cedars were the trees mentioned most in the Bible, symbolizing a source of protection, wisdom and abundance.

When I'm writing a book or recording an interview, I love to diffuse cedarwood, rosemary and peppermint to support creativity, memory and energy.

– Dr. Josh

RESEARCH STUDIES

One study found that cedarwood essential oil is a viable alternative to other anti-bacterial agents and is an effective module in controlling both bacteria and yeasts responsible for oral infections.[19]

A study found that using cedarwood oil on children could greatly improve their focus and learning capacity. The results showed cedarwood oil inhalation improved focus in children with ADHD by 65 percent.[20]

⊘ KEY BENEFITS

- Supports focus
- Promotes hair growth
- Reduces skin irritations
- Fights fungal infections

- Repels bugs
- May reduce cough
- Supports healthy menstruation
- Relieves tension

⛉ SAFETY

Cedarwood oil is not safe for internal use. Avoid using it during pregnancy. Dilution is recommended for topical use.

⬙ THERAPEUTIC COMPOUNDS

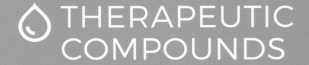

Alpha-cedrene Beta-cedrene

Cedrol Thujopsene

SUPER 7 RX CEDARWOOD USES

1. Improves Focus and Eases Symptoms of ADD/ADHD

Inhaling cedarwood oil may improve focus and ease symptoms of ADHD. For children with ADHD, an important study by Dr. Terry Friedmann proved that taking three deep inhalations of a blend that included cedarwood oil for 30 days showed significant improvements.

2. Improves Acne and Eczema

Cedarwood oil can treat inflammation that leads to irritating skin issues such as eczema. It reduces skin peeling and treats infections with its anti-fungal properties. To improve acne naturally, add 2 to 3 drops of cedarwood oil to lotion or massage it directly into your skin.

3. Sharpens Focus and Concentration

Add 2 to 3 drops to skin lotion or soap to enhance your focus. You can also inhale it directly from the bottle or diffuse it.

4. Provides Cough and Sinus Relief

Help remove phlegm from your respiratory tract and lungs by rubbing cedarwood oil onto your chest and throat. Inhaling the oil may also reduce congestion.

5. Repels Insects

Apply cedarwood oil topically to drive away mosquitoes, flies and other insects. It can also be added to water and sprayed on beds and couches. To keep moths away, add 3 drops to cotton balls and leave them around the house.

6. Helps Relieve Tension

Cedarwood oil has a soothing and calming effect on the mind and helps ease tight muscles. Add the oil to a diffuser, inhale it directly from the bottle or apply it topically.

7. Fights Fungal Infections

Applying cedarwood oil topically or diffusing it aids in protecting the body from fungal pathogens and internal and external infections.

CILANTRO

CORIANDRUM SATIVUM

The culinary uses and benefits of cilantro have been documented for millennia. Its seeds were found in caves dating back to ancient Israel. Cilantro has been featured in the cuisines of Europe, Asia, North Africa and the Middle East for centuries and provides not only a fresh boost of flavor but also many therapeutic properties, such as its ability to fight both fungus and bacteria. Today in America, cilantro and cilantro oils are often included in liver detoxification supplements due to their ability to cleanse the liver and potentially support the body in eliminating heavy metals such as mercury and lead.

Cilantro leaves are steam-distilled to create the essential oil, and it has a fresh and slightly citrusy aroma and flavor. Since cilantro oil is distilled from the leaf of *Coriandrum sativum*, the oil's aroma bears a striking resemblance to that of coriander oil, which is distilled from the seed of the same plant. Applied topically, cilantro is soothing and cooling to the skin, and it adds a fresh, herbal aroma to any essential oil blend when diffused.

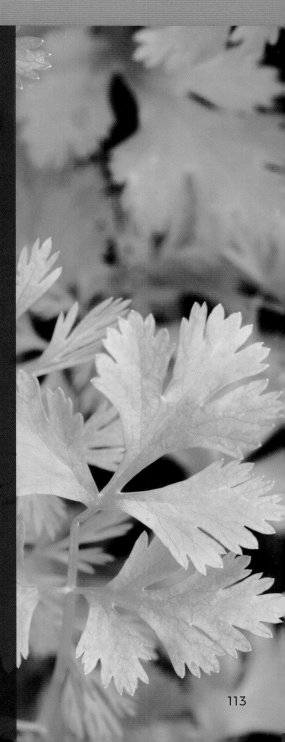

RESEARCH STUDIES

Researchers believe that *Coriandrum sativum* could be a remedy for diabetes, since it shows the ability in tests to support healthy liver function and balance blood sugar.[21]

One study found that *Coriandrum sativum* significantly accelerates the removal of stubborn heavy metal deposits from the body.[22]

⊘ KEY BENEFITS

- Fights inflammation
- Eases the mind
- May improve sleep
- Has anti-fungal and anti-bacterial properties
- Helps cleanse and detoxify the body

- Supports healthy blood sugar levels and is synergistic with conventional diabetes treatments
- Helps ease gas, indigestion and bloating
- Alleviates allergy symptoms

🛡 SAFETY

Cilantro oil is generally non-toxic, non-irritant and non-sensitizing.

💧 THERAPEUTIC COMPOUNDS

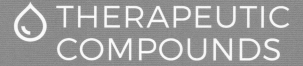

Dodecenal   Decenal

SUPER 7 RX CILANTRO USES

1. Supports Heavy Metal Detox

Cilantro essential oil has been shown to bind toxic metals together—loosening them from tissue and facilitating their elimination from the body. Ingest 1 to 2 drops at a time or diffuse the oil.

2. Supports Healthy Liver Function

To support healthy liver function, take 1 to 2 drops of cilantro internally in food or liquid, apply it topically to your abdomen or diffuse it.

3. Helps Settle the Stomach

Cilantro oil can help settle nausea, prevent gas and bloating, relieve indigestion and heartburn and ease stomach cramps. It may also protect the body against food poisoning because of its anti-microbial properties. Apply 3 to 5 drops topically to your stomach.

4. Supports Anti-Aging

Cilantro has antioxidant properties that protect the body against damage caused by free radicals. Diffuse cilantro oil around your home to support the reduction of oxidative stress.

5. Encourages Proper Blood Sugar Levels

Cilantro helps to balance blood sugar levels. As needed, ingest 1 to 3 drops of cilantro oil as a natural support for diabetes.

6. Supports Cardiovascular Disease Protection

Cilantro oil has polyphenolic content and natural cardio-protective nutrients responsible for preventing oxidative damage that is directly associated with cardiac damage. Ingest 1 drop of cilantro oil for protection.

7. May Prevent Urinary Tract Infections

Cilantro oil's anti-bacterial compounds help to keep the urinary tract healthy and free from germs that cause UTIs. Take internally or apply it to your abdomen.

CINNAMON BARK

CINNAMOMUM VERUM

As early as 2000 B.C., Egyptians employed cinnamon and cassia as perfuming agents during the embalming process, and cinnamon was even mentioned in the Old Testament as an ingredient in the holy anointing oil. Legend also has it that the Roman emperor Nero burned as much as he could find of the precious spice on the funeral pyre of his second wife Poppaea Sabina in A.D. 65 to atone for his role in her death.

Cinnamon bark oil is extracted by steam distillation from the outer bark of the cinnamon tree and has been touted for its medicinal properties for thousands of years. The warm and intense aroma of cinnamon bark can stimulate the appetite and ignite the senses. Cinnamon bark oil is highly concentrated with antioxidants, which makes it effective as a natural digestive aid, blood sugar stabilizer and circulation booster. It's also commonly used to combat cardiovascular diseases and to aid in fighting infections.

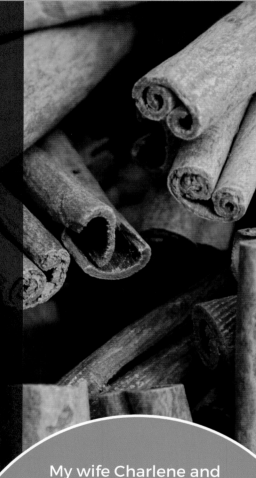

My wife Charlene and I diffuse cinnamon throughout our home during the holidays because we love the scent, and it's great for supporting the immune system.

– Ty

RESEARCH STUDIES

A 2011 study found that a 70 percent methanolic extract of cinnamon oil showed significant ability to enhance immune function by combatting oxidative stress.[23]

A 2012 study concluded that *Cinnamomum verum* volatile oil applied either separately or in combination with other oil extracts had the most effective anti-microbial activity against certain infectious diseases.[24]

KEY BENEFITS

- Helps decrease inflammation
- Increases circulation
- Contains anti-viral properties
- Fights free radicals

- May help relieve depression
- Stimulates the immune system
- Boosts libido
- Fights parasites

SAFETY

People with sensitive skin may experience skin irritation when using cinnamon oil topically or internally. Test a small amount first, mixed with a carrier oil.

THERAPEUTIC COMPOUNDS

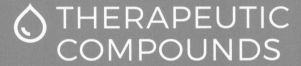

Cinnamaldehyde   Eugenol

Methyleugenol   Phellandrene

SUPER 7 RX CINNAMON BARK USES

SINGLE ESSENTIAL OILS

1. Boosts Heart Health

Because of its circulation-boosting abilities, cinnamon oil can support the cleansing of arteries. Apply 2 to 3 drops of cinnamon oil mixed with ½ teaspoon of coconut oil to your chest to promote warmth and increased blood flow.

2. Supports Healthy Blood Sugar and Insulin Release

Cinnamon oil may help keep blood sugar stable and prevent chronic fatigue, moodiness, sugar cravings and overeating. Inhale cinnamon essential oil, diffuse it or apply it to your chest and wrists.

3. May Help with High Cholesterol

One study revealed that a key constituent in cinnamon bark oil, cinnamate, lowers the activity of an enzyme that makes cholesterol in the body called HMG CoA reductase—the same enzyme targeted by statins. Take 1 to 2 drops of cinnamon essential oil internally to fight high cholesterol.

4. Helps Fight Infections

Diffusing cinnamon bark essential oil has shown an inhibitory effect against respiratory tract pathogens, including some penicillin-resistant strains. Diffuse it daily for protection against infection or to relieve a present infection.

5. Promotes Weight Loss

Because cinnamon oil can balance blood sugar levels and improve the taste of foods without added sugar, it's effective for curbing a sweet tooth. Add 1 to 2 drops to fruit, oats, baked goods or smoothies to help slow the rate at which glucose is released into the blood.

6. Fights Parasites

Studies have found that cinnamon oil inhibits the growth of certain harmful parasites. Ingest the oil to fight harmful parasites and impede parasite growth.

7. Soothes Sore Throat

Cinnamon oil can help prevent mucus buildup and clear nasal passages. Drink hot lemon water, honey and 1 drop of cinnamon oil in the morning to soothe a sore throat (plus curb cravings and support immune function).

CITRONELLA

CYMBOPOGON NARDUS

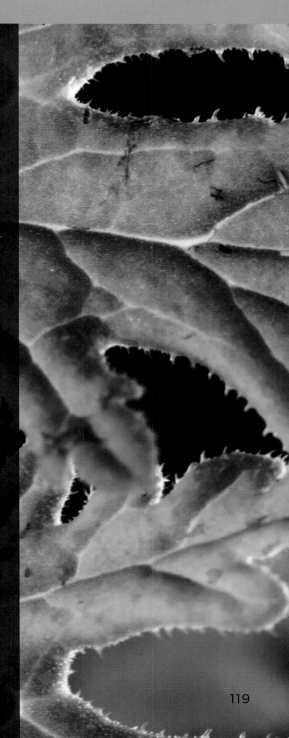

The first thing you may think of when you hear the word "citronella" is bugs flying away from a campsite thanks to your trusty citronella candle. It's true that citronella is extremely effective agent against mosquitoes and other pesky insects, but it also has a multitude of other uses. In Chinese medicine, citronella is prescribed to treat aches and pains in muscles and joints. It is also commonly used in soaps, detergents and cleaning products. Not only that, but citronella is also incredibly calming.

Citronella has a light citrus aroma, and it has anti-bacterial, anti-fungal and antiseptic properties. As a concentrated form of antioxidants and phytochemicals steam-distilled from the plant's stems and leaves, citronella oil has been used for centuries in China, Indonesia and Sri Lanka to help decrease rashes, inflammation, infections, pain and other conditions. Of course, the most popular use for citronella is as a constituent in homemade or commercially sold insect repellents.

RESEARCH STUDIES

A 2000 review found that many citrus volatile components, including the main type found in citronella (called geraniol), had high antioxidant capabilities for lowering inflammation and reducing cellular damage.[25]

A 2003 article found that citronella's geraniol has strong anti-helminthic activity, meaning it effectively expels parasitic worms, bugs and leeches from the body by either stunning or killing them without causing any damage to the host.[26]

⊘ KEY BENEFITS

- Repels insects
- Fights free radical damage
- Contains anti-bacterial and anti-fungal properties
- May reduce inflammation

- Promotes relaxation
- Helps fight respiratory infections
- Soothes muscle pain
- Helps control pets' behavior

🛡 SAFETY

Because citronella oil may irritate sensitive skin, dilution is recommended.

💧 THERAPEUTIC COMPOUNDS

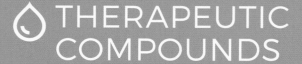

Citronellal

Citronellol

Geraniol

SUPER 7 RX CITRONELLA USES

1. Repels Insects

Citronella effectively repels mosquitoes, body lice, head lice and flies. Combine 3 to 5 drops of citronella oil with coconut oil and spread it on your body like a lotion, or add the oil to a spray bottle filled with water and spray it on your clothes, skin and furniture.

2. Helps Reduce Pain and Swelling

Due to its antioxidant properties and ability to increase blood flow, citronella is used as a natural support for arthritis. Massage 3 to 5 drops onto swollen joints, tissue and muscles, or soak in a warm bath with 5 drops of citronella oil.

3. Relaxes the Body and Mind

Citronella oil has relaxing properties that can help reduce stress and aid sleep. Diffuse citronella or massage citronella oil into your skin, specifically on the back of your neck.

4. Detoxifies the Body/Kidneys

Citronella oil can increase sweating and urination, which draws toxins out of the body. Combine 2 drops with a teaspoon of raw honey, 2 drops of lemon oil and hot water. Mix well and drink. This combination may improve the elimination of excess fats, sodium, uric acid and toxins.

5. Cleans and Deodorizes the Home

Deodorize the home and help kill bacteria and fungi with citronella oil. Add to a spray bottle filled with water and use the mixture on kitchen and household appliances. Adding citronella oil to the dishwasher, refrigerator and laundry machine is also effective.

6. Calms Pets

Combine 3 drops of citronella oil with coconut oil, and then massage the mixture into small areas on your pet's skin. Citronella oil can also be added to a clean cotton swab and applied topically to calm a nervous pet.

7. Supports Hair Health

Citronella oil can eliminate excess oil and greasiness from the hair while also adding shine and fighting dandruff. Add 5 to 7 drops to a bottle of shampoo or conditioner or combine with 1 teaspoon of coconut oil and massage the mixture into your hair and scalp.

CLARY SAGE

SALVIA SCLAREA

Clary sage has a surprising and fascinating history. Medieval authors called the herb "clear eye" and considered it beneficial in healing visual problems. In fact, "clary" is derived from the Latin word "clarus," which means clear. In the Middle Ages, it was known as "Oculus Christi," or the "eyes of Christ." In Chinese medicine, sage is used to strengthen the kidneys, adrenals and female reproductive organs. Clary sage is considered one of the top essential oils for balancing hormones, especially in women. It is highly beneficial when dealing with cramps, heavy menstrual cycles, hot flashes and hormonal imbalances.

The flower from the clary sage plant is steam-distilled, and it has a musky but feminine and balancing aroma. The main chemical component of clary sage oil is linalyl acetate, making it one of the most relaxing, soothing and balancing essential oils. Inhaling clary sage oil may promote feelings of relaxation, allowing for a restful night's sleep. It's also known for its ability to support healthy circulation, digestion and eye health.

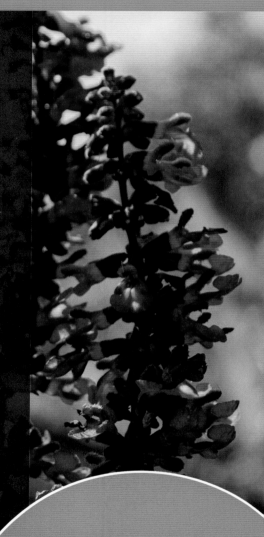

Clary sage is my favorite herbal oil to prescribe my female patients who are struggling with hormonal imbalances.

– Dr. Josh

RESEARCH STUDIES

Evidence suggests that aromatherapy can be effective in reducing maternal anxiety, fear and pain during labor. Of the essential oils that were tested, clary sage oil and Roman chamomile oil were the most effective in alleviating pain.[27]

Results of a 2015 study support the use of formulations containing clary sage oil as the active natural anti-microbial agent. Because of its anti-microbial properties, clary sage oil may be applied to wounds and skin infections.[28]

KEY BENEFITS

- Supports hormone balance
- May increase circulation
- Can improve mood
- Helps reduce stress

- Contains anti-fungal and antiseptic properties
- May relieve asthma symptoms
- Boosts eye, hair and skin health

SAFETY

Clary sage oil is not safe for use during pregnancy, especially during the first trimester or when using it on the abdomen, because it can cause uterine contractions.

THERAPEUTIC COMPOUNDS

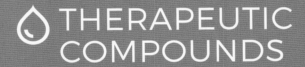

Germacrene-D   Linalool

Linalyl acetate

SUPER 7 RX CLARY SAGE USES

1. Supports Hormonal Balance

Clary sage oil contains natural phytoestrogens, which give it the ability to produce estrogenic effects. The oil can help regulate estrogen levels and support the long-term health of the uterus. To help balance hormones, apply 3 drops regularly to your abdomen, 2 drops to your neck or diffuse the oil.

2. Helps with Menstrual Discomfort

Clary sage oil has the power to alleviate some of the symptoms of PMS. It is also anti-spasmodic, meaning it can treat spasms and muscle cramps. To relieve menstrual discomfort, take it internally or apply it topically to your abdomen.

3. Promotes Restfulness

Clary sage oil is a natural sedative. To help relieve insomnia and feelings of anxiety, diffuse it at your bedside or rub 1 to 2 drops onto your neck and the soles of your feet.

4. Supports Healthy Circulation

By opening up the blood vessels and allowing for increased blood circulation, clary sage oil may be beneficial to the heart. It also naturally lowers blood pressure by relaxing the brain and arteries. Rub the oil onto your limbs and chest.

5. May Help Lower Cholesterol

The anti-inflammatory and antioxidant properties of clary sage oil may help to lower cholesterol naturally. Diffuse it or add 5 drops to a warm-water bath.

6. Contains Compounds Beneficial for Fighting Leukemia

A chemical compound found in clary sage oil, called sclareol, is able to kill leukemia cell lines through apoptosis. An insufficient amount of apoptosis results in uncontrolled abnormal cell proliferation, i.e. cancer. Take clary sage oil internally to promote apoptosis.

7. Boosts Skin Health

An important ester in clary sage oil, called linalyl acetate, has been shown to reduce skin inflammation and work as a natural remedy for rashes. Combine clary sage oil with jojoba oil and apply it to your skin.

CLOVE

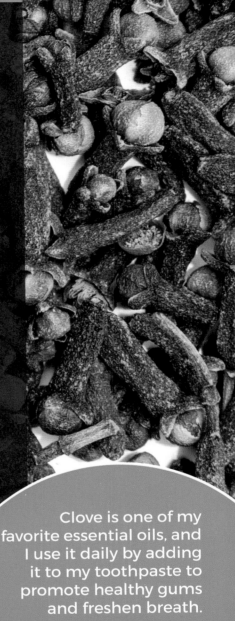

EUGENIA CARYOPHYLLATA

History tells us that clove has been used in China for more than 2,000 years as a fragrance and spice, and that it hit the international health scene several hundred years later. Since then, it has been applied in numerous products for pest control in agriculture and for cosmetic purposes. The Ancient Persians also used clove as a love potion. Today, we know that clove possesses an abundance of therapeutic properties due to its high antioxidant score (ranked No. 1 among herbs and spices).

Cloves can be found in nature as the unopened pink flower buds of the evergreen tree; the buds are steam-distilled for its essential oil, and it has a warm and spicy aroma. The most profound properties of clove oil are related to its widespread application in traditional medicine. Because it contains high levels of eugenol, clove essential oil has proven to be remarkably versatile and has been researched as an effective supplement or alternative to various modern remedies.

Clove is one of my favorite essential oils, and I use it daily by adding it to my toothpaste to promote healthy gums and freshen breath.

– Jordan

A 2007 study found that clove and rosemary essential oils have powerful bactericidal and fungicidal processes. Both oils proved to have significant anti-microbial effects against Staphylococcus epidermidis, Escherichia coli and Candida albicans.[29]

In a study, clove outperformed eugenol, eugenyl-acetate and fluoride in its ability to slow dental erosion. Not only did clove oil lead the pack by "significantly" decreasing erosion, it actually remineralized teeth.[30]

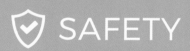 KEY BENEFITS

- May lessen symptoms of osteoporosis
- Supports blood circulation
- Contains anti-anemic properties
- Contains anti-fungal properties
- Promotes healthy gums
- Fights parasites
- Boosts energy
- Helps fight acne

SAFETY

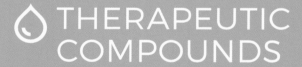 THERAPEUTIC COMPOUNDS

Dilution is recommended for topical use. If taking clove oil internally, do not use for more than two weeks consecutively. When taking it internally, we also recommend taking a probiotic supplement twice daily to restore beneficial flora.

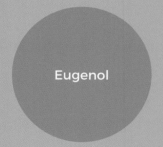

Eugenol

SUPER 7 RX CLOVE USES

1. Helps Fight Candida

Clove is an anti-fungal agent, and studies show that it is equally as effective as nystatin, a drug commonly prescribed to manage yeast infections of the mouth (thrush). Place 1 drop of clove oil in a capsule or mix it into your food or beverage and consume daily for up to two weeks to fight candida.

2. Promotes Oral Health

Clove is widely accepted as a reliable solution for dry sockets and to relieve the pain and discomfort associated with various dental disorders. It also slows tooth decalcification, or dental erosion. Dilute 1 to 2 drops with equal parts coconut oil and apply to the affected area.

3. Battles Parasites

Take clove oil internally for up to two weeks, either mixed with a carrier oil or in capsules, to rid the body of unwanted parasites.

4. Helps Prevent Oxidative Stress

Research has shown that clove contains an astounding amount of antioxidants that slow aging. To prevent damage caused by free radicals, diffuse it or dilute it with a carrier oil and apply it topically to your neck and chest.

5. May Improve Acne

Clove oil is a powerful anti-bacterial agent that can help eliminate acne and skin infections. Mix 3 drops of clove oil with 2 teaspoons of raw honey. Apply the mixture to your face, let it sit for a few minutes and then rinse off and pat dry.

6. Fights Cold and Flu Viruses

The anti-viral properties in clove essential oil help boost the immune system. Clove oil has the power to purify blood, thereby increasing the resistance to diseases and infections. To boost the immune system, diffuse clove oil or apply it topically with carrier oil.

7. Supports Healthy Blood Pressure Levels

To ease feelings of stress and uneasiness and to lower elevated blood pressure associated with stress, diffuse clove oil at home or dilute it with coconut oil and apply to your wrists.

CORIANDER

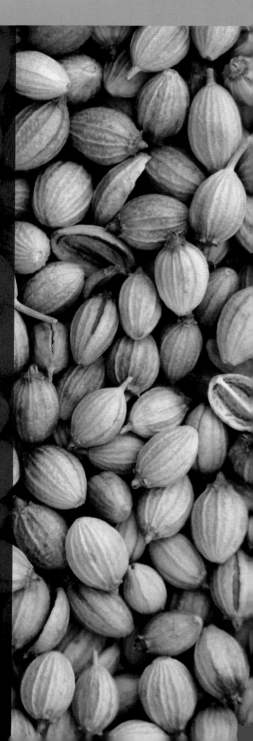

CORIANDRUM SATIVUM

Having deep historical roots, coriander seeds were found in the ancient Egyptian tomb of Ramses the Great. The seeds and leaves are a wonderful garnish or added spice. Coriander essential oil is steam-distilled from the seeds of the plant—the same plant used to make cilantro essential oil. It has a woody, spicy and sweet aroma, and it has been used for centuries to support the digestive and hormonal systems.

Modern life can often leave us more exhausted than encouraged. With such a hectic pace, we are blessed to have oils like coriander, with benefits that allow us to slow down as days speed up. Its pleasant and sweet aroma helps melt away stress. It is both calming and stimulating, helping to improve mood and boost energy levels.

RESEARCH STUDIES

A 2014 study found that coriander oil has the power to fight a fungal infection of the oral cavity. The study highlighted coriander's potential anti-fungal activity and suggested use for future toxicological research.[31]

Coriander oil can also effectively kill pathogenic bacteria related to foodborne diseases and hospital infections. Research showed that the oil displayed effective anti-microbial activity against all bacteria tested.[32]

KEY BENEFITS

- Contains anti-bacterial and anti-fungal properties
- Provides sedative and calming effects
- May help relieve migraine headaches

- Eases upset stomach
- Promotes digestion
- Promotes blood circulation
- Promotes healthy insulin response
- Helps alleviate muscle and joint pain

SAFETY

Those with sensitive skin should dilute coriander with a carrier oil before topical use.

THERAPEUTIC COMPOUNDS

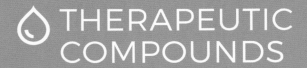

Linalool

Terpenes

SUPER 7 RX CORIANDER USES

1. Supports Healthy Blood Sugar Levels

Coriander contains compounds that lead to a wide array of pharmacological activities, including its ability to potentially assist with lowering cholesterol, blood pressure and blood sugar levels. To support healthy blood sugar, take 1 drop internally as needed.

2. Eases Gas, Nausea and Bloating

Coriander oil's digestive and anti-spasmodic properties aid in relieving gas and nausea; it helps to relax the digestive system and may ease irritability that can lead to nausea. Apply 2 to 3 drops topically to your abdomen, or take 1 drop internally.

3. Helps with Rashes and Skin Irritation

Coriander oil is considered an effective Ayurvedic remedy for rashes and itchy skin, due to its anti-irritant, soothing, anti-inflammatory and antiseptic properties. Apply 2 to 3 drops topically to the area of concern.

4. Eases Anxiety

Coriander oil is a mild stimulant, and it is capable of relaxing the mind—reducing feelings of stress and nervousness. Diffuse or apply a blend of coriander, lavender and Roman chamomile topically to the soles of your feet and the back of your neck.

5. Helps Alleviate Muscle and Joint Pain

Because of its anti-inflammatory and anti-spasmodic properties, coriander oil may reduce pain associated with arthritis, rheumatism, stiffness and gout. For soothing relief, apply it topically to the area of concern.

6. May Help with Adrenal Fatigue

To naturally support your adrenals and promote proper function, apply coriander to the back of your neck or the soles of your feet.

7. Stimulates Appetite

To boost appetite and help battle anorexia, take 1 drop of coriander oil internally or apply 2 to 3 drops to your palms, cup your nose and inhale deeply for 5 minutes.

CUMIN

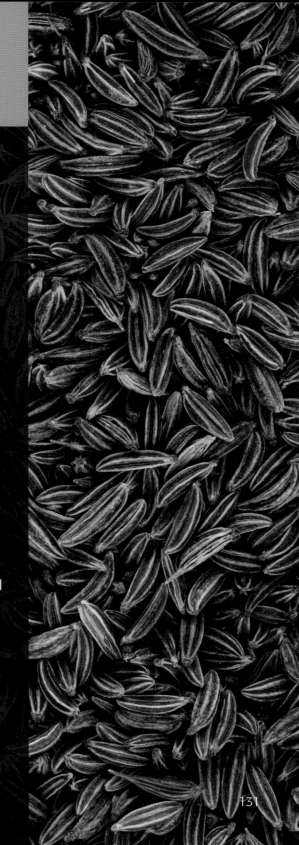

CUMINUM CYMINUM

The ancient Egyptians used cumin as a spice in foods as well as in the mummification process. The Greeks and Romans used cumin as both a spice and a medicine. Interestingly, it was also used to make the complexion paler. Cumin has been used as a traditional Middle Eastern spice and is one of the main ingredients of curry and often used to make hummus. In France, the oil is a preferred treatment for chronic viral diseases, since its main aldehyde, cuminal, combines anti-viral effects with a calming, sedative action.

Cumin oil is extracted from dried and crushed cumin seeds through steam distillation. This essential oil has been used to boost the cardiovascular, immune and nervous systems. It has a spicy and earthy aroma that can stimulate appetite and aid the digestive system by encouraging bowel movements. It is valued for its anti-bacterial, antioxidant, anti-parasitic, anti-viral and stimulating properties.

RESEARCH STUDIES

A 2005 study found that cumin oil could be used to help control bacterial diseases. The activity was particularly high against numerous harmful bacteria responsible for plant diseases worldwide.[33]

Another 2005 study suggests that cuminaldehyde, a component of cumin seeds, may be useful as a lead compound and a new agent within anti-diabetic medications because it helps improve glucose tolerance.[34]

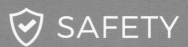 KEY BENEFITS

- Aids digestion
- Fights viral infections
- Helps detoxify the body
- Alleviates cramps and spasms
- Works to prevent gas

- Helps to regulate menstruation
- May ease anxiety and stress
- Assists in toning muscles, tissues and skin

SAFETY

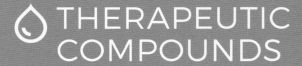 THERAPEUTIC COMPOUNDS

Do not use during pregnancy, as cumin oil is an emenagogue (stimulates blood flow in the uterus). Avoid direct sunlight for up to 12 hours after external application.

Cuminic acids

Cymene

Beta-Pinene

Alpha- and Y-Terpinenes

SUPER 7 RX CUMIN USES

1. Aids Digestion

Cumin oil promotes the discharge of bile and gastric juices when taken in small doses, which can help the digestive system. It can also prevent the formation of gas. Take 1 drop of cumin oil by adding it to food to help relieve digestive issues.

2. Assists in Detoxifying the Body

Cumin oil is a diuretic and may stimulate urination, which helps the body to flush out excess water, salt and toxins. Take 1 drop of cumin oil internally to detoxify your body.

3. May Prevent Infections

Cumin oil has antiseptic and anti-bacterial properties, so it may help to prevent infections and bacterial overgrowth. It can be used on both internal and external wounds and cuts. Dilute 2 to 3 drops and apply to the infection, or take 1 drop internally for infections.

4. Relieves Cramps and Spasms

Because of its anti-spasmodic properties, cumin oil can help to relieve cramps and spasms due to menstruation and issues such as digestive spasms and restless legs syndrome. Apply cumin oil topically to the area of concern.

5. Tones Skin, Muscles and Organs

Cumin works as a tonic, so it has the ability to tone various systems in the body, including the nervous, digestive, circulatory and excretory systems. Massage 2 to 4 drops of cumin oil and 1 teaspoon of coconut oil onto the soles of your feet to stimulate bodily organs.

6. Regulates Menstruation Cycle

Cumin oil works as an emmenagogue—meaning it helps to maintain a regular menstrual cycle by opening obstructed menses. Apply it topically over your uterus, inhale from the bottle deeply 10 times or take it internally.

7. Supports Nerve Tissue

Cumin oil is good for nerves and supports nervous disorders such as convulsions, anxiety and stress. Add 1 drop to your favorite dish for added flavor and benefit, or diffuse it.

CYPRESS

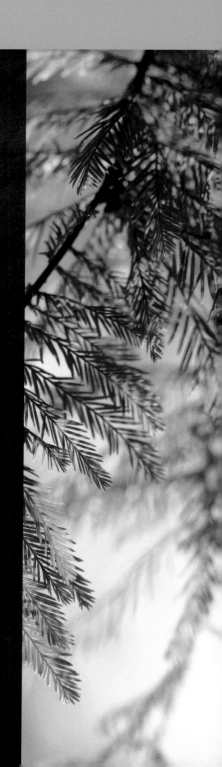

CUPRESSUS SEMPERVIRENS

During the early times, Phoenicians and Cretans used cypress to build houses and ships, while the Egyptians used it to make sarcophagi for burying their dead. The Greeks also used cypress wood to carve statues of their gods. The botanical name comes from the Greek word that means "ever living." Cypress trees are often cited in art and literature, and they are believed to be an emblem of death. In fact, legend has it that the cross upon which Jesus was crucified was made out of cypress.

Despite its somewhat sorrowful symbolisms, cypress is also well known for the fragrant and relaxing oil it produces. Cypress essential oil is valued because of its ability to fight infections, aid the respiratory system, help remove toxins from the body and work as a stimulant that can relieve anxiety. The young twigs, stems and needles of the cypress tree are steam-distilled, and the essential oil has a clean and energizing aroma that is slightly woody with evergreen undertones. Cypress contains monoterpenes, making it beneficial for oily skin conditions. Adding a few drops to a clay mask can help restore balance.

RESEARCH STUDIES

A 2004 study found that a component present in cypress oil, called camphene, inhibited the growth of nine bacteria and all yeasts studied.[35]

Compounds in cypress oil, including cosmosiin, caffeic acid and p-coumaric acid, have demonstrated powerful liver protective properties. Results indicate that cypress essential oil contains antioxidant compounds that can rid the body of excess toxins and inhibit free radical scavenging.[36]

✓ KEY BENEFITS

- Eases muscle pain
- Works as natural deodorizer
- Helps boost mood
- May improve carpal tunnel syndrome
- Assists in relieving restless legs
- Contains anti-bacterial and antiseptic properties
- May minimize varicose veins and cellulite
- Relieves feelings of anxiety

SAFETY

Avoid use during pregnancy. Do not take cypress oil internally.

THERAPEUTIC COMPOUNDS

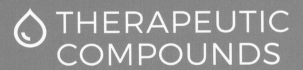

Carene

Limonene

Alpha-Pinene

SUPER 7 RX CYPRESS USES

1. Reduces the Appearance of Varicose Veins and Cellulite

Cypress essential oil stimulates blood flow and relieves fluid retention—alleviating the causes of varicose veins and cellulite. Apply 2 to 4 drops along with a carrier oil to the areas of concern.

2. Helps Diminish Hemorrhoids

Cypress essential oil is known as an effective oil for reducing and preventing hemorrhoids. Apply 3 to 4 drops with a cotton ball.

3. Eases Restless Leg Syndrome

When used topically, cypress oil may help reduce the discomfort associated with restless leg syndrome and could help increase blood circulation. Apply it topically to the area of concern.

4. Lessens Swelling from Sprains and Strains

Because of cypress oil's anti-spasmodic qualities, it helps inhibit problems associated with spasms, such as cramps and muscle strains. Apply it topically to areas of concern.

5. Supports a Healthy Prostate

Cypress oil may help reduce the size of an enlarged prostate. The applications most commonly used for prostate conditions are bath, massage blend or suppository. For suppository use, contact a clinically trained and registered aromatherapist.

6. Helps with Edema and Fluid Retention

Cypress oil is a diuretic, so it helps the body flush out internal toxins. It also increases sweat and perspiration, which allows the body to quickly remove toxins, excess salt and water. Apply it topically to your wrists, the back of your neck, abdomen and the soles of your feet.

7. Calms Respiratory Conditions

Cypress oil calms the respiratory system and works as an anti-spasmodic agent—helping to relieve respiratory conditions such as asthma and bronchitis. To remedy respiratory conditions, add 5 drops to a warm-water bath, or dilute it and apply the mixture to your chest to work as a vapor rub.

EUCALYPTUS

EUCALYPTUS RADIATA

According to English folklore, an early English settler had his thumb nearly severed by an ax. His father, who was well versed in Aboriginal folk medicine, advised that he apply a bandage of tightly bound eucalyptus leaves around the cut after it was sutured. Later, when a surgeon saw the wound, he remarked how amazed he was because the thumb healed so quickly and without any trace of infection.

The eucalyptus tree (also known as Tasmanian Blue Gum) is an evergreen tree native to Australia that's often thought of as the main food source of koala bears. While it provides amazing nutritional support for wildlife, the essential oil that is extracted from eucalyptus leaves also has powerful therapeutic properties. Eucalyptus has a cool, crisp aroma. The main chemical components of *Eucalyptus radiata* are eucalyptol and alpha-terpineol, making it an ideal oil to promote feelings of clear breathing and open airways and for creating a soothing massage experience.

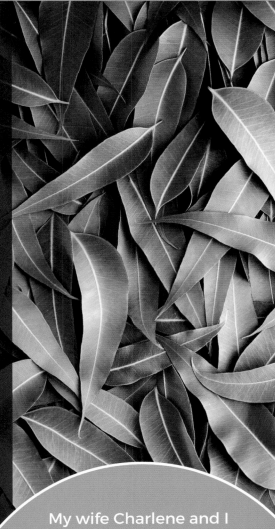

My wife Charlene and I use a blend of eucalyptus and peppermint to support our kids' health when they are sick.

– Ty

RESEARCH STUDIES

Eucalyptus oil has been found to be effective in reducing pain, swelling and inflammation. When used on patients who underwent a total knee replacement, eucalyptus inhalation significantly lowered blood pressure and pain levels.[37]

A 2015 research study concluded that topical application of 1,8-cineole (the primary active ingredient in eucalyptus) offers a novel therapeutic approach to reduce infection-induced mucus secretion.[38]

KEY BENEFITS

- Reduces earaches
- May reduce fever
- Fights infections
- Boosts mental clarity
- Relieves respiratory conditions

- Helps reduce pain and inflammation
- Aids in disinfecting house and clothes
- Serves as a remedy for skin irritations and insect bites

SAFETY

People with sensitive skin should dilute eucalyptus oil before topical use. Also, dilute it before using with children. Do not apply near the face of young children.

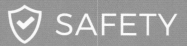 THERAPEUTIC COMPOUNDS

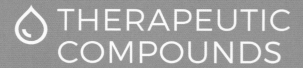

Alpha-Terpineol

Eucalyptol (1,8-cineole)

SUPER 7 RX EUCALYPTUS USES

1. Helps Ease Symptoms of Bronchitis and Pneumonia

Eucalyptus can ease symptoms of respiratory conditions by dilating the blood vessels and allowing more oxygen into the lungs. Mix 3 to 5 drops with equal parts of peppermint and coconut oil to make a homemade vapor rub; rub the mixture onto your chest.

2. Reduces Earaches

Eucalyptus can be an effective treatment for earaches. Add several drops of eucalyptus oil to a pan of boiling water, remove the pan from the heat, place a towel over your head and inhale the steam. Also try gently massaging the oil into the skin around your ear.

3. Helps Improve Asthma and Allergies

Studies show that eucalyptus oil is effective at treating sinusitis and that patients sometimes experience faster improvement when using the oil for allergies, breathing and sinus issues. Gargle with 1 to 2 drops of eucalyptus oil or apply it topically to your chest.

4. Promotes Energy and Focus

To feel energized, alert and focused,diffuse eucalyptus throughout your home or at work, or rub a few drops on your temples or neck.

5. Provides Relief from Shingles

Eucalyptus oil may help with the pain associated with shingles. Apply eucalyptus to your skin for instant relief from itching and pain.

6. Serves as a Cleaning Aid

Because of its anti-microbial properties, eucalyptus oil can help disinfect the home. Put 10 to 15 drops into home-care products such as laundry detergent and toilet cleaner. It can also be added to vacuums or a diffuser to inhibit the growth of mold and bacteria in the home.

7. Aids in Wound Care

Because of its anti-microbial and antiseptic properties, eucalyptus oil effectively treats wounds, burns, cuts, insect stings, abrasions, sores and scrapes. It also fights infections and may speed healing. Apply eucalyptus oil to the affected area twice daily.

FENNEL

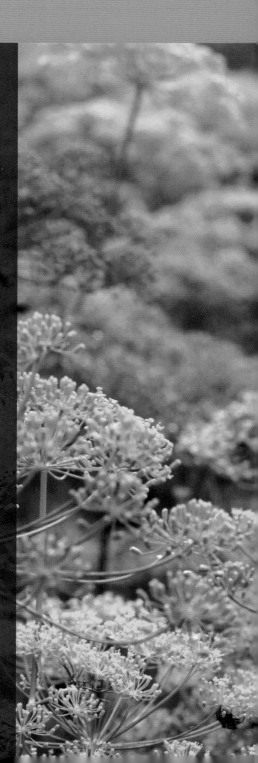

FOENICULUM VULGARE

The history of fennel use dates back to ancient times when Roman warriors were said to have consumed fennel to make them strong and ready for battle. Fennel seed oil has been used in many cultures for its medicinal properties. In ancient Chinese medicine, it was used to help with a variety of ailments—from relieving congestion to increasing the flow of breast milk.

Fennel is a celery-like winter vegetable with an interesting flavor and fragrance. Fennel oil is made by steam-distilling the crushed seeds, and the aroma is purifying and supportive. It can bring relief to exhausted muscles and joints, whether your workout is spending hours at the gym, chasing your children around the house or simply taking strides through the workday.

RESEARCH STUDIES

A 2003 study found that fennel seed oil emulsion was superior to a placebo in decreasing the intensity of infantile colic. Fennel seed oil is able to reduce intestinal spasms and increase motility of the small intestine.[39]

Researchers say that fennel essential oil might have remarkable anti-cancer potential against a breast cancer cell line and liver cancer cell line because of its strong free radical-scavenging activity.[40]

KEY BENEFITS

- Helps relieve digestive conditions
- Contains antiseptic and anti-toxic properties
- Alleviates cramps and spasms
- Eases respiratory conditions

- Promotes the flow of breast milk
- Aids in relieving menstrual issues and PMS
- May relieve nausea and colic
- Works as a natural antioxidant

SAFETY

Do not use during pregnancy. Also, do not use if you are prone to seizures or have epilepsy. Fennel oil is not intended for long-term internal use. To avoid skin irritation, dilute it before topical use.

THERAPEUTIC COMPOUNDS

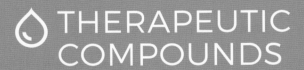

Anethole

Benzene

Limonene

SUPER 7 RX FENNEL USES

1. Aids Digestion

Fennel essential oil aids digestion by stimulating the secretion of digestive juices. It can also help balance the pH level within the stomach, thereby reducing acid reflux after meals. Fennel oil may also be used to treat intestinal parasites and sluggish bowels. Take 1 to 2 drops internally by adding the oil to water or tea, or take it in a capsule.

2. Improves Colic

Fennel seed oil has been shown to reduce colic pain and increase motility in the small intestine. The safest way to reduce colic pain is for a breastfeeding mother to drink fennel tea. Alternatively, 1 diluted drop can be applied topically to the baby's abdomen.

3. Prevents Edema and Fluid Retention

Fennel essential oil is a natural diuretic and can be used to prevent the retention of fluid within the body. Combine 1 to 2 drops of fennel oil with equal parts of grapefruit oil and rub the mixture onto the affected area.

4. Eases PMS and Menstrual Symptoms

Fennel essential oil is anti-spasmodic and may reduce uterine contraction frequency and intensity. Take 1 to 2 drops by adding it to tea or water. Fennel oil may also be applied topically to your abdomen to help tone female organs and support healthy menstruation.

5. Relieves Symptoms of Menopause

Research suggests fennel oil has potential in preventing bone loss in women with postmenopausal osteoporosis. It also helps to maintain emotional balance as well as promote healthy hormone levels. Take it internally, or apply it topically to your abdomen.[41]

6. Stimulates the Flow of Breast Milk

Fennel oil helps promote a healthy balance of hormones and may support the flow of breast milk in women with low milk supply. Take it internally or drink fennel tea.

7. Lessens Gas and Bloating

Taking fennel essential oil internally promotes healthy digestion and may help to relieve hunger pains.

FIR NEEDLE

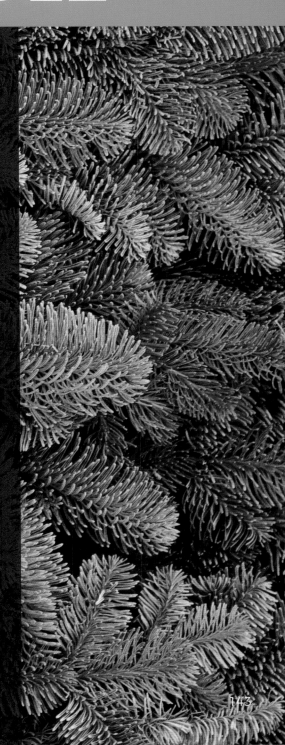

ABIES BALSAMEA

The mention of fir needle most likely conjures up scenes of a winter wonderland, but this tree and its essential oil are year-round sources of enjoyment as well as good health. Many cultures named the fir tree the "forest healer" because of its curative properties. Native Americans widely used fir needles for padding pillows for peaceful sleep, and they also used them as a sudatory (post-delivery disease prevention) for women after childbirth.

Fir needle essential oil is extracted through the process of steam distillation from fir needles, which are the soft, flat, needle-like "leaves" of the fir tree. The needles house the majority of the active chemicals and important compounds. The essential oil has a fresh, woody and earthy scent just like the tree itself. Most commonly, fir needle essential oil is used to fight sore throats and respiratory infections, fatigue, muscle aches and arthritis. It even aids in the repair of broken bones.

RESEARCH STUDIES

Modern studies have shown the many anti-tumor characteristics in fir needle essential oil, making it a promising natural cancer treatment. In one study, compounds in fir oil increased levels of glutathione, a powerful antioxidant that protects against cancer.[42]

Research results showed that three constituents of fir needle oil were active against multiple strains of bacteria, displaying the infection-fighting power of fir needle essential oil.[43]

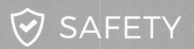 ## KEY BENEFITS

- Helps relieve arthritis pain
- Boosts respiratory function
- Combats cold and flu symptoms
- Soothes muscle aches

- May relieve rheumatic symptoms
- Helps with sinusitis
- Can prevent infections
- Improves bone health

SAFETY

THERAPEUTIC COMPOUNDS

Because possible skin sensitivity may occur, dilution is recommended before topical use.

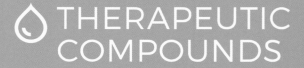

Alpha-Pinene

Camphene

Limonene

Tricyclene

SUPER 7 RX FIR NEEDLE USES

1. Helps with Respiratory Issues

Fir needle oil can be very helpful for respiratory issues that accompany the common cold and flu. Add 5 drops of fir needle oil to your diffuser and breathe in some natural relief.

2. Aids in Healing Broken Bones

Fir needle oil can assist in bone repair. Dilute it with a carrier oil (such as coconut oil) and apply it to the problematic area three times per day.

3. Helps with Ligament Tears

Fir needle oil may help speed the healing of ligament tears. Apply it topically to the affected area to help speed recovery.

4. Displays Anti-tumor Properties

Fir needle essential oil has been found to be an efficient anti-cancer agent, which may make it an effective supplement to take for cancerous tumors. Take 1 to 2 drops internally, or massage the oil onto the affected area to support beneficial tumor and anti-cancer response.

5. Provides Pain Relief

Fir needle essential oil makes an excellent analgesic. To help relax muscles and soothe body aches—important for muscle recovery—apply it topically to aching muscles and body aches.

6. Cleans and Sanitizes the House

Fir needle makes an excellent addition to homemade cleaning solutions. The next time you're creating an all-purpose cleaner, add a few drops of fir needle oil for a natural yet powerful disinfecting boost.

7. May Help Prevent Osteoporosis

When applied topically, essential oils such as fir, cypress and helichrysum may help to increase bone density. Dilute it with a carrier oil and apply to the area of concern.

FRANKINCENSE

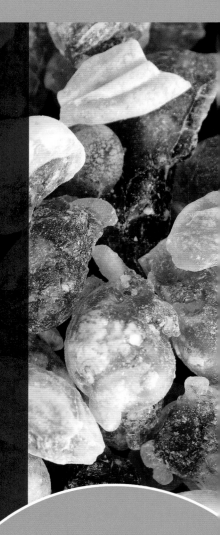

BOSWELLIA FREREANA, BOSWELLIA CARTERII, BOSWELLIA SACRA

Often called the "king of oils," frankincense is powerful, effective and incredibly therapeutic. For thousands of years, religious followers have used frankincense during worship, meditation and spiritual practices. The word frankincense appears 17 times in the Bible, and the word incense is mentioned 113 times; in such cases, incense is often assumed to imply frankincense along with myrrh and other spices. A beautiful small tree or shrub with abundant pinnate leaves and white or pale pink flowers, frankincense yields a natural oleo gum resin that is collected by making incisions into the bark. Its essential oil is collected from the resin through steam distillation.

One of the most prized and precious essential oils, frankincense has extraordinary health benefits. It is used to help relieve chronic stress and anxiety, reduce pain and inflammation, boost immunity and even combat tumors. The sesquiterpenes in frankincense enable it to go beyond the blood-brain barrier. It also increases the activity of leukocytes, which help the body fight infections. We wonder if the magi from the East knew of frankincense's healing properties when they presented it to young Jesus?

Frankincense is an oil I will never be without. I apply it to areas of pain and inflammation—including blemished skin and painful joints.

– Jordan

🔬 RESEARCH STUDIES

Frankincense oil has been shown to induce breast cancer cell death, suggesting that it is effective against breast cancer. Frankincense represses signaling pathways and cell cycle regulators that have been proposed as therapeutic targets for breast cancer.[44]

A 2011 study found that frankincense essential oil has anti-inflammatory effects in the treatment of gingivitis. After frankincense treatment, participants showed significant decreases in gingivitis index, plaque index and probing pocket depth.[45]

✓ KEY BENEFITS

- Combats negative emotions and stress
- Supports immunity and helps prevent illness
- Contains anti-tumor properties
- Heightens spiritual awareness

- Lessens the signs of aging skin
- Encourages healthy hormone levels
- May ease digestion
- Helps relieve inflammation and pain

✓ SAFETY

Frankincense is known to have blood-thinning effects, so people with problems related to blood clotting should not use before consulting with their health care provider.

💧 THERAPEUTIC COMPOUNDS

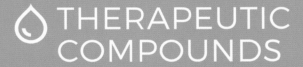

Alpha-Pinene

Alpha-Thujene

Limonene

SUPER 7 RX FRANKINCENSE USES

1. Serves as a Powerful Addition to Cancer-Fighting Protocols

Frankincense essential oil has been shown to help fight specific types of cancer cells. Take 2 to 3 drops internally, use as a suppository (under the supervision of a health practitioner) or massage the oil onto the affected area to support healthy immune system response.

2. May Relieve Joint Inflammation and Pain

To improve circulation and help relieve symptoms of joint or muscle pain related to conditions such as arthritis, digestive disorders and asthma, massage frankincense oil onto the painful area or diffuse.

3. Boosts the Immune System

Studies have demonstrated that frankincense has immune-enhancing abilities. It can be used to prevent germs from forming on the skin, in the mouth or in the home. Diffuse it, take it internally or rub onto your temples, wrists and the soles of your feet.

4. Promotes Relaxation During Meditation and Prayer

Frankincense oil may help induce a feeling of peace and relaxation, making it ideal for prayer time and meditation. Diffuse it during meditation and anoint your family with this ancient, powerful oil.

5. Relieves Cold and Flu Symptoms

Frankincense oil can help eliminate phlegm in the lungs and acts as an anti-inflammatory agent in the nasal passages. To treat respiratory conditions, add 5 drops of frankincense oil to a diffuser and breathe in deeply for 5 minutes, or rub 2 to 3 drops onto your chest.

6. Reduces the Appearance of Stretch Marks and Wrinkles

Frankincense oil can help minimize stretch marks, scars and wrinkles. Mix 2 to 3 drops of the oil with equal parts of coconut or jojoba oil and apply to the affected areas.

7. Helps Those with Brain Injury and Alzheimer's

Because it improves cognitive health and responses, frankincense oil may be used on people with Alzheimer's disease, dementia and brain injury. Take it internally, diffuse it, or apply it topically to the back of your neck and under your nose.

GERANIUM

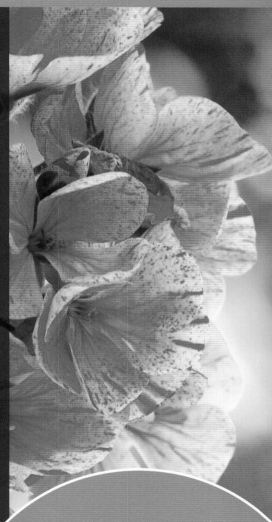

PELARGONIUM GRAVEOLENS

The uses of geranium essential oil date back to ancient Egypt, where Egyptians used the oil to beautify their skin. Native Americans drank a tea made from the powdered roots of geranium as a natural medicine. In the Victorian era, fresh geranium leaves were placed at dining tables as decorative pieces and to be consumed if desired; in fact, the edible leaves and flowers of the plant were often used in desserts, cakes, jellies and teas.

Today, geranium is commonly used as a holistic treatment to improve various aspects of physical, mental and emotional health, as it has antidepressant, antiseptic and wound-healing properties. It is often used to treat acne, eczema and psoriasis, as well as help with anxiety and encourage the balance of hormones. The leaves of the geranium plant are steam-distilled to produce the essential oil, which has a sweet, citrus-rosy and strengthening aroma.

Geranium is an essential oil that Charlene and I love to add to body lotions and facial moisturizers to give us healthy skin and to promote anti-aging.

– Ty

RESEARCH STUDIES

When mice received geranium essential oil intravaginally, it significantly decreased the amount of candida cells in the vaginal cavity. This suggests that vaginal application of geranium oil or its main component, geraniol, can suppress Candida cell growth.[46]

A 2013 study measured the effects of geranium oil on hemorrhage episodes. With no adverse side effects, geranium oil proved to be a compound that significantly reduced the number of hereditary hemorrhage episodes that occurred in the tested patients.[47]

⊘ KEY BENEFITS

- Helps balance hormones
- Assists in relieving stress
- Helps fight depression
- Minimizes inflammation
- Benefits skin health
- May reduce blood pressure
- Contains anti-yeast properties
- May reduce menopause symptoms

⊘ SAFETY

Since geranium oil influences certain hormone secretions, avoid using it during the first trimester of pregnancy, and use in topical dilutions only thereafter. Also, geranium oil may irritate sensitive skin.

◊ THERAPEUTIC COMPOUNDS

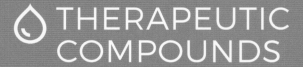

Citronellol   Geraniol

SUPER 7 RX GERANIUM USES

1. Promotes Radiant, Youthful Skin

Because geranium oil is an astringent, it induces contractions, which improves skin tone. It has the power to minimize the appearance of wrinkles and can help slow down the effects of aging. Add 2 drops to facial lotion or equal parts of coconut oil and apply it twice daily.

2. Helps Balance Hormones

Geranium can regulate hormone levels and help ease the symptoms of PMS and menstruation. Apply 1 to 2 drops topically to your abdomen along with clary sage oil, orange oil and a carrier oil just prior to the onset of your menstrual cycle.

3. Aids in Cleaning the Kidneys

Geranium oil is a natural diuretic, meaning it may increase urination, thereby helping to eliminate toxins from the body. Take it internally, or apply it topically to your abdomen.

4. Promotes Healthy Muscle Toning

Geranium oil helps to tighten and contract muscles. As a result, it can help prevent muscles and skin from sagging, and its use may result in a more toned abdomen. Create a massage oil by mixing 5 drops of geranium oil with 1 tablespoon of jojoba oil.

5. Reduces the Appearance of Eczema and Psoriasis

Geranium oil has anti-inflammatory and moisturizing properties that can aid in the repair of red, dry, flaking skin. Mix geranium oil with shea butter and apply it to any damaged skin.

6. Induces Blood Clotting

Geranium oil causes the contraction of blood vessels and helps to stop blood flow; it also speeds up the formation of blood clots. This aids in healing wounds or incisions, and it keeps toxins from entering the body.

7. May Help Prevent Alzheimer's and Dementia

Geranium oil works with the natural chemistry of the brain to help prevent conditions that can lead to memory loss. Rub the oil onto your temples, wrists and the back of your neck.

GINGER

ZINGIBER OFFICINALE

Today, ginger is easily accessible in local grocery stores and markets, but back in the 14th century, its cost was about the same amount as a live sheep or other livestock—thanks to its widespread use as a tonic to treat many ailments. A featured ingredient in many Asian dishes, ginger has a hot, fragrant flavor when used as a kitchen spice. In Western tradition, ginger is most used in sweets such as gingerbread and ginger snaps, and the spice often evokes warm feelings of Christmastime. The root is steam-distilled, and it has a warming and stimulating aroma.

In Chinese medicine, ginger is one of the most used herbs because of its warming properties, which help reduce internal dampness of the body. The most potent form of ginger is the essential oil because it contains the highest levels of gingerol, which has powerful anti-inflammatory properties and numerous other health benefits. Ginger oil is used to treat nausea, digestive distress, menstrual disorders, arthritis, chronic pain and respiratory conditions. It is also known to bring on feelings of courageousness and self-assurance, which is why it's often referred to as "the oil of empowerment."

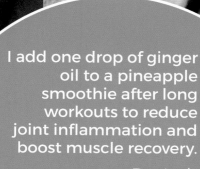

I add one drop of ginger oil to a pineapple smoothie after long workouts to reduce joint inflammation and boost muscle recovery.

– Dr. Josh

RESEARCH STUDIES

A scientific review reported that when ginger essential oil was inhaled, it was effective in reducing nausea after surgery. Ginger essential oil also demonstrated analgesic activity, helping to relieve pain immediately after surgery.[48]

A 2013 study concluded that ginger essential oil possesses antioxidant activity as well as significant anti-inflammatory and antinociceptive (pain-blocking) properties.[49]

KEY BENEFITS

- Contains anti-inflammatory properties
- May help relieve nausea and vomiting
- Encourages blood circulation
- Provides immune system support
- Helps improve mood
- Can aid digestion
- Stimulates libido
- Treats respiratory conditions

SAFETY

Dilution is recommended for those with sensitive skin.

THERAPEUTIC COMPOUNDS

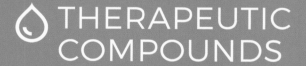

Alpha-Zingiberene

Gingerol

SUPER 7 RX GINGER USES

1. Helps Ease Nausea and Morning Sickness

Ginger essential oil is effective as a natural remedy for nausea and vomiting. To relieve nausea and vomiting, diffuse 2 to 3 drops or apply 1 to 2 drops topically onto your stomach.

2. Promotes Digestion

Ginger essential oil is one of the best natural remedies for colic, indigestion, diarrhea, spasms and stomachaches. Rub a few drops of ginger oil with a carrier oil on your abdomen, inhale it directly or add 1 drop to your food or beverage.

3. Aids in Healing Infections

Ginger oil is an antiseptic, fighting a broad spectrum of infections. This includes intestinal infections, bacterial dysentery and food poisoning. For external infections, apply 2 to 3 drops topically to the affected area. For internal infections, consume it by adding it to tea, water or food. Add one drop at a time, tasting between drops for tolerance.

4. Eases Colds and Sore Throats

Ginger essential oil helps remove mucus from the throat and lungs. It also naturally aids in relieving coughs, asthma and bronchitis and helps with loss of breath. Add 1 drop of ginger essential oil to a cup of green tea twice daily. It can also be applied topically to your chest.

5. Reduces Inflammation and Joint Pain

A component of ginger essential oil, called zingibain, is responsible for the oil's anti-inflammatory properties. This component provides pain relief and treats muscle aches, arthritis, headaches and migraines. To reduce inflammation, take 1 to 3 drops of ginger oil internally once a day, or apply 2 drops topically to the affected area.

6. Helps Relieve Anxiety

Ginger oil may be able to relieve feelings of anxiety, depression and exhaustion. The warming quality of ginger oil acts as a sleep aid and stimulates feelings of courage and ease. Use the oil aromatically by diffusing 3 to 5 drops, or add 5 drops to a warm-water bath.

7. May Alleviate Pain from Sprains and Strains

Research suggests that consuming ginger essential oil daily is more effective in treating muscle and joint pain than some prescription painkillers. Apply to the affected area or add to warm bath water.

GRAPEFRUIT

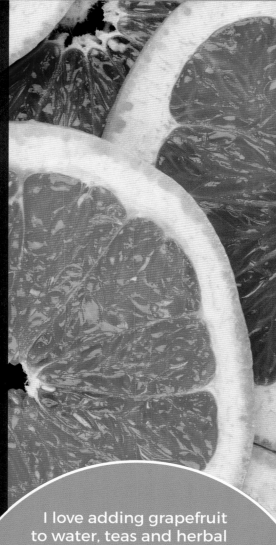

CITRUS X PARADISE

Referred to as a "forbidden fruit" and one of the "Seven Wonders of Barbados, " grapefruit was first documented in 1750 by Welshman Rev. Griffith Hughes. The name "grapefruit" is attributed to the fruits growing in clusters that resemble those of grapes. The earliest records of grapefruits were found in the West Indies during the early 18th century, and Florida was home to the first planted grapefruit trees in 1820.

Grapefruit oil has been used for centuries to help fight inflammation, weight gain, sugar cravings and even hangover symptoms. As one of the most versatile essential oils, the aroma of grapefruit oil is clean, fresh and a little bitter, just like the actual fruit itself. It has the signature taste and smell of citrus fruits, which is why many people like to use it in natural household cleaning products and homemade body care and cosmetics, including lotions, soaps and shampoos.

I love adding grapefruit to water, teas and herbal infusions to improve nutrient absorption and support natural cleansing and detoxification.

– Jordan

RESEARCH STUDIES

A 2002 study reported that grapefruit oil significantly affected brain activity and relaxation. Adults who inhaled the oils experienced improved mood and reduced feelings of stress. They also experienced a noticeable reduction in systolic blood pressure.[50]

Researchers found that grapefruit has a refreshing and exciting effect when inhaled, which suggests there is an activation of sympathetic nerve activity that helps control body weight.[51]

✓ KEY BENEFITS

- Helps disinfect surfaces
- May reduce symptoms of depression
- Stimulates the immune system
- Helps decrease fluid retention

- Curbs sugar cravings
- May boost weight loss
- Promotes toxin elimination
- May lessen fatigue

🛡 SAFETY

Avoid direct sunlight for up to 12 hours after external application. Grapefruit oil cannot be taken with certain medications, as it may have drug interactions.

💧 THERAPEUTIC COMPOUNDS

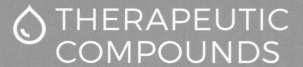

D-Limonene   Myrcene

SUPER 7 RX GRAPEFRUIT USES

1. May Boost Weight Loss

Grapefruit oil can support metabolism and may reduce appetite. Mix grapefruit oil with patchouli oil and diffuse it. To boost your metabolism, add 2 drops to water, a smoothie or sparkling beverage. Also massage the oil onto your chest and wrists when a craving strikes.

2. Curbs Food Cravings

Grapefruit is known to lower sugar cravings and help kick sugar addiction when inhaled. Add several drops to a cotton ball along with a touch of coconut oil; then rub it onto your wrists, neck or chest, or inhale it directly to stave off cravings.

3. Promotes Lymphatic Drainage

Grapefruit oil is an excellent diuretic and lymphatic stimulant, making it effective for shedding excess water weight; it can also help eliminate toxins and excess salt. Take 1 to 2 drops internally, or apply it topically over your kidneys.

4. Helps with Gallbladder Function and Fat Digestion

By increasing blood to the digestive organs, grapefruit oil helps with detoxification. It has a positive effect on digestion, can help reduce fluid retention and fights microbes within the intestines, gut and other digestive organs. Make a homemade massage lotion with grapefruit and coconut or jojoba oil, and then rub the mixture onto your abdomen.

5. Fights Candida

Grapefruit essential oil has anti-fungal abilities and is able to reduce yeast and bacteria. Research shows that grapefruit is also effective at fighting urinary tract infections. Diffuse 5 drops, or take 1 to 2 drops internally.

6. Freshens the Air

To get rid of unpleasant odors, diffuse grapefruit oil along with other citrus scents such as lemon oil and orange oil. Additionally, use grapefruit oil on wooden surfaces, countertops, floors or household appliances to help kill bacteria and mask odor.

7. Helps Reduce the Appearance of Cellulite

Grapefruit essential oil helps to reduce inflammation and increase blood flow, which may lessen the appearance of cellulite. Rub a mixture of grapefruit oil and coconut oil onto areas of concern daily.

HELICHRYSUM

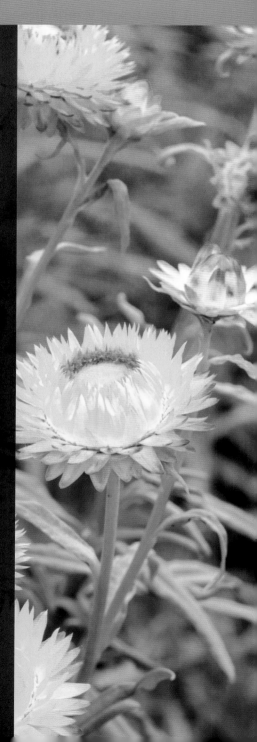

HELICHRYSUM ITALICUM

In traditional Mediterranean medicine, helichrysum oil has been used for centuries. Helichrysum is often referred to as "The Everlasting Flower" because of its rejuvenating benefits for the skin and ability to improve the complexion. It is an all-natural alternative to many expensive, high-end facial creams and serums. By adding a few drops helichrysum to your favorite carrier oil, you may benefit from an array of therapeutic properties without the harsh chemicals of many over-the-counter products.

Helichrysum is considered a medicinal plant with many promising pharmacological activities because it operates as a natural antibiotic, anti-fungal and anti-microbial agent. One of the most unique properties of helichrysum is its ability to support the health of neurological tissues. There are more than 500 species of helichrysum. Its flowers and leaves are the most useful parts of the plant; they are steam-distilled to extract the essential oils, which have a sweet, fruity and rich aroma.

RESEARCH STUDIES

In 2014, researchers found that helichrysum oil has anti-microbial and anti-inflammatory properties that make it effective against bacteria (such as Staphylococcus aureus). It also displayed anti-fungal action against Candida.[52]

Researchers found that the ethanolic compounds present in the extract of helichrysum flowers elicits anti-spasmodic actions inside an inflamed digestive system, helping to reduce gut swelling, cramping and digestive pain.[53]

KEY BENEFITS

- Helps relieve allergy symptoms
- May ease nerve pain
- Fights skin inflammation
- May relieve indigestion and acid reflux
- Supports the liver and gallbladder
- Fights inflammation of the muscles and joints
- Inhibits Candida growth
- Aids in wound healing

SAFETY

Helichrysum is generally well tolerated.

THERAPEUTIC COMPOUNDS

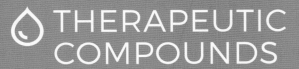

Italidione

Neryl acetate

L-Limonene

Y-Curcumene

SUPER 7 RX
HELICHRYSUM USES

1. May Ease Nerve Pain

Helichrysum, especially when combined with frankincense oil, may support the neurological system and can alleviate some of the symptoms of multiple sclerosis. Apply 2 drops of each oil to your temples, wrists and the soles of your feet every day for three weeks. Take one week off and repeat the cycle.

2. Diminishes Bruising and Bleeding

Helichrysum's anti-inflammatory and anti-spasmodic properties help to reduce pain, bruising and swelling. Apply 2 to 3 drops topically to the back of your neck or any area of pain; repeat several times daily.

3. Reduces the Appearance of Wrinkles

Helichrysum hydrates the skin and can decrease signs of aging and block UV damage that can lead to skin cancer. Use helichrysum topically by combining 2 to 3 drops with a carrier oil, and apply it where you are most prone to wrinkles.

4. Acts as a Natural Digestive Aid and Diuretic

Helichrysum helps stimulate the secretion of gastric juices to break down food and prevent indigestion. It also reduces bloating. Rub onto your abdomen or take internally.

5. Detoxifies Liver and Kidney

Known to be an anti-spasmodic agent, blood purifier and anti-inflammatory, helichrysum has been used as a liver and kidney stimulant and detoxifier for centuries. Take internally to promote healthy liver and pancreas function and heavy metal chelation.

6. May Stop Cancer Cell Growth

Helichrysum contains flavonoid antioxidant compounds that inhibit oxidative stress and cancer growth in lab experiments. It may protect cells against radiation-induced DNA damage, cell mutation and death, and cancerous tumor growth. Take it internally by adding the oil to a glass of water or cup of tea.

7. Boosts the Immune System

Because of its gut-healing and anti-inflammatory properties, helichrysum may boost immunity. It inhibits the growth of harmful bacteria, fungi and viruses. Diffuse it or take it internally to promote gut health and immunity.

HOLY BASIL
(TULSI)

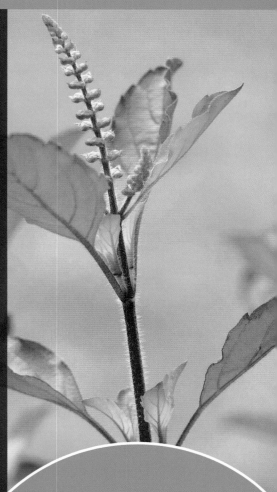

OCIMUM SANCTUM

Holy basil has a rich history as both a therapeutic and sacred plant, with its use dating back over 3,000 years. Holy basil goes by another name, "Tulsi," which means "incomparable one." The sacredness of holy basil was celebrated in the Puranas—Hindu religious texts that are part of the ancient Hindu scriptures known as the Vedas—and it is highly regarded in Ayurvedic medicine. According to Ayurveda, the herb has an effect on the spiritual aspects, facilitating expanded states of awareness. Tulsi is also an ancient sacred plant in India, where it is often called "The Elixir of Life."

Known as an adaptogen, Tulsi can be stimulating or sedating, depending on the body's needs. Holy basil oil is extracted from the leaves, and it is used as an anti-stress agent that promotes health throughout the entire body. Both in Western and Chinese medicine, holy basil oil is used to remedy adrenal fatigue, anxiety, high cortisol levels and many hormonal conditions. It has a sharp, fresh and minty aroma that has anti-inflammatory and analgesic properties.

Holy Basil is one of my personal favorites. I love to use it topically and consume it internally. I call it my mind and muscle booster.

– Jordan

RESEARCH STUDIES

When compared with a control group, holy basil treatment proved to be an effective dietary therapy in noninsulin-dependent diabetes mellitus.[54]

Tulsi essential oil, at concentrations of 4.5 percent and 2.25 percent, completely inhibited the growth of Staphylococcus aureus (including MRSA) and Escherichia coli.[55]

KEY BENEFITS

- **Supports hormone balance**
- **May reduce anxiety**
- **Aids hypothyroidism**
- **Contains antioxidant and antibiotic properties**
- **Remedies acne**
- **Promotes healthy blood sugar levels**
- **Proves useful for lung disorders**
- **Helps improve adrenal fatigue**

SAFETY

Oils high in eugenol should be used with caution on those with impaired liver function. People who have clotting disorders should avoid use of holy basil, as eugenol is an anticoagulant.

THERAPEUTIC COMPOUNDS

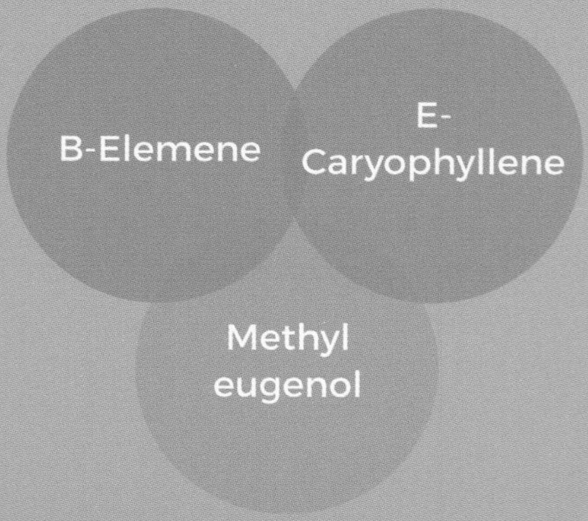
B-Elemene
E-Caryophyllene
Methyl eugenol

SUPER 7 RX HOLY BASIL USES

1. Supports Thyroid Function

Holy basil acts as an adaptogen (helps the body adapt to stress and exerts a normalizing effect upon bodily processes) to modulate the stress response and fight adrenal fatigue. To support proper thyroid function, take 1 to 2 drops internally with a carrier oil or in a glass of water.

2. May Lessen Anxiety

As stated above, holy basil has been traditionally used to support people through times of stress, working as an adaptogen and anxiolytic (decreasing anxiety). Take it internally or rub on your temples to help decrease stress and elevate your mood.

3. Supports the Nervous System

Holy basil has been shown to improve memory and cognition, anxiety and depression, insomnia, migraines and headaches. Apply it topically to your wrists, temples or the soles of your feet to benefit from its many therapeutic properties.

4. Helps Reduce Inflammation

Holy basil possesses anti-inflammatory and immune-boosting properties that can protect the body against fever, pain, stress and inflammation. Make holy basil tea by adding 2 to 3 drops to hot tea, or apply it topically to areas of pain and discomfort.

5. Supports Healthy Blood Glucose Levels

Holy basil is known for its ability to affect blood glucose levels; in fact, many people use it to manage or even help reverse diabetes. Drink holy basil tea once daily to positively influence blood sugar levels and support diabetes management.

6. Can Regulate Cortisol Levels

Holy basil is able to regulate cortisol levels in the body, which are the stress hormones that can hinder learning, memory, immune function, bone density, weight loss and cardiovascular function. Drink holy basil tea or apply it topically.

7. Treats Respiratory Conditions

Components of holy basil leaves provide relief from congestion and other symptoms of respiratory disorders. To treat respiratory conditions, add 2 to 3 drops of holy basil oil to hot water, or apply it topically to the back of your neck, chest and the soles of your feet.

HYSSOP

HYSSOPUS OFFICINALIS

Hyssop is a rare oil with many therapeutic properties. For thousands of years, hyssop has been used as a purifier and cleanser; the Romans revered hyssop because they believed it helped protect them against plagues. Its reputation as a protector has led people to hang dried hyssop around their homes in order to keep out the "evil eye" or negativity. It has also been left at gravesites to protect the dead.

The Bible mentions hyssop several times, mostly in the Old Testament. In Leviticus, God commanded His people to use hyssop in the ceremonial cleansing of people and houses. In one example, God tells the priests to use hyssop together with cedarwood, scarlet yarn and the blood of a clean bird to sprinkle a person recently healed from a skin disease (likely leprosy). The essential oils are extracted from the leaves of the plant, and with its pleasing herbal, minty aroma, it can lift the spirits.

RESEARCH STUDIES

A 2002 study found that hyssop oil has muscle-relaxing activity. The oil reduced spontaneous movements and decreased the basal or vascular tone, which is the degree of constriction experienced by a blood vessel relative to its maximally dilated state.[56]

A study concluded that hyssop oil may be a promising treatment for herpes type 2 virus.[57]

KEY BENEFITS

- Works as an anti-bacterial and anti-viral agent
- Promotes emotional balance
- May help with wound healing
- Promotes mental alertness

- Helps reduce anxiety
- Helps detoxify the body
- Fights inflammation
- Provides relief from respiratory conditions

SAFETY

Avoid using while pregnant because it may cause the uterus to contract. Do not exceed 30 drops of hyssop oil in a day, as it is a convulsant and may increase your risk of seizure.

THERAPEUTIC COMPOUNDS

Cispino-champhone

Trans-Pinocamphone

Beta-Pinene

SUPER 7 RX HYSSOP USES

1. Helps Relieve Respiratory Conditions

Hyssop relieves spasms in the respiratory system and soothes coughs. It's also an expectorant, loosening phlegm that has been deposited in the respiratory tract. Hyssop may also reduce lung inflammation. Add 2 to 3 drops to tea, or apply it to your throat and chest.

2. May Prevent Infections

Because of its antiseptic properties, hyssop helps prevent infections from developing in wounds and cuts. Hyssop also aids in the healing process of deep cuts, scars, insect bites and acne. Apply it topically to the area of concern.

3. Fights Parasites

Hyssop is a vermifuge, which means it has the ability to fight parasites such as tapeworms, hookworms and flukes. Take hyssop oil internally to help rid the body of internal parasites.

4. Encourages Healthy Circulation

By increasing circulation, hyssop can work as a natural treatment for gout, rheumatism, arthritis and swelling. The heart rate lowers when blood circulates properly, thereby relaxing the muscles and regulating blood pressure levels. Consume hyssop oil in tea or hot water to improve circulation.

5. Reduces Muscle Pain and Spasms

Hyssop oil has muscle-relaxing activity, and it may inhibit contractions and spasms that can lead to cramps. Apply 3 to 5 drops topically to the area of concern, or add 5 to 10 drops to a warm-water bath with Epsom salts.

6. Supports a Healthy Immune System

By improving circulation, aiding digestion and helping to prevent infection, hyssop oil supports a healthy immune system. Consume hyssop oil in tea or hot water to boost the immune system.

7. Promotes Skin Health

Hyssop promotes cellular regeneration and the growth of new skin, thereby minimizing the look of scars, stretch marks and wounds. It also helps fight bacteria on the skin. Dilute 2 to 3 drops with a carrier oil and apply it topically to the area of concern.

JASMINE

JASMINUM GRANDIFLORUM

Jasmine is a very famous and fascinating flower. This flower blooms only at night and fills the surroundings with its unmistakable and alluring fragrance. It has a strong yet sweet, pleasing and romantic fragrance, which is common in flowers that bloom only at night. Women are sometimes named "Jasmine," primarily in the Middle Eastern region and the Indian Subcontinent, but also in other parts of the world. The jasmine flower is often associated with romance and love. Jasmine has been inspiring poets for ages as well.

Jasmine oil is extracted from the fragrant flowers of jasmine, and it is a popular natural remedy for improving mood, overcoming stress and balancing hormones. Jasmine oil has been used for hundreds of years in parts of Asia as a natural treatment for depression, anxiety, emotional stress, low libido and insomnia.

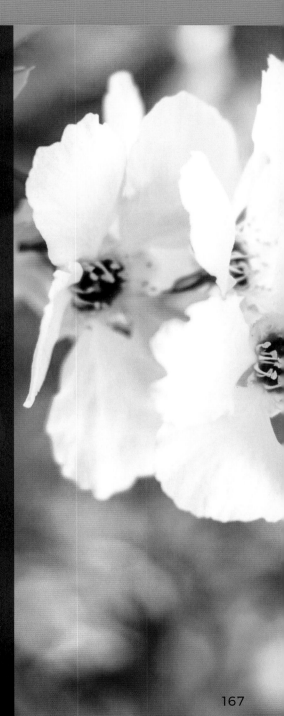

RESEARCH STUDIES

Jasmine oil can cause significant increases in breathing rate, blood oxygen saturation and systolic and diastolic blood pressure. In a 2010 study testing the effects of using jasmine in an aromatherapy massage, participants in the jasmine oil group rated themselves as more alert, more vigorous and less depressed than subjects in the control group.[58]

Researchers found that aromatherapy and massage with phytoestrogen-rich oils, such as jasmine oil, helped decrease symptoms of menopause and PMS without any negative side effects.[59]

⊘ KEY BENEFITS

- Helps relieve stress
- May reduce anxiety
- Promotes restful sleep
- Serves as an aphrodisiac
- Aids pain relief

- Enhances alertness and energy
- May help with menopausal symptoms
- Proves useful for PMS symptoms and cramps

🛡 SAFETY

💧 THERAPEUTIC COMPOUNDS

Jasmine oil is not intended for use during pregnancy, as it is an emmenagogue (stimulates blood flow in the pelvic area).

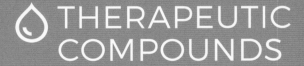

Benzyl acetate

Benzyl benzoate

Phytol

SUPER 7 RX JASMINE USES

1. Acts as an Aphrodisiac

Jasmine oil causes increases of the physical signs of arousal, such as breathing rate, body temperature, blood oxygen saturation and systolic and diastolic blood pressure. Diffuse 5 drops of jasmine oil, or apply it topically to the soles of your feet as well as your wrists.

2. Helps Fight Depression and Anxiety

Jasmine oil can improve mood and boost energy levels because of its regenerating and stimulating properties. The oil also has the power to boost concentration and brain activity. Diffuse it, or apply 1 or 3 drops topically to your temples, wrists, the back of your neck or the soles of your feet. Jasmine oil can also be added to a warm bath.

3. Fights Wrinkles and Aging Skin

Jasmine oil displays both antibiotic and anti-viral properties, giving it the ability to help calm skin irritation and inflammation and promote youthful, radiant skin. Mix 1 to 3 drops of jasmine oil into a lip balm, face wash or lotion to fight wrinkles.

4. Acts as a Sleep Aid

Jasmine oil exhibits a calming effect and can act as a natural sedative and help with sleep. Combine jasmine oil with other soothing oils, such as lavender and frankincense, and diffuse it or apply it topically.

5. Eases Feelings of Being Overwhelmed

Jasmine can help ease postpartum symptoms, including anxiety, depression, muscle pain and low energy. It also helps balance hormones naturally and has been used traditionally to increase the production of breast milk. Diffuse jasmine oil or apply it topically.

6. Promotes Hormone Balance

Using jasmine oil may help reduce hot flashes. Diffuse jasmine oil or apply it topically to the back of your neck or the soles of your feet to reduce PMS symptoms, including headaches, stomach cramps, acne and restlessness.

7. Serves as a Mood-Lifting Perfume

Jasmine oil has a warm, flowery smell, similar to many women's perfumes. Apply 1 to 2 drops topically to your wrists, mixed with a carrier oil to tone down the smell. Jasmine oil blends well with vanilla, lavender and orange when making a homemade perfume.

JUNIPER BERRY

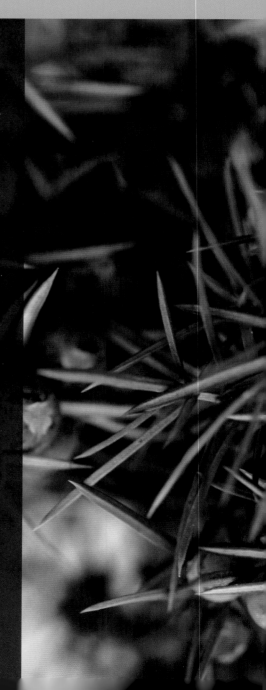

JUNIPERUS COMMUNIS

Herbal uses of juniper berry dates back to early Greek and Arabian physicians. During the Bubonic Plague, cautious people kept a few berries in their mouths to produce an antiseptic aura and prevent infection. Juniper tea was once used to disinfect surgeon's tools. Juniper berries were also used as food and medicine by the Indians of the American plains.

Interestingly, juniper berry is not a berry at all but a cone with unusually fleshy and merged scales, which give it a berry-like appearance. The essential oil is steam-distilled from the "berries" of the plant and has a sweet, balsamic aroma. Known as a powerful detoxifier and immune system booster, juniper berry essential oil is commonly used as a natural treatment for sore throats and respiratory infections, fatigue, muscle aches and arthritis. It can also help soothe skin flair-ups, boost the immune system, fight insomnia and improve digestion.

RESEARCH STUDIES

Research states that juniper berry oil possesses a wide spectrum of pharmacological compounds that act as natural anti-bacterial and anti-fungal agents.[60]

Juniper berry essential oil demonstrated the ability to aid digestive health in a 2007 study. Researchers found that cows given daily juniper and garlic supplementation experienced generally improved digestion.[61]

KEY BENEFITS

- Contains anti-bacterial and anti-fungal properties
- Helps detoxify the body
- Supports healthy circulation
- Works as a diuretic
- Treats skin conditions
- May help with insomnia
- Aids digestion
- Boosts the immune system

SAFETY

Those with sensitive skin should dilute juniper berry oil before applying it topically.

THERAPEUTIC COMPOUNDS

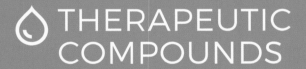

Alpha-Pinene   Sabinene

SUPER 7 RX JUNIPER BERRY USES

1. Soothes and Protects Skin

Juniper berry oil supports healthy skin, helps reduce the appearance of stretch marks and may treat skin conditions caused by hormone imbalances. Add 1 to 2 drops to face or body wash, or dilute 2 to 3 drops with a carrier oil and apply it to the areas of concern.

2. Assists in Cleansing the Liver

Juniper can help stimulate digestive enzymes and make it easier to break down and absorb protein, fats and nutrients from foods. For a natural digestive aid or liver cleanse, add a few drops to a smoothie or glass of water.

3. Boosts Kidney and Urinary Health

Juniper berry oil helps speed up urination and elimination—drawing out toxins, waste and irritants from the digestive tract. Apply 1 to 3 drops to your abdomen or take it internally.

4. Helps Reduce Bloating and Gas

Juniper berries serve as a natural diuretic, which helps the body flush out excess fluids from the bladder and urethra. This process helps reduce bloating and gas. Apply 1 to 3 drops to your abdomen or take it internally.

5. Serves as a Household Cleaner

As a natural antiseptic that can keep certain bacterial strains from spreading within the home, use juniper berry oil on kitchen and bathroom surfaces or appliances. Add 5 drops to the washing machine as a natural alternative to harsh anti-bacterial commercial detergents.

6. Acts as a Sleep Aid

Juniper berry essential oil may relieve muscle tension and prevent restlessness, helping you fall asleep. Diffuse 5 drops before bed, or apply 1 to 3 drops to your neck, chest and the soles of your feet.

7. Soothes Sore Muscles

Juniper berry oil can reduce pain and inflammation, as well as help alleviate pain from injuries and strenuous physical activity. Massage it into the area of concern. It can also be added to bath water, along with lavender oil and Epsom salts.

LAVENDER

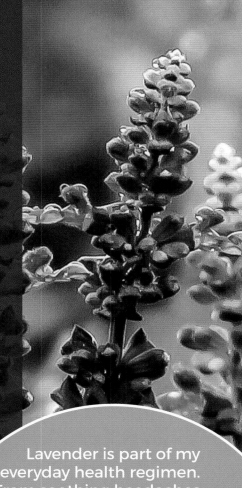

LAVANDULA ANGUSTIFOLIA

Ancient texts tell us that lavender has been used for medicinal and religious purposes for over 2,500 years. The Egyptians used it for mummification and as perfume. The Romans used it for cooking and scenting the air. They also added lavender to their bath water, hence the name from the Latin "lavare" meaning "to wash."

In quite possibly the most famous usage of all, Mary may have applied lavender with her hair to anoint Jesus. Interestingly, many researchers claim that 2,000 years ago lavender was referred to as spikenard or simply "nard" from the Greek name for lavender, naardus, after the Syrian city of Naarda. According to John 12:3, "Mary then took a pound of very costly perfume of pure *nard*, and anointed the feet of Jesus and wiped His feet with her hair; and the house was filled with the fragrance of the perfume."

Today, lavender oil is the most commonly used essential oil in the world. It is often considered a "must-have" oil to keep on hand at all times due to its versatile uses, including relaxing properties that promote peaceful sleep and ease feelings of tension. The lavender flowers are steam-distilled for their essential oil, and the aroma is floral, sweet and calming.

Lavender is part of my everyday health regimen. From soothing headaches to acting as first aid for my family, lavender is a "go-to" health booster in the Rubin household.

– Jordan

RESEARCH STUDIES

A 2014 study found lavender oil not only lessened the severity of lab-induced diabetes, but also improved body weight and protected the liver and kidneys from degeneration in laboratory animals.[62]

A 2013 study found that taking 80 milligrams of lavender essential oil internally via capsules alleviated insomnia, anxiety and depression, and also improved Alzheimer's symptoms. Another study found that lavender oil reduced depression by 32.7 percent in people suffering from post-traumatic stress disorder (PTSD).[63] [64]

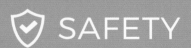 KEY BENEFITS

- Helps improve sleep
- May reduce anxiety and depression
- Serves as first aid for burns and wounds
- Improves skin and reduces acne
- Proves helpful for eczema and psoriasis
- Helps relieve headaches
- Promotes balanced blood sugar
- Helps lower blood pressure

SAFETY

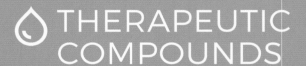 THERAPEUTIC COMPOUNDS

For most people, lavender oil is well tolerated.

Alpha-Terpineol

Beta-Ocimene

Linalool

Linalyl acetate

SUPER 7 RX LAVENDER USES

1. Promotes Sleep

To help get a good night's rest, diffuse 5 drops of lavender oil beside your bed, or apply 2 to 3 drops to the back of your neck, as well as your chest and temples.

2. Soothes Burns, Sunburns and Cuts

Lavender has been shown to be highly soothing to skin cuts and irritations. Mix lavender oil with coconut oil and apply it to the areas of concern twice daily.

3. Helps Relieve Anxiety and Stress

Lavender oil is known to bring on feelings of peace and relaxation. Diffuse lavender oil, add it to a warm-water bath or apply it to your temples, wrists and the soles of your feet.

4. Combats High Blood Pressure

Diffuse lavender oil beside you during your workday to help soothe stressed behaviors and promote healthy blood pressure.

5. Stimulates Healthy Blood Sugar Balance

Lavender oil shows promise in protecting the body from increases in blood glucose. Apply it to the back of your neck and your chest, diffuse it or add 1 drop to a glass of water or cup of tea.

6. Helps Relieve Headaches and Migraines

For relief from headache pain, inhale lavender oil for 15 minutes. You can also mix 2 drops of lavender oil with 2 drops of peppermint oil and apply it to the back of your neck and your temples for a tension and pain relief aid.

7. Encourages Healthy Skin

Lavender oil can be applied directly on the skin or mixed with coconut oil for those with sensitivities. Mixing lavender oil with equal parts frankincense oil will help boost skin health.

LEMON

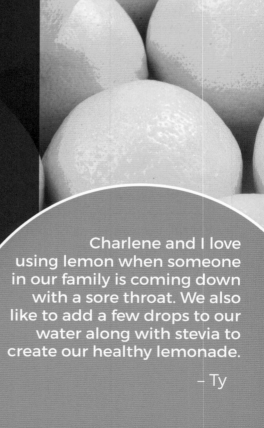

SINGLE ESSENTIAL OILS

CITRUS LIMON

Ayurvedic medicine practitioners have been using lemon essential oil to treat a wide spectrum of health conditions for at least 1,000 years. In Traditional Chinese Medicine, lemon peel oil has the ability to combat conditions related to dampness such as the common cold, candida, infections, loose stools, respiratory conditions and sore throats. Also, it has been used throughout history to support the health of the liver and as a natural remedy for gallstones. Lemon oil contains the compound d-limonene, which also has powerful anti-cancer properties.

Lemon oil is known for its ability to help cleanse toxins from any part of the body; it is widely used to stimulate lymph drainage, rejuvenate energy, purify skin and repel insects. The rind of the lemon is cold-pressed for the extraction of its essential oil, which has a sweet, citrusy and sharp aroma that is uplifting and refreshing. Lemon is a powerful cleansing agent that purifies the air and surfaces, and it can be used as a non-toxic cleaner throughout the home. When added to water, lemon oil provides a refreshing and healthy boost throughout the day.

Charlene and I love using lemon when someone in our family is coming down with a sore throat. We also like to add a few drops to our water along with stevia to create our healthy lemonade.

– Ty

RESEARCH STUDIES

A 2014 study found that lemon oil aromatherapy reduced nausea and vomiting during pregnancy. The nausea and vomiting intensity in the lemon oil group were significantly lower than the control group.[65]

Lemon essential oil has proven strong anti-stress effects. In a study, mice were exposed to three behavioral tasks. After utilizing lemon oil, the results suggested that it possessed notable antidepressant-like effects on the mice during these tasks.[66]

KEY BENEFITS

- Helps purify the body
- Freshens breath
- Aids in cough suppression
- Supports fat digestion
- Fights cancer
- Stimulates lymphatic drainage
- Promotes weight loss

SAFETY

Avoid direct sunlight for up to 12 hours after external application.

THERAPEUTIC COMPOUNDS

Alpha-Pinenes

Beta-Pinenes

D-Limonene

SUPER 7 RX LEMON USES

1. Promotes Lymphatic Drainage

Lemon oil is beneficial for improving blood flow and reducing swelling in lymph nodes. Apply 1 to 2 drops topically directly to your lymph nodes or diffuse it.

2. Helps Clear Mucus and Phlegm

Lemon oil helps to relieve congestion and eliminate mucus. It can also slow a runny nose and reduce the symptoms of allergies. Inhale lemon oil directly from the bottle or apply it topically, mixed with a carrier oil, to your chest and nose.

3. May Improve Mood

Help lift mood, improve concentration, fight depression and combat addiction by diffusing lemon essential oil, or apply it topically to your wrists and chest.

4. Assists in Gallbladder Health and Gallstone Removal

To help pass painful gallstones, mix 1 quart of sauerkraut juice, 1 quart of tomato juice, 10 drops of lemon oil and 10 drops of peppermint oil. Divide the mixture into two jars. Drink one jar the first morning, and the second jar the following morning.

5. Boosts the Immune System

Lemon essential oil has anti-bacterial properties, and it helps the body get rid of toxins that could lead to illness. Research shows that lemon oil protects the body against human pathogens such as E. coli and salmonella. To boost the immune system, take it internally.

6. Proves Effective for Cleaning Multiple Surfaces

Disinfect and degrease your home, car or office with lemon oil. Add it to a spray bottle of water to clean tables, countertops and other surfaces. Lemon oil also makes a great furniture polish; simply add a few drops to olive oil to clean, protect and shine wood.

7. Lessens Allergy Symptoms

Lemon oil can help to combat seasonal allergies and asthma attacks. It works as a natural antihistamine, relieves excess mucus and cools down inflammation. Take 1 to 2 drops internally mixed with equal parts of peppermint and lavender for allergy relief.

LEMONGRASS

CYMBOPOGON FLEXUOSUS

Besides being a delectable citrusy seasoning in Thai cooking, most of us would never guess that this delicious grass holds so much therapeutic power. Traditionally, lemongrass parts as well as its oil have been used to treat circulatory issues, behavioral problems, headaches, infections, nervous system disorders and menstrual irregularities. In some cultures, it is known as "fever grass" due to its ability to bring down a fever. This particular remedy is made even more effective when it is combined with black pepper oil.

Lemongrass essential oil is used in aromatherapy to help relieve muscle pain, fight bacteria, ward off insects, reduce body aches and aid digestion. It can also be used for flavoring teas and soups—and it adds fragrance to cosmetics, soaps and homemade deodorizers. The leaves of the herb are steam-distilled to extract the essential oil, which has a light and fresh lemony aroma with earthy undertones. Lemongrass essential oil is stimulating, relaxing, soothing and balancing.

After a hard workout, I rub lemongrass and frankincense on sore joints and muscles to speed recovery.

– Dr. Josh

179

RESEARCH STUDIES

When the effects that lemongrass had as an anti-bacterial agent were tested, results indicated that lemongrass oil disrupted bacterial growth and replication and worked as an anti-microbial (bacteria-killing) agent.[67]

A 2008 study showed that lemongrass oil has the power to reduce fungal infections. Early research suggests that drinking lemongrass infusion for 10 days may decrease the symptoms of thrush in people with HIV/AIDS.[68]

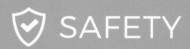 ## KEY BENEFITS

- Helps relieve headaches
- Can reduce stomachaches
- Supports ligaments and tendons
- Contains anti-fungal and anti-yeast properties
- Aids in fever reduction
- Serves as a natural insect repellent
- Boosts energy
- Eases digestive tract spasms

SAFETY

Because lemongrass can stimulate menstrual flow, women who are pregnant should not use it. Also, it is not recommended for children or nursing mothers.

THERAPEUTIC COMPOUNDS

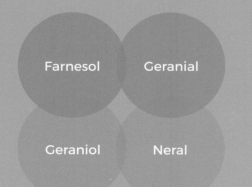

Farnesol

Geranial

Geraniol

Neral

SUPER 7 RX LEMONGRASS USES

1. Repels Bugs

Lemongrass oil is a natural repellant with a mild smell. Add 10 to 15 drops to water and use the mixture as bug spray, or diffuse it to repel insects. Lemongrass oil can also be used to help repel fleas by adding 5 drops of the oil to water and applying it to the pet's coat.

2. Promotes Skin Health

Lemongrass oil's antiseptic and astringent properties make it perfect for getting even and glowing skin. Add lemongrass oil to shampoos, conditioners, deodorants, soaps and lotions.

3. Acts as a Natural Deodorizer

Use lemongrass oil as a natural and safe air freshener or deodorizer. Add 5 to 10 drops of lemongrass oil to water and use it as a mist, or diffuse it. You can customize the fragrance by adding lavender or peppermint oil.

4. Treats Gastric Ulcers

Lemongrass has been known for centuries as a treatment for stomach distress, gastritis and gastric ulcers. Add lemongrass oil or infused lemongrass water to tea, soup or a smoothie to treat stomach pains, nausea and diarrhea.

5. Acts as a Fever Reducer

Consuming lemongrass oil or a lemongrass infusion has been known to reduce fevers. Lab studies have shown that a lemongrass infusion is effective in relieving feverish symptoms.

6. Lowers Cholesterol

Consumption of lemongrass oil has been shown to sustain healthy levels of triglycerides and reduce LDL cholesterol in the body. To lower cholesterol levels, take 1 to 2 drops of lemongrass oil internally in a capsule or glass of water.

7. Treats Candida/Yeast Infections

Lemongrass oil can decrease the severity of yeast infections. Take 1 to 2 drops internally.

LIME

CITRUS AURANTIFOLIA

No one is exactly sure where limes originated, but they are said to have come from the Indonesian archipelago or perhaps the nearby mainland of Asia. The Arabs may have taken lemons and limes from India to the eastern Mediterranean countries and Africa around A.D. 1000. Limes were introduced to the western Mediterranean countries by returning crusaders in the 12th and 13th centuries. Columbus took citrus-fruit seed, probably including limes, to the West Indies on his second voyage in 1493, and lime trees soon became widely distributed in the West Indies, Mexico and Florida.

Of course, you may be most familiar with lime's culinary uses as a citrusy delight. However, as an essential oil, it offers a wave of therapeutic benefits. It boosts mental clarity and has an invigorating and stimulating effect with its tart, sweet and lively aroma. It also supports the immune system by fighting infections and helps to cleanse the body. The entire peel is put through a steam distillation method to extract the essential oil. Try blending lime oil with bergamot or a bright floral oil, and diffuse it in a space that needs uplifting.

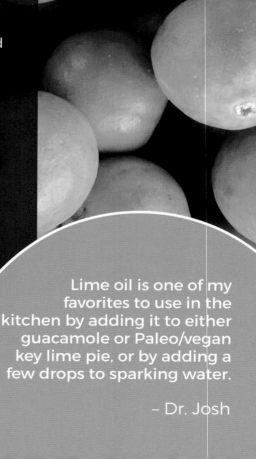

Lime oil is one of my favorites to use in the kitchen by adding it to either guacamole or Paleo/vegan key lime pie, or by adding a few drops to sparking water.

– Dr. Josh

RESEARCH STUDIES

A 2010 study found that lime essential oil plays an important role in weight loss and could be used in the treatment of drug-induced obesity and related diseases.[69]

A 2006 study evaluated 21 essential oils for their anti-bacterial activity against six bacterial species. Nineteen oils, including lime essential oil, showed anti-bacterial activity against one or more strains.[70]

KEY BENEFITS

- Proves useful for respiratory conditions
- Fights acne and skin irritations
- May relieve stress and anxiety
- Supports emotional balance
- Serves as a natural disinfectant
- Boosts skin and hair health
- Contains anti-bacterial and antiseptic properties
- Can improve mental clarity

SAFETY

Avoid direct sunlight for up to 12 hours after topical application.

THERAPEUTIC COMPOUNDS

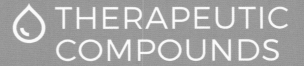

Alpha-Pinenes   Beta-cedrene

D-Limonene   Gamma-Terpinene

SUPER 7 RX LIME USES

1. Eases a Sore Throat

Lime oil's powerful anti-bacterial, antiseptic and anti-viral properties help protect the body against infections that may lead to a sore throat. Take 1 to 2 drops internally by placing the oil under your tongue, or apply 2 to 4 drops topically, along with peppermint, on your throat.

2. Cleanses Water

Because it can help kill bacteria that cause diarrhea, food poisoning, cholera and typhoid, lime oil is an excellent addition to help cleanse drinking water. It also helps treat internal and external bacterial infections. Add a few drops to 8 ounces of water before consuming.

3. Encourages Lymphatic Drainage

Lime oil helps remove wastes and toxins from your body—improving immunity against pathogens. To support lymphatic flow, mix equal parts of lime oil, geranium oil and rosemary oil with coconut oil. Apply directly to your lymphatic pathways.

4. Aids Gallbladder Function and Fat Digestion

Lime oil can help clear a congested gallbladder. Mix lime oil, lemon oil and rosemary oil with a carrier oil. Add it to a compress or bath water, or massage it over your gallbladder.

5. Lifts Mood and Promotes Balance

Lime oil is stimulating and invigorating; it helps reduce anxiety and stress. Add 5 to 10 drops of lime oil to a warm-water bath, or apply it topically to your wrists, temples, abdomen, the back of your neck and the soles of your feet.

6. Repels Insects

Lime oil repels insects such as mosquitoes and ants. It can even be used to repel head lice. As a natural bug repellant, add 5 to 10 drops to a spray bottle filled with water and spray on your clothes, skin and furniture. To kill head lice, combine 5 to 10 drops of lime oil with equal parts of tea tree oil and coconut oil and massage into your hair for 10 minutes before rinsing.

6. Fights Acne and Skin Conditions

Because of its anti-bacterial and antiseptic properties, lime oil can be used on the skin to help prevent acne and skin issues. Dilute it with coconut oil or jojoba oil, and apply it to the area of concern twice daily.

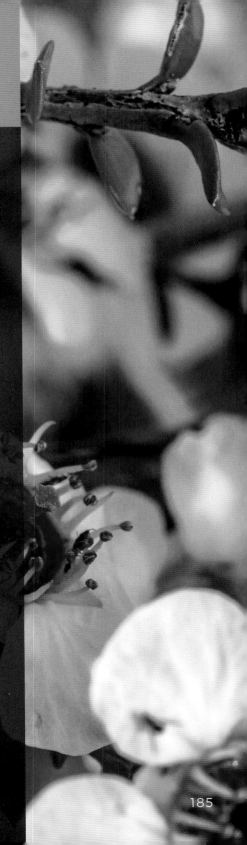

MANUKA

LEPTOSPERMUM SCOPARIUM

Legend has it that when Captain Cook sailed into Mercury Bay in 1769, his crew was sick with scurvy and infection. He was greeted by the local Māori people of New Zealand, who offered him a medicinal decoction of boiled manuka leaves known for its unique healing powers. The manuka tree had long been treasured by the Māori people, who used the bark and leaves to treat colds, dysentery, fever and numerous other skin aliments.

Today, when people think of manuka, they think of honey—and manuka honey does indeed have some amazing benefits. Manuka essential oil is yet another powerful remedy that comes from this small shrub. In fact, it is still being used around the world as an effective plant-based remedy for a variety of skin conditions, including ringworm, chronic sores, athlete's foot, eczema, psoriasis and dermatitis. The oil is a natural healing agent, with anti-bacterial, anti-fungal and anti-inflammatory properties; it is also a strong antioxidant. Its properties are often compared to those of tea tree oil, yet it is even gentler on sensitive skin and has a more honey-like, floral scent. The oil is made by steam-distilling the leaves of the manuka tree.

RESEARCH STUDIES

A 2016 study concluded that the potent anti-microbial and anti-inflammatory properties of manuka essential oil make it a strong candidate for use in helping combat infections and immune-related disease.[71]

In clinical studies, manuka oil showed significant adhesion-inhibiting activity against periodontopathic bacterial strains (oral pathogens).[72]

⊘ KEY BENEFITS

- Contains powerful anti-bacterial and anti-fungal properties
- Supports relaxation and sleep
- Serves as an acne scar treatment
- Serves as a remedy for skin irritation

- Contains anti-microbial and antiseptic properties
- Acts as a natural fever reducer
- Provides allergy relief
- Fights infections

🛡 SAFETY

Avoid use during pregnancy because of its spasmolytic (muscle relaxing) activity.

💧 THERAPEUTIC COMPOUNDS

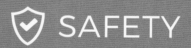
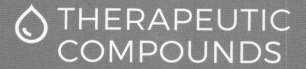

Cadina Calamenene

Leptospermone Pinene

SUPER 7 RX MANUKA USES

1. Serves as a Remedy for Eczema, Acne and Psoriasis

The anti-inflammatory properties of manuka oil may improve red, dry and flaking skin and conditions such as eczema, psoriasis, acne, dermatitis and cracked heels. Make a soothing cream by mixing manuka oil with shea butter for body care and honey to address acne.

2. Calms Allergy Symptoms

For anyone who suffers from allergic reactions to dust, pollen or pet hair, manuka oil can be used to help calm those reactions. Apply manuka oil to any area of your skin that reacts to an allergen, or diffuse 6 to 8 drops for allergy relief.

3. Helps Heal Scars and Reduce Age Spots

Manuka has cicatrisant properties, meaning that using it is an effective way to promote the healing of damaged skin and scarring. It can also aid in the growth and regeneration of new cells while protecting wounds from infection. Add a few drops to any face or body lotion.

4. Aids in Relaxation and Sleep

Manuka has the ability to combat stress and anxiety due to its remarkable calming and soothing effects on the heart and mind. To help relax your mind, diffuse manuka at home, at the office or by your bed to promote a good night's sleep.

5. Serves as a Natural Remedy for Athlete's Foot

Manuka oil can help eliminate a variety of fungi and bacteria that thrive on the feet and toes. Create a foot soak by adding 6 drops of manuka oil to warm water and soaking your feet for 20 minutes each day.

6. Calms Respiratory Conditions

Inhaling manuka oil can help treat respiratory conditions, such as sinus congestion, asthma and cold and flu symptoms. Diffuse it, or add 6 to 8 drops to boiling water and breathe in its vapors for 5 minutes.

7. Promotes Oral Health

Manuka has been clinically demonstrated as a potential remedy for the bacteria responsible for gum and tooth disease.[73]

MARJORAM

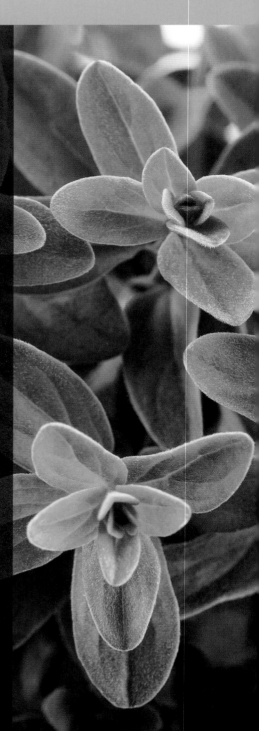

ORIGANUM MAJORANA

In ancient Egypt, marjoram was used to heal, disinfect and preserve. Aphrodite, the goddess of love, was said to treasure this herb. The Greeks called marjoram "joy of the mountain" and used it to make wreaths and garlands for weddings and funerals. During the Middle Ages, European women used marjoram in bouquets known as nosegays.

Marjoram essential oil is made by steam-distilling the plant's leaves. It is a calming oil with a spicy and woody aroma. Oregano is a common marjoram substitute, and vice versa, because of their likeness, but marjoram has a finer texture and a milder flavor profile. Marjoram has a warming effect on the body and mind, helps ease muscle tension and benefits the nervous system. It has powerful anti-bacterial, anti-infectious and antiseptic properties as well.

RESEARCH STUDIES

In patients suffering from arthritis, a blend of marjoram, lavender, eucalyptus, rosemary and peppermint combined with a carrier oil reduced perceived pain and depression compared to the control group.[74]

A 2014 study reported that a blend of essential oils including marjoram, black pepper, lavender and peppermint could affect neck pain. The essential oil group showed significant improvement in 10 areas of pain compared to the control group.[75]

KEY BENEFITS

- Relaxes tense muscles
- Aids the digestive system
- Lessens cramps and spasms
- Boosts skin health

- Can relax the mind and calm nerves
- Treats respiratory conditions
- Works as an immune stimulant
- May reduce neck and back pain

SAFETY

Avoid use during pregnancy, as marjoram oil is an emmenagogue. Dilute marjoram oil before applying it topically.

THERAPEUTIC COMPOUNDS

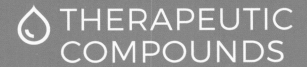

Alpha- & Y-Terpinenes

Linalool

SUPER 7 RX MARJORAM USES

1. Prevents and Improves Gastric Ulcers

Marjoram oil has shown an ability to prevent and help gastric ulcers. Take 1 to 2 drops of marjoram oil internally until symptoms subside. The herb can also be taken as a tea or supplement.

2. Helps Alleviate Headaches, Neck Pain and Back Pain

Marjoram oil can help reduce the pain that often comes with tension headaches and neck pain. Marjoram relaxes tense muscles and improves circulation, which can have pain-reducing effects for conditions caused by tight muscles. Apply it topically to areas of pain.

3. Relieves Muscle Pain and Spasms

Marjoram oil works to relieve muscle tension and pain due to overexertion. It may also alleviate some of the pain associated with the common cold, fevers, inflammation and toothaches. Dilute 3 to 5 drops and apply it topically to the area of concern twice daily.

4. Helps Prevent Infections

Due to its anti-bacterial, antiseptic and anti-viral properties, marjoram oil may help prevent infections and ailments such as the common cold, influenza, measles, mumps and cold sores. Dilute 2 to 5 drops and apply it topically twice daily.

5. Aids in Stress and Anxiety Relief

Marjoram oil has sedative properties and works to help create a calming and peaceful feeling. Diffuse marjoram oil or inhale it directly from the bottle. For topical use, dilute and apply it to the back of your neck and wrists.

6. Helps with Stomach Cramps and Flatulence

Marjoram oil helps to treat constipation, flatulence and colic by relaxing the digestive system with its sedative properties. Take it internally by placing 1 drop under your tongue, or dilute and apply it topically to your abdomen and lower back.

7. May Regulate Blood Pressure

Marjoram oil has the ability to widen and relax the blood vessels, which may ease the flow of blood and reduce high blood pressure. Take it internally by placing it under your tongue, or dilute and apply it topically over your heart.

MELALEUCA
(TEA TREE)

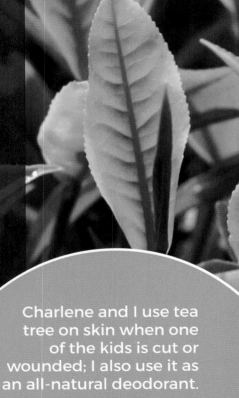

MELALEUCA ALTERNIFOLIA

Melaleuca, or tea tree oil, has been passed down for thousands of years by the native indigenous Bundjalung aborigines of Australia. While their healers tended to use spiritual medicine to heal serious illnesses, they also used the leaves of the tea tree plant to treat more common medical concerns. As legend has it, there was one "mystical" lake where the tea tree leaves had been falling for hundreds of years and that the mud became saturated with the tea tree oil. This mud was applied to skin for medicinal purposes.

Melaleuca essential oil is well known for its powerful antiseptic properties and ability to treat wounds. For over 70 years, tea tree oil has been documented in numerous medical studies for its ability to kill many strains of bacteria, viruses and fungi. The leaves of the melaleuca plant are steam-distilled to extract the essential oil. Tea tree has a fresh, woody, earthy and medicinal aroma that has powerful cleansing and purifying properties. The Earth is rich with natural healing power, and there may be no better example of this than melaleuca. It purifies as it heals and is a must for any home medicine cabinet.

Charlene and I use tea tree on skin when one of the kids is cut or wounded; I also use it as an all-natural deodorant.

– Ty

RESEARCH STUDIES

A 2007 study used a 5 percent tea tree oil topical gel to treat acne lesions. The results found that those who used tea tree oil had approximately a 5-times greater improvement in acne than those who did not use the treatment.[76]

Tea tree oil was found to inhibit 301 different types of yeast isolated from the mouths of patients, demonstrating the effectiveness of using tea tree oil in treating oral yeast in cancer patients and the use in oral hygiene products.[77]

⊘ KEY BENEFITS

- Treats acne
- Helps treat chickenpox
- Provides relief for cold sores
- Can ease earaches

- Serves as a remedy for bad breath
- Prevents and helps kill head lice
- Works as a natural deodorant
- Inhibits mold growth

⊘ SAFETY

Melaleuca (tea tree) oil should not be taken internally for any reason. If using tea tree in the mouth (as in a mouthwash or toothpaste), spit out the oil afterwards to prevent potential side effects such as digestive issues, hives or dizziness.

⬡ THERAPEUTIC COMPOUNDS

Alpha- & Y-Terpinenes

Terpinen-4-ol

P-Cymene

SUPER 7 RX MELALEUCA USES

1. Treats Acne

Tea tree oil is considered one of the most effective home treatments for acne. It is reportedly just as effective as benzoyl peroxide but without the associated negative side effects that many people experience. Create a gentle and effective face wash by mixing 5 drops of tea tree oil with 2 teaspoons of raw honey.

2. Helps with Dandruff

Tea tree oil soothes dry, flaking skin and can be used as a natural treatment for head lice. Add 5 drops of tea tree oil to shampoo or conditioner, or make a natural shampoo by combining 5 to 10 drops of tea tree oil with aloe vera gel, coconut milk and lavender oil.

3. Disinfects the Home

Tea tree oil has powerful anti-microbial properties, allowing it to fight bad bacteria in the home. Combine tea tree oil with water, vinegar and lemon essential oil, and add it to a spray bottle to use on countertops, kitchen appliances, showers, toilets and sinks.

4. Helps Treat Psoriasis and Eczema

Use tea tree oil to relieve skin inflammation associated with conditions such as psoriasis and eczema. Make an anti-inflammatory and soothing lotion by combining 5 drops of tea tree oil, 5 drops of lavender oil and 1 teaspoon of coconut oil. Apply it topically twice daily.

5. May Remedy Toenail Fungus and Ringworm

Because of its ability to kill fungi, tea tree oil is a great choice to use on toenail fungus, athlete's foot and ringworm. Apply it topically to the affected area. For stubborn fungi, mix tea tree with oregano oil.

6. Acts as a Natural Deodorant

Because of its anti-microbial properties, tea tree oil can destroy the bacteria on the skin that causes body odor. Combine 5 drops of tea tree oil with 1 teaspoon each of coconut oil and baking soda. Apply the mixture to your armpits or even in your shoes or sports gear.

7. Cleans Infections and Cuts

The antiseptic and anti-bacterial properties of tea tree oil make it a natural treatment for cuts, wounds, burns and skin infections or irritations. Combine 2 drops of tea tree oil with 2 drops of lavender oil, and apply it directly to the area of concern.

MELISSA
(LEMON BALM)

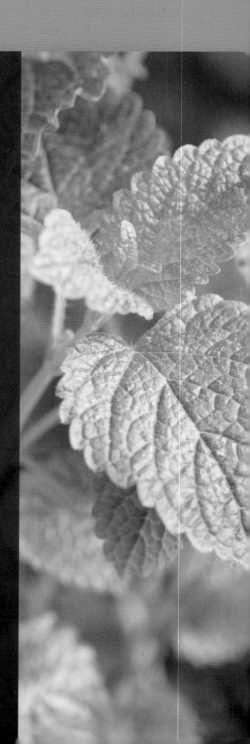

MELISSA OFFICINALIS

Although it's not one of the better-known essential oils, melissa oil has been used therapeutically for hundreds of years. In the 14th century, melissa oil was included in tonic water made by the French Carmelite nuns. In the 16th century, famed philosopher, physician and botanist Paracelsus called the herb "The Elixir of Life," while 17th century writer and gardener John Evelyn described it as "sovereign for the brain, strengthening the memory and powerfully chasing away melancholy."

Melissa essential oil, also known as lemon balm, is a member of the mint family, and the oils are extracted by steam-distilling the leaves and flowers. Melissa oil is known for its anti-bacterial, anti-viral, anti-spasmodic and antidepressant properties. It has a delicate and lemony aroma that promotes emotional balance and boosts skin health.

🔬 RESEARCH STUDIES

A 2004 study found that melissa essential oil has potential as an anti-tumor agent, as evidenced by a reduction of human cancer cell lines when evaluated in an in vitro study.[78]

A study suggested that ingesting melissa oil could have beneficial metabolic effects. When used on mice, melissa oil slowed fatty acid synthesis (a process that creates fatty buildups in the body).[79]

⊘ KEY BENEFITS

- May prevent infections
- Boosts skin health
- Can boost mood
- Relieves PMS and menstrual symptoms

- Aids in fighting depression
- May help reduce high blood pressure
- Encourages hormone balance
- Soothes respiratory conditions

🛡 SAFETY

Avoid use during pregnancy, as melissa oil is an emmemagogue. If using it on sensitive skin, dilute it with a carrier oil before application.

💧 THERAPEUTIC COMPOUNDS

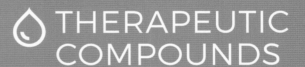

Citronellal   Geranial

Germacrene   Neral

SUPER 7 RX MELISSA USES

1. May Help Prevent Dementia

Melissa is probably the most studied of the essential oils for its affect on people with Alzheimer's disease, and it is very likely one of the most effective. Diffuse it daily to potentially prevent the onset of dementia.

2. Treats Eczema

Melissa oil is used for treating eczema and acne, as it contains anti-bacterial and anti-fungal properties. Use 5 drops per ounce of carrier oil, especially for use on the face. Alternatively, you can add it to moisturizer or a spray bottle with water and spritz on your face.

3. Treats Cold Sores and Herpes

Melissa is often the herb of choice for treating cold sores, as it is effective at fighting viruses in the herpes virus family. Apply 2 to 3 diluted drops topically to the area of concern.

4. May Help Improve Hypoglycemia

Studies suggest that melissa oil is an efficient hypoglycaemic agent, probably due to enhanced glucose uptake and metabolism in the liver as well as adipose tissue and the inhibition of gluconeogenesis in the liver. Take a few drops internally to promote healthy glucose levels.

5. Can Relieve Feelings of Depression and Anxiety

Melissa essential oil has antidepressant and sedative properties, and it may create a feeling of peace and warmth. It can promote emotional balance and has uplifting compounds. Diffuse or apply it topically to your wrists, ears and the back of your neck.

6. May Reduce Vertigo and Nervousness

Melissa serves as a tonic and helps the body avoid nervous disorders. Apply 2 to 3 drops topically to your ears or the back of your neck to alleviate nervousness, nausea, vomiting and dizziness. It can also be taken internally by adding 1 drop to water or tea.

7. Promotes Healthy Blood Pressure

Melissa oil has the power to reduce blood pressure levels because of its hypotensive properties. To help relieve hypertension, apply it topically to your chest or the back of your neck, or take 1 to 2 drops internally.

MYRRH

COMMIPHORA MYRRHA

Discovered more than 3,700 years ago, myrrh was used by the Ancient Egyptians during the embalming process and in perfumes and cosmetics. Ancient records show that myrrh was deemed so valuable that at times it was valued at its weight in gold. Myrrh essential oil is well known because it was mentioned 152 times in the Bible, serving as a spice, natural remedy, means to purify the dead and, of course, as a gift from the magi to baby Jesus.

Myrrh essential oil has potent antioxidant activity and has been researched as a potential cancer treatment. The resin of the myrrh tree is dried and steam-distilled; the essential oil has a smoky, sweet and sometimes bitter aroma. An ancient healer and treatment for a multitude of ailments and symptoms, myrrh is a remarkable essential oil that you will likely run out of quickly.

An essential part of Chelsea's and my skincare routine, we use myrrh oil daily on our skin because it protects against UV radiation and supports youthful, glowing skin.

– Dr. Josh

RESEARCH STUDIES

A 2013 study reported the anti-cancer effects of myrrh essential oil. The cell death rate was higher in the myrrh essential oil group compared with that of the other tested groups, including frankincense. The results also indicated that breast cancer cells exhibited increased sensitivity to myrrh oil.[80]

A study identifies myrrh oil as an anti-inflammatory and wound-healing product. Treatment with myrrh induced an initial increase in white blood cell levels that persisted through the post-injury healing period.[81]

⊘ KEY BENEFITS

- Has anti-cancer properties
- Serves as a potent antioxidant
- Contains anti-bacterial and anti-fungal properties
- Fights parasites

- Boosts skin health
- Aids relaxation
- Helps relieve congestion
- Can fight infections and support wound healing

🛡 SAFETY

Do not use it during pregnancy, as myrrh oil is fetotoxic (poisonous to a fetus). Myrrh oil may lower blood sugar levels, so it is not recommended for people with diabetes or other blood sugar conditions. For topical use, dilute it with a carrier oil and test it on a small area.

🜄 THERAPEUTIC COMPOUNDS

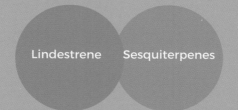

Lindestrene   Sesquiterpenes

SUPER 7 RX MYRRH USES

1. Acts as an Anti-inflammatory

Myrrh has healing, anti-bacterial, anti-fungal and anti-inflammatory properties that may reduce swelling and treat infections. Add 2 to 3 drops of myrrh oil to a cold compress and apply it directly to the infected or inflamed area.

2. Promotes Awareness During Prayer and Meditation

Because of its significance in the Bible, using myrrh is ideal during prayer and meditation. Diffuse it to help promote awareness and connect with God during meditation, and anoint others with the oil.

3. Helps Treats Vaginal and Oral Yeast

To treat Candida overgrowth, take 1 drop of myrrh oil internally, or dilute 2 to 3 drops with equal parts of a carrier oil and apply it topically to affected areas. For oral thrush, add 1 to 2 drops to natural mouthwash and gargle several times a day.

4. May Alleviate Gum Disease and Mouth Infections

Myrrh oil may help to relieve inflammation of the mouth and gums caused by diseases such as gingivitis and mouth ulcers. Add to mouthwash or toothpaste to help prevent gum disease and mouth infections.

5. Fights Parasites and Fungal Infections

Myrrh is a natural treatment for parasites, and it can also help to reduce fungal infections such as athlete's foot or ringworm. To fight infection, take 1 to 2 drops internally with water or in a capsule, or apply it directly to the fungal infection site.

6. Displays Cancer-Fighting Qualities

Myrrh is being studied for its potential anti-cancer benefits. Apply it directly to a skin cancer site twice daily. Myrrh oil is also an astringent, so it strengthens the body's cells, helps to stop bleeding and may prevent hair loss by strengthening hair roots.

7. Treats Wounds and Ulcers

Myrrh oil has the power to increase the function of white blood cells, which are critical for wound healing. It can decrease the incidence of ulcers and improve their healing time. Apply 2 to 3 drops, diluted with a carrier oil, to the affected area twice daily.

ORANGE

CITRUS SINENSIS

Orange (often known as sweet orange) has a fascinating historical and even mythical background. The Japanese believed citrus blossoms represented chastity. Ancient Arab women used it to color gray hair. Nostradamus wrote about how to use its blossoms and fruit to make cosmetics. Hercules so valued it that he stole the golden fruit from Hesperides, who protected it as the primary food of the ancient Roman and Greek gods.

Interestingly, sweet orange does not occur as a wild plant anywhere in the world, and is thought to be a natural hybrid of the pummelo (*Citrus maxima*) and the mandarin (*Citrus reticulata*). Orange essential oil is cold-pressed from the outer peel of the common orange fruit. It is used for its anti-cancer, antidepressant, digestive and sedative properties. Possessing a citrusy and tart aroma, orange oil uplifts your emotions while sweeping away stress. It can also work as a secret weapon in the kitchen against stubborn grease stains.

Orange oil is awesome in recipes like orange pancakes and orange chocolate cake. I also like using it to flavor water and tea. And I like to diffuse it in my office while I'm working to keep me in a good mood and keep my office smelling fresh.

– Ty

RESEARCH STUDIES

A 2010 study found that orange oil could effectively help stop the growth of human lung and colon cancer cells. This is due to orange oil's PMFs (flavonoid antioxidants) that have been shown to halt cancer proliferation and trigger cancer cell death.[82]

A recent study showed that orange and rose essential oil may relax the brain. After half of a test group was exposed to diffused orange and rose oil for 90 seconds, they experienced notable increases in "comfortable," "relaxed" and "natural" feelings.[83]

KEY BENEFITS

- Eases cold and flu symptoms
- Demonstrates anti-tumor activity
- Helps reduce appearance of wrinkles
- Acts as a natural anti-bacterial agent

- Aids in easing anxiety
- May increase circulation
- May improve blood pressure
- Supports lymphatic drainage

SAFETY

THERAPEUTIC COMPOUNDS

Avoid direct sunlight for up to 12 hours after external application. Orange oil can cause reactions on sensitive skin, so test on a small area first.

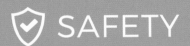

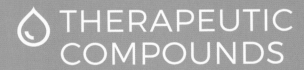

Limonene   Myrcene

SUPER 7 RX ORANGE USES

1. Provides Immune System Support

Orange oil has virus- and bacteria-fighting abilities. To boost the immune system and fight free radical damage, take 1 to 2 drops of orange oil internally. Place it under your tongue or add it to a glass of water or your favorite beverage.

2. Displays Cancer-Fighting Properties

The anti-cancer activity of orange oil is largely due to the presence of limonene. There are now over 200 research articles on limonene, supporting its effective chemo-preventive agents against cancer cells. Put 1 to 2 drops of orange oil into your favorite tea, juice or sparkling water.

3. Encourages Lymphatic Drainage

Orange oil may stimulate the lymphatic system, liver, kidneys and bladder—drawing out toxins, excess sodium and waste from the digestive tract. Dilute 2 to 4 drops of orange oil with coconut oil and gently rub it onto your lymph nodes, chest and lymphatic pathways.

4. Fights Anxiety

Orange essential oil is an anxiety-reducing oil thanks to its calming properties. Diffusing orange oil, adding some to your body wash or inhaling it directly may fight anxiety and lower stress levels.

5. Improves Mood

Orange oil has a direct effect on the brain's olfactory system that quickly evokes emotional responses—lifting moods and promoting relaxation. Diffuse orange oil or apply it topically.

6. Boosts Digestion

As an anti-inflammatory agent, relaxant and circulation-enhancer, orange oil promotes better digestion and may help ease cramps or constipation. Apply 2 to 3 drops to your abdominal area to boost digestion. To improve detoxification, take 1 to 2 drops internally; this encourages an increase in urine production and may prevent bloating.

6. Serves as a Natural Household Cleaner

Orange oil has a fresh and citrusy smell, and it has the power to fight bacteria and microorganisms in your home. Add orange oil to a spray bottle filled with water and use it on countertops, appliances, showers, toilets and sinks.

OREGANO

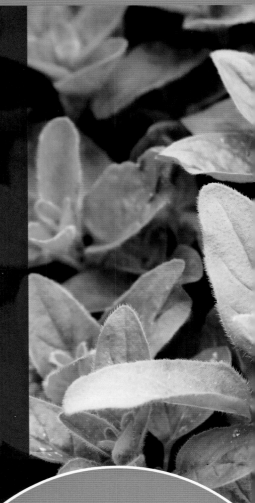

ORIGANUM VULGARE

Oregano has been a precious commodity for over 2,500 years and a popular folk medicine remedy. Hippocrates, the ancient Greek physician and the father of Western medicine, used oregano as an antiseptic for treating respiratory and digestive diseases. Ancient Greeks believed oregano was a useful poison antidote and used it extensively to treat skin infections, sore throats, wounds and viral infections. Traditional Chinese Medicine practitioners have also used oregano for generations to treat diarrhea, parasites and fungal infections.

The oregano plant is known for its potent flavor, as well as its therapeutic properties. The oregano leaves are steam-distilled, and the essential oil has a sharp and herbaceous aroma. Oregano essential oil is an incredible natural antibiotic because it contains carvacrol and thymol, two powerful compounds with anti-bacterial and anti-fungal properties. Dozens of studies confirm that oregano oil can be used along with or as an alternative to antibiotics for a number of health concerns. The research supports the fact that oregano is more than just an antibiotic—it's the *ultimate* natural antibiotic!

Oregano oil is a powerful blemish fighter and is great for stubborn skin conditions. I combine oregano oil with coconut oil and clay, and then apply it to affected areas.

– Jordan

RESEARCH STUDIES

Twenty clinical strains of bacteria were tested on patients with different clinical conditions. Oregano oil was active against all tested strains. It proved to be an effective means for the prevention of antibiotic-resistant strain development.[84]

A 2014 study found that oregano oil has powerful anti-viral properties against non-enveloped murine norovirus, a human norovirus surrogate, in some cases inactivating the virus within an hour of exposure.[85]

✓ KEY BENEFITS

- Contains anti-bacterial and anti-fungal properties
- Helps prevent and treat viral infections
- Fights inflammation
- Helps relieve allergy symptoms
- Has shown promising anti-tumor properties
- Boosts the immune system
- Aids the respiratory system

🛡 SAFETY

Avoid use during pregnancy—as oregano oil may cause embryotoxicity—or on infants and small children. It may cause skin irritation when used topically, so dilute it with a carrier oil and test on a small patch of skin first. If using internally, do not use for more than 10 days. After 10 days, take a break for one week.

THERAPEUTIC COMPOUNDS

Carvacrol   Thymol

SUPER 7 RX OREGANO USES

1. Acts as a Natural Antibiotic

Oregano oil has anti-bacterial properties that are powerful enough to kill different types of bad bacteria, including E. Coli. It can prevent bacterial overgrowth and colonization in the large intestine, and it helps protect the body from toxicity. Dilute it with a carrier oil and apply it topically to the soles of your feet or take it internally for 10 days at a time and then cycle off.

2. Battles Candida and Fungal Overgrowth

Oil of oregano can be used to treat fungi and yeast such as candida. Oregano can also treat toenail fungus when used topically. For internal use, take 2 to 4 drops twice daily for up to 10 days.

3. Helps Fight Pneumonia and Bronchitis

Oregano oil can help prevent or fight pneumonia, bronchitis and other types of bacterial infections. For external infections, apply 2 to 3 diluted drops to the affected area. To prevent internal bacterial overgrowth, ingest 2 to 4 drops twice daily for up to 10 days.

4. Proves Effective Against MRSA and Staph Infection

Oregano is the oil of choice for acute MRSA and other staph infections. Add 3 drops of oregano oil to a capsule or to the food or beverage of your choice along with a carrier oil; take it twice daily for up to 10 days.

5. Fights Intestinal Worms and Parasites

Because oregano oil has anti-parasitic and anti-viral properties, it can be used internally to combat parasitic infections. Take oregano oil internally for up to 10 days.

6. Helps Removes Warts

One of the more common uses of oregano oil is its ability to safely diminish and possibly remove warts. When using oregano oil for removing warts, make sure to dilute it with another oil or mix it with clay.

7. Cleanses Mold From the Home

Oregano is effective at eradicating mold growth around your home. Add 5 to 7 drops to a homemade cleaning solution along with tea tree oil and lavender.

PATCHOULI

POGOSTEMON CABLIN

Perhaps due to its power as a moth repellent, the aroma of patchouli was pervasive in cloth and clothing exported from India in the 19th century. In fact, the scent became an indicator of true "Oriental" fabric, so much so that English and French garment makers scented their imitation products with patchouli to ensure their acceptance in the domestic marketplace. Patchouli oil has also been used for centuries in traditional medicine in Malaysia, China and Japan. As a cell rejuvenator, it has been used to help heal wounds and reduce the appearance of scars. It was also considered an excellent remedy for insect and snakebites.

Patchouli leaves are put through a steam distillation process to extract the essential oil. The strong scent of patchouli oil has been used for centuries in perfumes; more recently it's been used in incense, insect repellents and natural remedies. Patchouli is considered a great balancer, relaxing yet stimulating, particularly relevant for conditions of weak immunity. Patchouli is known to treat various skin conditions, such as acne and inflammation. It also has anti-fungal, digestive and antiseptic properties.

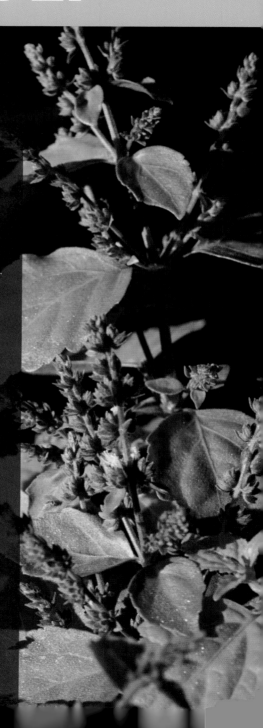

RESEARCH STUDIES

After comparing the scoring result of 26 compounds in patchouli oil, researchers found that there was anti-bacterial activity in all 26 compounds in patchouli oil—proving that it has strong anti-microbial activity.[86]

A study found that patchouli alcohol has anti-inflammatory activities and is able to suppress the production of inflammatory mediators, which may make it useful in preventing cancer initiation and progression.[87]

KEY BENEFITS

- Works as a bug repellent
- Boosts the immune system
- Works as a natural deodorant
- Impedes fungal growth

- May reduce inflammation
- Strengthens hair and skin
- Treats dandruff
- May Improve depression

SAFETY

Patchouli oil may inhibit blood clotting, and therefore poses a drug interaction risk. Check with your healthcare practitioner before use if you are taking any prescription medications.

THERAPEUTIC COMPOUNDS

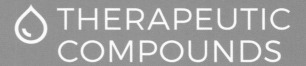

Alpha-Pinene

Sabinene

SUPER 7 RX PATCHOULI USES

1. Helps Ease Anxiety and Fight Depression

Patchouli oil has antidepressant properties; when used aromatically, it encourages the release of serotonin and dopamine, which help to ease feelings of anger, anxiety and anxiousness. Diffuse 5 drops of patchouli oil, or add 5 to 10 drops to a warm-water bath.

2. May Reduce Inflammation

Patchouli oil has anti-phlogistic properties, meaning it has the power to soothe inflammation in the body. Patchouli oil can address internal inflammation and conditions such as arthritis and gout. Rub 3 to 5 drops onto your feet, stomach, lower back and any other inflamed area.

3. Fights Infections

With antiseptic properties, patchouli oil can protect wounds or sores from becoming infected. It can also fight athlete's foot or other fungal infections. To fight infections, apply patchouli oil directly on the affected area, or add it to a warm-water bath.

4. May Help Erectile Dysfunction

Patchouli oil has the power to increase libido. It also serves as a natural supplement for helping with impotency and erectile dysfunction. Diffuse 5 drops of patchouli oil, or apply 1 to 3 drops topically to your temples, the back of your neck and the soles of your feet.

5. Strengthens Hair and Skin

Patchouli oil may prevent hair loss and regenerate new skin cells. For hair, massage it into your scalp or add it to conditioner. For your skin, dilute patchouli oil with equal parts of coconut or jojoba oil and apply it topically, or add it to face wash or lotion.

6. Repels Insects

Patchouli oil repels mosquitoes, fleas, ants, lice, moths and flies. Add 5 to 10 drops to a spray bottle filled with water and spray on your clothes, skin, sheets or furniture.

7. Acts as a Natural Deodorant

Patchouli oil has a sweet, musky and spicy aroma; it can be used to mask body odor. It also makes a great home deodorizer. Apply it under your arms, or add it to your favorite lotion.

PEPPERMINT

MENTHA PIPERITA

Peppermint is one of the oldest European herbs used for medicinal purposes, and historical accounts date its use to ancient Egyptian, Chinese and Japanese folk medicine. In ancient Greece, mint was used in funerary rites, together with rosemary and myrtle, and not simply to offset the smell of decay. In the Bible, mint is referenced along with anise and cumin to be given as a tithe to the Lord, demonstrating its value during that time.

A cross between a variety of wild mints, peppermint was more widely discovered in the 17th century. The essential oils are gathered by steam distillation of the fresh aerial parts of the flowering plant. Peppermint essential oil is used for its anti-nausea benefits and soothing effects on muscles, the colon and the gastric lining. It has a sharp, minty and intense aroma that serves as a stimulating and invigorating agent. Peppermint oil gives a cooling sensation and has a calming effect on the body, which can help relieve sore muscles and ease headaches when used topically. It also has anti-microbial properties, so it can help freshen bad breath and soothe digestive issues.

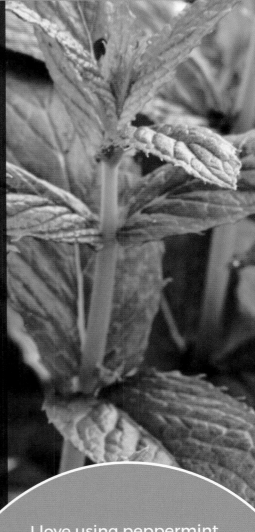

I love using peppermint oil as an addition to my toothpaste to fight bacteria that cause tooth decay and to promote healthy gums.

– Jordan

RESEARCH STUDIES

A 2007 study used peppermint oil to treat irritable bowel syndrome. After four weeks, patients reported an average 50 percent reduction in symptoms, including abdominal bloating, abdominal discomfort, diarrhea, constipation and pain during elimination.[88]

A 1994 study found that a combination of peppermint and eucalyptus oil has significant effects on mechanisms associated with the pathophysiology of headaches.[89]

⊘ KEY BENEFITS

- Soothes digestive issues
- Freshens breath
- Helps relieve headaches
- Provides mental focus

- Promotes respiratory cleansing
- Boosts energy
- Eases tight muscles
- Helps relieve nausea and vomiting

🛡 SAFETY

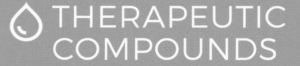

💧 THERAPEUTIC COMPOUNDS

Some medications may adversely interact with peppermint oil, so consult a physician with concerns about drug interactions.

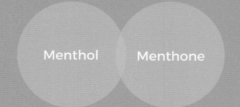

Menthol   Menthone

SUPER 7 RX PEPPERMINT USES

1. Helps Relieve Muscle Pain

Peppermint oil may help reduce pain and relax muscles. It is especially helpful in soothing an aching back, sore muscles and tension headaches. Dilute 2 to 4 drops and apply it topically to the area of concern.

2. Soothes Respiratory Conditions

Peppermint oil acts as an expectorant and may relieve some symptoms of a respiratory illness. Dilute 2 to 4 drops and apply it topically to your chest and the back of your neck. Alternatively, you can add 10 drops to boiling water, put a towel over your head and breathe in the aroma for 5 minutes.

3. Boosts Energy

Because peppermint is invigorating and stimulating, it can help fight chronic fatigue and improve concentration. Diffuse it, or apply it to your temples, wrists and the back of your neck. It can also be inhaled directly for a quick energy boost.

4. Helps Reduce Allergy Symptoms

Peppermint helps relax the muscles in the nasal passages and clear out mucus and pollen during allergy season. Diffuse 5 drops, inhale it directly from the bottle or dilute 2 to 3 drops and apply it topically to your forehead, neck and chest.

5. Aids in Headache Relief

Peppermint oil may improve circulation, soothe the gut and relax tense muscles. It can also help clear your nasal passages when you're suffering from a sinus headache. Apply it to your forehead and temples for pain relief.

6. Eases Digestive Conditions

Peppermint oil helps to relax the muscles in the intestines and reduce bloating, gas and nausea. It may also serve as a natural remedy for irritable bowel syndrome. Diffuse it, apply it topically to your abdomen, or take 1 to 2 drops internally.

7. Freshens Breath and Fights Cavities

Peppermint oil has anti-microbial properties that will freshen breath and may kill bacteria that lead to cavities and gum disease. Add 1 drop to toothpaste or mouthwash, or place the oil under your tongue before drinking a glass of water.

ROMAN CHAMOMILE

CHAMAEMELUM NOBILE

Although it is called "Roman" chamomile, its history as a celebrated and widely used herb extends far beyond Ancient Rome. Hieroglyphic records show that Roman chamomile was used cosmetically for at least 2,000 years. Greek physicians prescribed it for fevers and female disorders. And although "Roman chamomile" was not the official name of the plant at the time, the term was given after it was seen sprouting around the Roman Colosseum in the 19th century. Also, historically, Roman chamomile has been the essential oil of choice for mothers to use with their children because of its gentle and calming properties.

Roman chamomile essential oil is steam-distilled from the plant's flowers and has a sweet, fresh, apple-like and fruity aroma. Considered to be one of the most ancient and versatile essential oils, Roman chamomile has been used to treat a variety of conditions because of its anti-spasmodic effects due to its high esters content. Today, it is commonly used in the natural treatment of nervous system problems, eczema, fever, heartburn, gout, anxiety and insomnia.

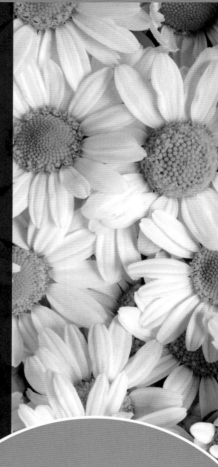

When it's time for bed, Chelsea and I love to diffuse a blend of Roman chamomile and lavender to help us wind down and get a great night's sleep.

– Dr. Josh

🔬 RESEARCH STUDIES

A 2006 case study explored the inhalation effects of Roman chamomile on mood and sleep. The results found that volunteers experienced more drowsiness and calmness when breathing in Roman chamomile, demonstrating its potential to improve sleep and help to enter a restful state.[90]

A 2013 study found that an aromatherapy essential oil blend including lavender, Roman chamomile and neroli reduced anxiety levels in ICU patients. The essential oil also improved sleep quality in patients.[91]

✓ KEY BENEFITS

- Fights anxiety and depression
- Serves as a natural allergy reliever
- Helps alleviate PMS symptoms
- Reduces symptoms of insomnia
- Improves rashes and eczema
- Supports digestive health
- May relieve arthritic pain
- Soothes hemorrhoids

🛡 SAFETY

It is not recommended for use during pregnancy, as Roman chamomile oil is an emmenagogue (stimulates blood flow in the pelvic area). Use Roman chamomile internally for up to two weeks at a time.

💧 THERAPEUTIC COMPOUNDS

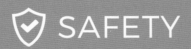
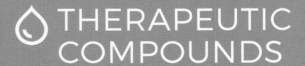

Angelate

Esters

Isobutyrate

SUPER 7 RX ROMAN CHAMOMILE USES

1. Helps Fight Anxiety and Depression

Roman chamomile fights stress and promotes relaxation. Inhaling Roman chamomile is a natural remedy for anxiety; the fragrance is carried directly to the brain and serves as an emotional trigger. Diffuse 5 drops, or inhale it directly from the bottle.

2. May Improve Digestion and Leaky Gut

Roman chamomile oil contains anodyne compounds that are antispasmodic and can be used to remedy various gastrointestinal disturbances, from gas to leaky gut to acid reflux. Use in low doses for children with colic and diarrhea. Apply 2-4 drops topically to the abdomen.

3. Encourages Restful Sleep

The relaxing properties of Roman chamomile promotes healthy sleep and fights insomnia. Diffuse next to bed, rub onto temples or inhale directly from the bottle.

4. Calms and Soothes Children

For centuries, mothers have used Roman chamomile to calm crying children, reduce fevers, eliminate earaches and soothe upset stomachs. It even helps children with ADD/ADHD. Either diffuse it or apply it topically.

5. Boosts Skin Health

Roman chamomile promotes smooth, healthy skin because of its anti-inflammatory and anti-bacterial properties. Use to fight acne, various skin conditions and signs of aging. Add 2 to 3 drops to a cotton ball and apply it to the area of concern, or add 5 drops to a face wash.

6. Promotes Heart Health

Roman chamomile provides cardiovascular protection because of its high levels of flavonoids. It may lower blood pressure and relax the heart. Apply 2 to 4 drops topically over your heart, or take it internally by placing it under your tongue.

7. Eases Nausea

Because of its relaxing properties, Roman chamomile can relieve nausea associated with pregnancy or motion sickness. Inhale directly from the bottle, or combine it with ginger, peppermint and lavender oil and diffuse. It can also be used topically on your temples for nausea.

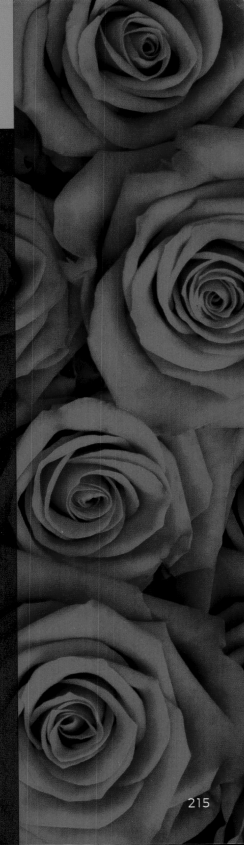

ROSE

ROSA DAMASCENA

Rose has been adored and revered throughout history as both a plant and an essential oil. Both Cleopatra and Joséphine de Beauharnais (wife of Napoleon I) were fans of rose, as were the Romans who used it lavishly in their banquets and parties. Rose was reputedly amongst one of the first plants to be distilled by Avicenna after his introduction of the refrigerated coil into the distillation process.

Rose essential oil is extracted by the steam distillation of the flower pedals. The essential oil has a floral, rich, deep, spicy and sensual aroma. Rose oil certainly has an indulgent and delightful scent, but its uses extend far beyond fragrance. It has been used to support multiple health conditions and in natural beauty treatments for thousands of years. Rose oil has the power to improve acne, balance hormones, boost libido and lift the spirit. It contains several therapeutic compounds that fight infection, aid digestion and promote healing in the body.

RESEARCH STUDIES

A 2009 study found that treatment with rose oil caused significant decreases in breathing rate, blood oxygen saturation and systolic blood pressure. The study's participants also rated themselves as calmer and more relaxed than control group subjects.[92]

Rose oil may be a useful treatment for depression because it contains flavonoids, which include free radical-reducing antioxidant compounds. Researchers found that treatment with rose oil vapor induced protective effects on oxidative stress in depression.[93]

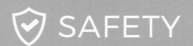

KEY BENEFITS

- Improves skin conditions
- Helps balance hormones
- May relieve anxiety
- Helps fight depression

- Can increase libido
- Aids digestion
- Promotes blood circulation
- Eases menstrual symptoms

SAFETY

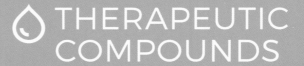

THERAPEUTIC COMPOUNDS

Avoid using it during pregnancy, as rose oil is an emmenagogue (stimulates blood flow in the pelvic area).

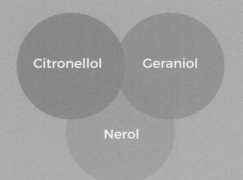

Citronellol

Geraniol

Nerol

SUPER 7 RX ROSE USES

1. Helps Fight Depression

Rose essential oil has sedative properties that can create a relaxing and peaceful feeling. Combine rose oil with lavender oil and diffuse it, or apply 1 to 2 drops topically to your wrists and the back of your neck.

2. Can Boost Libido

Because it acts as an anti-anxiety agent, rose essential oil can help treat sexual dysfunction related to feelings of anxiety and stress. It helps to balance hormones and can increase sex drive. Diffuse it, or apply 2 to 3 drops topically to your neck and chest.

3. Promotes Skin Health

The anti-microbial properties of rose oil make it a powerful treatment for skin conditions, including acne. It can also help prevent scarring, minimize the look of wrinkles and alleviate poison ivy rashes. Apply it topically or add to face wash, body wash or lotion.

4. Aids Digestion

Because of the relaxing properties present in rose essential oil, it can help improve digestive issues that are related to stress and anxiety.

Apply 2 to 3 drops topically to your abdomen to help ease stomachaches.

5. Helps with PMS and Menstrual Symptoms

Due to its anti-spasmodic properties, rose essential oil may relieve cramps associated with PMS and menstruation. It also fights feelings of moodiness and anxiety. Diffuse it, or apply it topically to your abdomen.

6. May Relieve Seizures

The anti-spasmodic and sedative properties of rose oil can help people who experience seizures. Diffuse it, or apply it topically to your wrists and the back of your neck.

7. Serves as a Fragrant Perfume

The sweet, inviting smell of rose essential oil serves as a superior alternative to synthetic perfumes. Simply dab 1 to 2 drops behind your ears or on your wrists. A little goes a long way!

ROSEMARY

ROSMARINUS OFFICINALIS

As a member of the mint family, rosemary has long been used as a powerful natural health booster. A tea made from rosemary leaves was once used to quiet nerves and strengthen memory, and the leaves are also used in perfumery and cooking. As early as 1584, rosemary was used as a symbol of remembrance on particular occasions such as funerals and weddings, or even as a decoration for brides. Shakespeare made reference to rosemary in *Hamlet* where Ophelia, decked with flowers, says to Laertes: "There's rosemary, that's for remembrance."

Rosemary's history extends further back than Shakespeare. The Ancient Egyptians, Romans and Greeks all considered it sacred, and it was widely used to cleanse the air and prevent sickness from spreading. It was used in folk medicine to improve memory, soothe digestive issues and relieve muscle aches and pains. More recently, it has been shown to boost nerve growth factor and support the healing of neurological tissue as well as boost brain function. Rosemary essential oil has a woody, evergreen-like scent and is steam-distilled from the leaves of the plant.

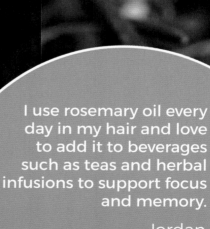

I use rosemary oil every day in my hair and love to add it to beverages such as teas and herbal infusions to support focus and memory.

– Jordan

RESEARCH STUDIES

A 2012 study evaluated rosemary oil's effect on cognitive performance and mood. Twenty healthy volunteers performed tasks in a cubicle diffused with rosemary. Test results showed improved performance at higher concentrations of rosemary essential oil.[94]

Rosemary was found to be active against certain pathogenic bacteria and drug-resistant mutants of E. coli. Similarly, it was found to be highly active against pathogenic fungi and drug-resistant mutants of Candida albicans.[95]

KEY BENEFITS

- Relieves muscle aches and pains
- Contains anti-inflammatory properties
- Promotes hormone balance
- Soothes respiratory conditions
- Improves alertness
- Regenerates nerve tissue
- Thickens hair
- May improve memory

SAFETY

Use rosemary oil minimally during pregnancy. Do not use it if you have high blood pressure or if you've been diagnosed with epilepsy.

THERAPEUTIC COMPOUNDS

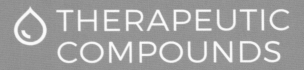

1,8-cineole

Linalool

Terpinen-4-ol

SUPER 7 RX ROSEMARY USES

SINGLE ESSENTIAL OILS

1. Increases Hair Growth

Rosemary essential oil stimulates hair growth and can help prevent baldness, slow graying and treat dandruff or dry scalp. Apply 3 to 5 drops to your scalp, rub it in and allow the oil to sit for 5 minutes before rinsing, or add 5 to 10 drops to shampoo or conditioner.

2. May Improve Memory

Studies show that rosemary oil improves cognitive performance, increases alertness and enhances overall quality of memory. Add it to a diffuser, or apply it topically under your nose or across your forehead.

3. Acts as a Natural Diabetes Remedy

Over time, incorporating rosemary oil into your daily routine can help to supplement and assist in the body's balance and regulation of hormones and blood sugar levels. Take 1 to 2 drops in a glass of water.

4. Helps Reduce Pain

Because of rosemary oil's anti-inflammatory properties, it has the power to reduce joint and muscle pain. Mix 2 drops of rosemary oil, 2 drops of peppermint oil and 1 teaspoon of coconut oil and rub it onto sore muscles and painful joints.

5. Promotes Liver Detox and Gallbladder Function

Using rosemary oil topically can enhance the performance of the bile-producing gallbladder and help to prevent toxin buildup in the body. Mix 3 drops of rosemary oil with ¼ teaspoon of coconut oil and rub it over your gallbladder area twice daily.

6. Aids in Detoxifying the Body

Rosemary oil boosts nutrient absorption and helps to reverse or prevent toxic overload. Take it internally, or apply 2 to 3 drops to your abdomen to detoxify your body.

7. Fights Respiratory Issues

Rosemary oil works as an expectorant—reducing mucus and relieving some of the symptoms of bronchitis, cold and other respiratory infections. Apply it topically to your chest, or diffuse it, to thin and expel mucus.

SANDALWOOD

SANTALUM ALBUM

Intoxicating and exotic with woody and earthy notes, sandalwood has an aroma that is one of a kind. Legendary poet, writer and singer Rabindranath Tagore once wrote, "As if to prove that love would conquer hate, the sandalwood perfumes the very axe that lays it low." For thousands of years, Hindus have used sandalwood during significant religious ceremonies. The ancient Egyptians imported the wood and used it in medicine, for embalming the dead and in ritual burning to venerate the gods.

Native to the Asian tropics, sandalwood, also known as East Indian sandalwood, is an evergreen tree that can grow up to 30 feet. Younger trees are not as fragrant or as high-quality as mature sandalwood trees are. Sandalwood essential oil can help one achieve more clarity and calmness due to its extensive therapeutic benefits. The wood is steam-distilled to extract the powerful essential oils that have been used throughout history to enhance meditation and support the cardiovascular system. Sandalwood is calming and balancing when used aromatically.

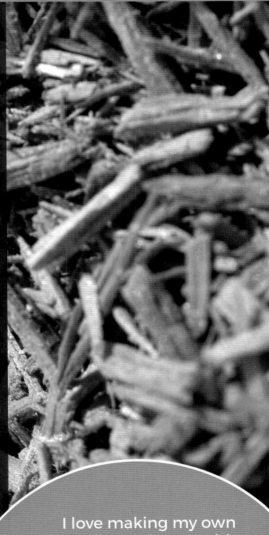

I love making my own homemade deodorant with coconut oil, baking soda, sandalwood, bergamot and black pepper oil.

– Dr. Josh

RESEARCH STUDIES

Sandalwood oil could be an effective chemo-preventive agent. The results indicate that sandalwood oil pre-treatment decreased papilloma incidence and multiplicity.[96]

Animal studies reported that sandalwood oil and alpha-santalol (its active compound) produced anti-cancer effects without causing toxic side effects.[97]

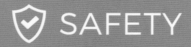 ## KEY BENEFITS

- Improves mental clarity
- Supports hormone balance
- Enhances memory
- May lower blood pressure

- Contains anti-inflammatory properties
- Treats respiratory conditions
- Serves as a natural aphrodisiac
- Soothes muscle cramps

SAFETY

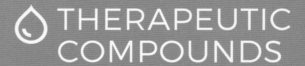 ## THERAPEUTIC COMPOUNDS

For areas of sensitive skin, dilute sandalwood oil with a carrier oil before application.

Alpha-Santalene

Alpha-Santalol

Beta-Santalene

Beta-Santalol

SUPER 7 RX SANDALWOOD USES

1. Promotes Mental Clarity and Memory

Sandalwood essential oil is frequently used in meditation and prayer because of its ability to promote mental clarity. May help Alzheimer's disease sufferers. Diffuse or apply 2 to 3 drops topically to your wrists and under your nose.

2. Can Boost Low Testosterone

For men with low testosterone, adding a few drops of sandalwood oil to homemade deodorant or homemade lotion is a great way to get some extra health benefits by promoting hormone balance.

3. Acts as an Aphrodisiac

Sandalwood oil is a natural anti-inflammatory agent that helps reduce swelling and bloating. Santalol, an active ingredient in sandalwood oil, can decrease cytokines (inflammation markers in the body). Apply 3 to 5 drops to the area of concern.

4. May Reduce Inflammation

Sandalwood oil is a natural anti-inflammatory agent that will help reduce swelling and bloating. Santalol, an active ingredient in sandalwood oil, can decrease cytokines (inflammation markers in the body). Apply 3 to 5 drops to the area of concern.

5. Supports Healthy Blood Pressure

Studies have found that sandalwood oil may decrease systolic blood pressure when applied directly to the skin. This can be due to its calming and sedative properties. Apply it topically to your chest, wrists and the back of your neck.

6. Inhibits Tumor Growth

Studies suggest that sandalwood oil has anti-cancer and chemo-protective effects when used internally. It may inhibit the growth of cancer cells and can be used as a natural anti-cancer agent. Take 1 to 2 drops of sandalwood oil internally.

7. Acts as a Natural Deodorant and Cologne

With its rich, woodsy aroma, sandalwood makes an excellent deodorant and cologne. To make your own deodorant, mix 10 drops of sandalwood, 4 tablespoons of coconut oil, 4 tablespoons of baking soda and 4 tablespoons of cornstarch. Store in the fridge.

SPIKENARD

NARDOSTACHYS JATAMANSI

In ancient times, spikenard essential oil (also known as "nard") was regarded as one of the most precious oils. Many say that Solomon prophesied a thousand years earlier of Christ's victory over death using a reference to spikenard. Song of Solomon 1:12 says, "While the king sat at his table, my spikenard sent forth its fragrance." According to some scholars, the seated position of the King is symbolic of His finished work at Calvary's tree. He is inviting His bride (the church) to come and join Him at the marriage supper feast. The bride's fragrance emanates out of her spirit in worship and adoration for the King's provision.

Spikenard was also used in Greek and Roman healing and ceremonies, and it was even used in medieval cookery. Used in Ayurveda, it's great for both healing and a deep connection to spirit. For those suffering from anxiety, spikenard can soothe the nerves and quiet the mind. Spikenard oil is used to treat insomnia, stress, digestive problems and infections. The roots of the plant are steam-distilled to extract the essential oil, which has a heavy, sweet, woody and spicy aroma— said to resemble the smell of moss.

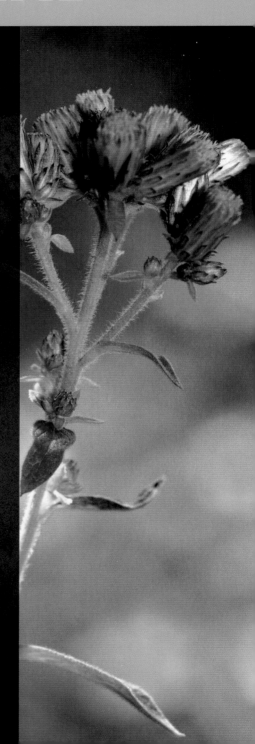

🔬 RESEARCH STUDIES

A 2008 study done on mice found that spikenard extract had sedative and calming benefits.[98]

Study results indicate that spikenard oil shows a positive response in hair growth promotion activity, showing that spikenard may work as a hair loss remedy.[99]

✓ KEY BENEFITS

- May reduce inflammation
- Fights bacteria and fungi
- Can relax the body and mind
- Boosts the immune system
- Helps protect the uterus and ovaries
- May improve insomnia
- Boosts skin and hair health

🛡 SAFETY

Do not use during pregnancy since spikenard oil can stimulate the uterus.

💧 THERAPEUTIC COMPOUNDS

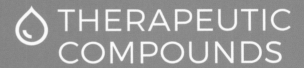

Bornyl acetate

Valeranone

Alpha-Patchoulene

SUPER 7 RX SPIKENARD USES

1. Displays Antibiotic Properties

When applied topically to wounds, spikenard can fight bacteria. Inside the body, spikenard helps treat bacterial infections in the kidneys, bladder and urethra. Apply 3 to 5 drops topically to the area of concern, or take 1 to 2 drops internally for infection and diffuse.

2. Can Reduce Inflammation

Spikenard oil relieves inflammation, which is at the root of many conditions and diseases such as asthma, arthritis, Crohn's disease, Alzheimer's disease, cancer, cardiovascular disease, diabetes, high blood pressure, high cholesterol and Parkinson's disease. Apply 3 to 5 drops topically twice daily, diffuse the oil or take 1 drop internally each day.

3. Helps Reduce Stress and Anxiety

Spikenard oil is relaxing and soothing for the skin and mind; it's often used as a sedative and calming agent. Diffuse spikenard oil or apply it topically.

4. Boosts the Immune System

Spikenard oil is an immune system booster because it calms the body, enabling it to function properly. To boost your immune system, diffuse spikenard or apply it topically to the soles of your feet or the back of your neck.

5. Promotes Hair Growth

Spikenard oil is known for promoting hair growth, helping to retain its natural color and slowing down the process of graying. Add 5 to 10 drops to a bottle of shampoo or conditioner, or combine 5 drops of spikenard oil with 1 teaspoon of coconut oil and massage the mixture into your scalp; let it sit for 5 minutes before rinsing.

6. Treats Insomnia

Spikenard's sedative and relaxing properties can be helpful to those with insomnia or sleep deprivation. Diffuse or apply 2 to 3 drops topically to your temples and the back of your neck.

7. Helps with Constipation

Spikenard oil is a natural laxative, and it stimulates the digestive system, helping to naturally relieve constipation. Apply spikenard oil onto your stomach and the soles of your feet.

THYME

THYMUS VULGARIS

You may not realize it when you walk past thyme in the grocery store, but it has been an herbal superhero for thousands of years. A symbol of courage throughout the ages, thyme was added to the bathwater of Roman soldiers to empower them for battle. The soldiers also exchanged sprigs of thyme as a sign of respect. Romans believed that eating thyme either before or during a meal would protect you from poison; this made the herb a particular favorite of the emperors. Greeks and Romans burned bundles of thyme to purify their temples and homes, and to evoke a spirit of courage in those who inhaled it.

The widespread use of thyme continued throughout the ages. When the Black Death struck in the late 1340s, millions of people turned to thyme for relief and protection. In the days before refrigeration, including thyme in recipes provided some protection against spoiled meat and foodborne disease. The oil has a fresh, herbaceous and medicinal aroma that, among its other mighty super powers, can aid concentration and relieve feelings of depression. The flowering tops and leaves are steam-distilled to capture an essential oil that has antiseptic, anti-bacterial, anti-spasmodic and calming properties.

In order to boost my immune system during the holidays, I make a chicken bone broth soup and add in several drops of thyme oil.

– Dr. Josh

RESEARCH STUDIES

Scientists investigated 120 strains of bacteria isolated from patients with various infections from hospital environments. The results of the experiments showed that thyme oil exhibited extremely strong activity against all strains, including antibiotic-resistant strains.[100]

A study examined the anti-inflammatory effects of thyme and oregano essential oils. Results showed that appropriate concentrations of thyme and oregano essential oils could reduce inflammation and potentially improve colitis.[101]

⊘ KEY BENEFITS

- Boosts the immune system
- Fights infections
- Improves respiratory conditions
- Aids digestion
- May relieve feelings of depression
- Inhibits fungal growth
- Helps relieve insomnia
- Supports healthy skin

⛨ SAFETY

◊ THERAPEUTIC COMPOUNDS

Avoid use during pregnancy, as thyme oil is an emmenagogue (stimulates blood flow in the pelvic area). People who have high blood pressure or epilepsy should avoid high doses of thyme oil.

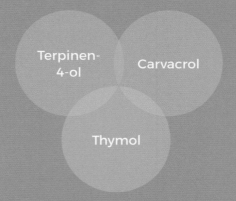

Terpinen-4-ol

Carvacrol

Thymol

SUPER 7 RX THYME USES

1. Improves Respiratory Conditions

Thyme oil is anti-bacterial, anti-fungal, spasmolytic and expectorant, so it helps quell bronchitis and a spasmodic cough. Diffuse it, apply it topically to your chest and neck, take 1 to 2 drops internally or add 5 to 7 drops of thyme oil to boiling water and breathe in the steam.

2. Battles Bacteria and Parasites

Thyme oil helps treat intestinal infections and bacterial infections in the genitals and urethra. It's useful in treating bacteria that build up in the respiratory system. Apply 2 to 4 drops directly to the affected area, or take 1 drop internally with water to battle bacteria and parasites.

3. Boosts Skin Health

Thyme oil protects the skin from harmful bacteria and fungal infections, so it can treat acne, wounds, cuts, rashes and scars. A powerful antioxidant, it can help slow the aging process as well. Apply 2 to 4 drops of thyme oil topically to the area of concern.

4. Calms Inflammatory Bowel Diseases (IBD)

Thyme can help calm IBD, Crohn's disease and colitis. Mix 1 drop each of thyme, Roman chamomile, peppermint, ginger and frankincense with a teaspoon of coconut oil. Consume this mixture with breakfast and again just before dinner until your symptoms subside, and then continue taking it twice daily for another week.

5. Serves as Insect Repellent

Thyme oil helps keep away pests and parasites that feed on the body, such as mosquitoes, fleas, lice and bed bugs. Apply it topically or diffuse it. A few drops of thyme oil placed in the closet or kitchen can also repel moths and beetles.

6. Promotes Healthy Hormone Balance

With progesterone-balancing effects, thyme oil may also relieve symptoms of menopause, including mood swings, hot flashes and insomnia. Diffuse it, or apply it to the back of your neck, on your wrists and on the soles of your feet.

7. Fights Uterine Fibroids

Uterine fibroids are caused by high levels of estrogen and low levels of progesterone. To help break them up, rub 2 drops each of thyme, clary sage and frankincense oils over your lower abdomen twice daily.

TURMERIC

CURCUMA LONGA

Turmeric is enjoying its time in the spotlight in recent years. This ancient spice, recognized for centuries as a food, medicine and coloring agent, has experienced a surge of popularity thanks to curcumin, the therapeutic compound that supplies its brilliant yellow color. But don't be fooled by its newfound fame—the use of turmeric dates back nearly 4,000 years to the Vedic culture in India, where it was used in cooking as well as religious ceremonies. In Ayurvedic medicine, turmeric is known as strengthening and warming to the whole body.

The plant was called Indian saffron during the Middle Ages because of its orange-yellow color. Turmeric essential oil, which is steam-distilled from the plant's root, is an extremely impressive natural health agent—one that has some of the most promising anti-cancer properties around. Turmeric oil also displays anti-allergic, anti-bacterial, anti-microbial, anti-fungal, anti-parasitic and anti-viral properties.

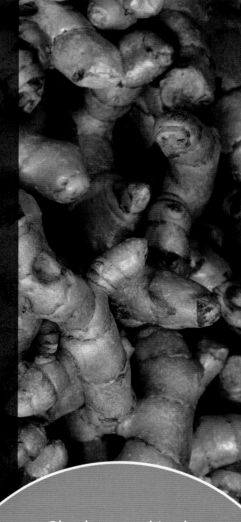

Charlene and I rub turmeric on our joints to relieve inflammation, and we also rub it on our kids' stomachs to support digestion.

– Ty

RESEARCH STUDIES

A 2013 study showed that two compounds in turmeric (curcumin and turmerone) displayed the ability to fight colon cancer. The combination of curcumin and turmerone given by mouth at both low and high doses abolished tumor formation in animals.[102]

Recent research has shown that aromatic turmerone has anti-convulsant properties. The turmerone was also able to lessen expression patterns of two seizure-related genes in zebrafish.[103]

KEY BENEFITS

- Aids digestion
- May improve certain cancers
- Acts as an anti-convulsant (helps prevent seizures)
- Fights depression and anxiety
- Supports neurological health
- Encourages healthy liver function
- Helps fight cold and flu
- Contains anti-inflammatory properties

SAFETY

Turmeric can easily stain clothes and skin, whether you use the spice or the oil, so be careful around fabrics and dilute it before topical use.

THERAPEUTIC COMPOUNDS

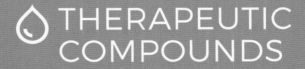

Alpha-Atlantone

Alpha-Turmerone

Curcumin

Ar-Turmerone

Beta-Turmerone

SUPER 7 RX TURMERIC USES

SINGLE ESSENTIAL OILS

1. Helps Relieve Arthritis and Joint Pain

Turmeric contains the active ingredient curcumin, which is an antioxidant that demonstrates anti-inflammatory properties in conditions such as arthritis, muscle sprains and other injuries. Add a few drops directly to the source of pain.

2. Serves as a Digestive Aid

Turmeric may help reduce symptoms of digestive conditions such as irritable bowel syndrome (IBS). Add 1 drop to your favorite tea for a spicy and beneficial kick to your beverage. Also apply it topically to your abdomen with a carrier oil.

3. Displays Promising Anti-Cancer Properties

Turmerone and curcumin in turmeric oil both displayed the ability to fight colon cancer in animal models, which may make it an effective supplement during cancer treatment. Take 1 drop internally in the morning and evening, mixed in your food or beverage. You can also mix it with a culinary carrier and consume this mixture in a capsule.

4. Fights Neurologic Diseases

Turmeric oil's aromatic turmerone is believed to be a promising way to support the regeneration necessary to improve neurologic diseases such as Parkinson's disease, Alzheimer's disease, spinal cord injury and stroke. Diffuse it, apply it topically or take it internally.

5. Relieves Depression and Anxiety

Turmeric essential oil is considered to be a strong relaxant and balancer, and studies show that it can help fight against two extremely common mood disorders, depression and anxiety. Diffuse it throughout the day to improve mood and encourage positive feelings.

6. May Help with Epilepsy

The anti-convulsant properties of turmeric oil may reduce or prevent some seizures. To aid in the prevention of seizures, take 1 to 2 drops internally or regularly drink hot turmeric tea.

7. Promotes Liver Detox

Studies have shown that turmeric is liver-protective, which is partly due to turmeric's anti-inflammatory activity. To encourage liver detoxification and help improve liver health, take it internally or apply it topically.

VETIVER

VETIVERIA ZIZANIOIDES

Vetiver and its essential oil have been used in many cultures across the globe for thousands of years. The massive use of this sacred herb is often attributed to its uplifting, soothing, healing, calming and shielding properties. In fact, vetiver is known as the "oil of tranquility" in India and Sri Lanka. In India, it has been used to make window blinds that help to keep out intense heat. When the blinds are sprinkled with water, they emit the vetiver scent, which cools the air and body in extreme temperatures. In Java, the root has been used for centuries in weaving mats and thatching huts.

Vetiver is native to India, and both its leaves and roots have wonderful uses. The roots of the perennial grass are steam-distilled to extract the essential oil, which has an earthy, balsamic, smoky and slightly sweet aroma. Modern vetiver oil is used to aid in the treatment of many conditions, including heat stroke, headaches, muscle aches, joint disorders and skin problems. Using vetiver oil is also a way to boost energy levels when you're exhausted.

When studying up on the latest clinical research, I use a blend of vetiver and rosemary to improve my focus and mental sharpness.

– Dr. Josh

RESEARCH STUDIES

A study found that vetiver oil is effective in treating children with ADHD. Lavender increased overall classroom performance by 53 percent, cedarwood increased performance by 83 percent and vetiver increased performance by an astonishing 100 percent.[104]

A 2015 study suggested that vetiver oil had antioxidant activity and protective effects against chemically-induced toxicity in laboratory animals. Vetiver oil treatment resulted in an improvement in kidney and liver function.[105]

KEY BENEFITS

- Helps boost energy levels
- Improves focus
- Relieves skin conditions
- May reduce feelings of anxiety and nervousness

- Provides anti-aging benefits
- May relieve joint and muscle pain
- Boosts cardiovascular health
- Supports neurological conditions

SAFETY

Those with sensitive skin should dilute vetiver oil with a carrier oil before topical use.

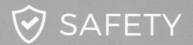 THERAPEUTIC COMPOUNDS

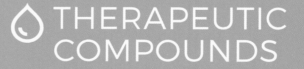

Delta-Selinene

Beta-Vetivenene

Khusimene

SUPER 7 RX VETIVER USES

1. Helps Fight Insomnia

Vetiver is calming and relaxing, and is therefore ideal for those suffering from insomnia. Diffuse it next to your bed, inhale it directly or add a few drops to a warm bath just before bedtime.

2. Serves as a Study Aid

Vetiver inspires a harmonious state while promoting deep concentration. Diffuse vetiver oil while studying for exams or working late hours to promote clear thinking and increased concentration.

3. Fights Aging and Free Radical Damage

Vetiver oil has a strong free radical scavenging activity that helps to slow the aging process, promote healthy and glowing skin, reduce the risk of cancer and boost detoxification. Diffuse it, or apply it topically.

4. Promotes Scar Healing

Vetiver oil is a cicatrisant, meaning it heals scars by promoting the regeneration of skin and tissue. By rejuvenating the skin, vetiver oil helps to remove dark spots along with acne scarring. Apply 2 to 4 drops of vetiver oil topically to the area of concern.

5. May Help People with ADD/ADHD

An important study has shown that vetiver oil is effective in children with ADHD and ADD because of its ability to relax and calm. Combine 2 drops of vetiver oil and 2 drops of lavender oil and diffuse it, or apply it topically.

6. Can Improve Nervous Tremors

Vetiver oil has been found to reduce tremors and boost the immune and nervous systems. Diffuse 5 drops or apply 2 to 3 drops topically to your wrists, the soles of your feet and the back of your neck to help reduce tremors such as those associated with Parkinson's disease.

7. Soothes Anxiety and Nervousness

Vetiver oil has been used in aromatherapy for relaxation and alleviating emotional stress, panic attacks, trauma, anxiety, insomnia, hysteria and depression. Diffuse the oil, apply it topically or add it to a warm-water bath to relieve feelings of anxiety and stress.

WINTERGREEN

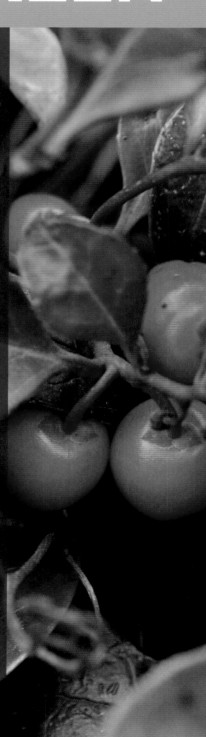

GAULTHERIA PROCUMBENS

Sometimes referred to as "Nature's Aspirin," wintergreen is an exceptional plant with many therapeutic qualities and has been known to treat various forms of pain for ages. In Ayurveda, wintergreen was used in many spiritual ceremonies where the sacred plant was trusted to bring harmony between the Earth and its inhabitants through its healing powers. The Native Americans used wintergreen to treat all kinds of musculoskeletal problems, arthritis among them. The Colonials had their share of aches and pains and quickly learned of this plant from the Native Americans.

Wintergreen essential oil is steam-distilled from the leaves of the plant. Wintergreen leaves themselves are actually odorless and tasteless, but after a compound present in the leaves is broken down to methyl salicylate, the signature minty aroma develops. Research shows that wintergreen oil has the ability to act like a natural analgesic, anti-arthritic, antiseptic and astringent. Wintergreen oil's active ingredient is methyl salicylate, and the oil is one of the best sources of this inflammation-fighting compound in the world. Furthermore, wintergreen is believed to be one of only several plants that naturally supply enough to form an extract. Wintergreen oil can help treat fatigue as well as lung, sinus and respiratory illnesses.

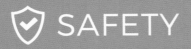 RESEARCH STUDIES

A study evaluated the use of wintergreen essential oil against inflammatory responses within damaged and infected tissue. Tests revealed that treatments of infected tissue led to a 60 percent reduction of pathogen development.[106]

The main constituent of wintergreen oil, methyl salicylate, was analyzed in a study. The results indicated that wintergreen can be used for pain management, as well as a way to numb skin and sore muscles.[107]

⊘ KEY BENEFITS

- Fights inflammation
- Lessens headache tension
- May improve PMS symptoms
- Supports the urinary system

- Helps improve alertness and senses
- Aids in relieving respiratory conditions
- May relieve muscle and joint pain
- Can reduce swelling and irritation

🛡 SAFETY

◌ THERAPEUTIC COMPOUNDS

Do not take it internally. Wintergreen oil consumption is dangerous due to the presence of menthyl salicylate. Diluted topical use is recommended.

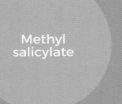

Methyl salicylate

SUPER 7 RX WINTERGREEN USES

SINGLE ESSENTIAL OILS

1. Battles Joint and Muscle Pain

Wintergreen oil may reduce swelling and irritation that occurs around painful muscles and tissue. It can relieve sore muscles, neck pain and lower back pain. Dilute 3 to 5 drops with equal parts of a carrier oil and apply it to the areas of concern.

2. Helps Improve Respiratory Conditions

Wintergreen contains an aspirin-like chemical that helps to reduce pain, congestion, swelling and fever associated with common illnesses. Combine 1 to 3 drops of wintergreen with coconut oil and rub it on your chest and upper back to help open your nasal passages.

3. Helps Fight and Prevent Infections

Wintergreen oil helps to combat bacterial growth, viruses and fungi because of its antiseptic and disinfectant properties. Dilute it before topical application. Add 5 to 10 drops to a spray bottle filled with water and use it on your clothes, furniture and any hard surface.

4. Addresses Gout Symptoms

Wintergreen oil stimulates the organs in the urinary system and the filtration of water by the kidneys, increasing the frequency and quantity of urine. This speeds up the removal of toxins like uric acid. Combine it with coconut oil and apply it to areas of concern.

5. Promotes Skin Health

As a natural astringent and antiseptic, wintergreen is able to fight inflammation from blemishes and skin disorders like acne. Add 1 to 2 drops to a face wash or apply it to the areas of concern.

6. Combats Fatigue

Respiratory-improving wintergreen oil may increase stamina, alertness and endurance. Inhale wintergreen oil directly from the bottle before a workout, or dilute and apply it topically to your neck, chest and wrists to fight sleepiness and fatigue.

7. Serves as a DIY Mouthwash and Toothpaste

Wintergreen oil fights germs in the mouth and is able to freshen breath and prevent mouth irritants and the growth of bacteria. Add a few drops to a glass of water and gargle for 30 to 60 seconds before rinsing. Do not swallow.

YLANG YLANG

CANANGA ADORATA

Ylang ylang has an interesting and extensive history of use in both the East and the West. In Indonesia, petals of ylang ylang flowers are scattered over the bed of couples on their wedding night. In the Philippines, healers have used ylang ylang in salves to treat insect bites, snakebites, cuts, burns and scrapes for centuries. The medicinal properties of ylang ylang were first recognized at the beginning of the 20th century by French chemists Garnier and Rechler. They discovered that the oil made an effective treatment for all types of diseases including malaria, typhus and intestinal infections. The chemists also noted the oil's calming effect on the heart during times of distress. In Oriental medicine, in fact, it is ylang ylang's calming effect on the heart that accounts for its primary therapeutic action.

Ylang ylang essential oil is steam-distilled from the flower petals of the large tropical tree, and its exquisite aroma is flowery and sweet in a way that will delight your senses. Ylang ylang means "flower of flowers," and it was given this name because of its sweet, floral aroma. It is considered an effective antidepressant, antiseptic and anti-spasmodic. It has a positive effect on immune health, blood flow and emotions, making it a natural remedy for disorders affecting the endocrine, cardiovascular, reproductive and digestive systems.

My wife Chelsea uses a blend of ylang ylang, jasmine and vanilla as a natural perfume, which I absolutely love!

– Dr. Josh

RESEARCH STUDIES

A 2006 study found that ylang ylang essential oil has the power to relieve feelings of depression and stress when used aromatically. It caused a significant decrease of blood pressure, and participants rated themselves as more calm and more relaxed than subjects in the control group.[108]

Ylang ylang essential oil significantly decreased systolic and diastolic blood pressure when it was used in an investigation involving 29 men. Ylang ylang also decreased heart rate and proved to have sedative effects when inhaled.[109]

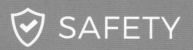 ## KEY BENEFITS

- Encourages blood flow
- May reduce inflammation
- Promotes regular heartbeat
- Improves cardiovascular conditions
- Boosts mood
- Can relieve stress
- Promotes healthy skin
- Enhances sexual energy

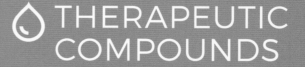 ## SAFETY

THERAPEUTIC COMPOUNDS

Some cases of sensitivity, nausea and headache have been observed when ylang ylang is used in excessive amounts.

Alpha-Farnesene

Beta-Caryophyllene

Caryophyllene

Germacrene

SUPER 7 RX YLANG YLANG USES

1. Helps Regulate Blood Pressure

Ylang ylang supports a healthy circulatory system. It's considered one of the most helpful essential oils for controlling blood pressure and preventing heart arrhythmia. Dilute it and apply 1 drop topically over your heart, or add 2 drops to a cup of water or warm tea.

2. Promotes Skin Health

When applied to the skin, ylang ylang oil may help prevent signs of aging. It may even help fight the development of skin cancer cells, including melanoma. Combine 2 drops with equal parts of coconut or jojoba oil and apply it topically to the area of concern twice daily.

3. Boosts Mood and Energy

Acting directly on the olfactory system of the brain, inhaling ylang ylang oil can have immediate, positive effects on your mood and act like a mild, natural depression remedy. Combine 3 to 5 drops with a carrier oil and massage it onto your temples and the back of your neck.

4. Helps Balance Hormones

Ylang ylang oil helps to reduce the cramps, tension and stress associated with PMS. Combine 2 drops of ylang ylang and 2 drops of lavender, and apply the mixture topically to the back of your neck and on your lower abdomen.

5. May Lessen Frustration and Anger

Ylang ylang oil aids in releasing negative emotions, including anger, low self-esteem and jealousy. Diffuse it, or inhale it directly from the bottle to help wash away frustration.

6. Encourages Self-Confidence

Inhaling ylang ylang can have immediate, positive effects on your self-confidence. It can empower you and help you take on life's challenges with greater confidence and optimism. Inhale it directly, diffuse it or apply it to your wrists and the back of your neck.

7. Serves as a Natural Aphrodisiac

Ylang ylang has been shown to act like a natural impotence remedy and help increase the libido of both men and women. It boosts energy and creates feelings of relaxation. Diffuse it, or apply it topically to your temples, wrists or the back of your neck.

CARRIER OILS

Carrier oils are used to dilute essential oils when they are being used topically; they help to *carry* the essential oils into the skin. Many lotions and skin care products are made with carrier oils, which are vegetable oils derived from the fatty portion of the plant, like the nuts, kernels or seeds. Unlike essential oils, carrier oils do not evaporate easily and do not give off strong aromas. Unfortunately, carrier oils often have a defined shelf life and will become rancid over time.

Each carrier oil offers a different combination of nourishing properties, benefits and characteristics. Some are more aromatic than others, and the color and shelf life will differ as well. The following pages will provide you with some of the most widely used carrier oils that can be combined with essential oils in aromatherapy.

ALMOND

Almond oil presents a variety of health benefits: It addresses bad cholesterol, helps prevent inflammation, hydrates dry skin and supports cardiovascular health. This oil has even been presented as an alternative, renewable biofuel source. When used topically, it is known for its ability to soften and soothe inflamed skin. It absorbs into the skin fairly quickly, leaving a slight hint of oil.

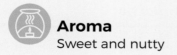 **Aroma**
Sweet and nutty

 Key Benefits
» Nourishes skin and hair
» Contains powerful antioxidants
» Protects skin from UV damage
» Fights acne
» Reduces inflammation

APRICOT KERNEL

The kernels of the apricot fruit are cold-pressed to extract the beneficial oils. This oil works great as a massage oil because it is very light and soothing to the skin. In Traditional Chinese Medicine, apricot kernel oil is used to treat tumors and ulcers. It has also been used to relieve digestive issues and boost skin health.

 Aroma
Light, sweet and nutty

 Key Benefits
» Stimulates the immune system
» Helps relieve pain
» Works to reduce swelling and inflammation
» Fights acne
» Soothes and nourishes dry or inflamed skin
» Improves skin conditions

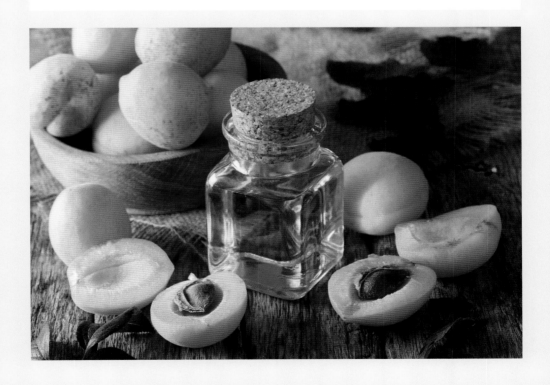

ARNICA

Arnica oil has been used for medicinal purposes since the 1500s. It contains helenalin, a potent anti-inflammatory agent, which is why arnica oil is commonly used on the skin in the form of an oil, cream, ointment, liniment or salve. This carrier oil needs to be diluted before topical use. When purchased from a store, arnica oil should already be diluted and ready for use, but make sure to read the label carefully. When applied to the skin, it helps to reduce pain caused by inflammation, while also treating bruises, aches, sprains and even arthritis flare-ups.

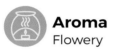 **Aroma**
Flowery

 Key Benefits
» Helps reduce inflammation
» Soothes sprains and muscle pain
» Boosts hair growth
» Fights bacteria
» Helps reduce swelling

ARGAN

For generations, natives of the Argan Forest in Morocco have pressed the argan nut to extract this precious oil to use as a dietary supplement for wound healing and rash relief, and to nourish skin and hair. Argan oil is rich in vitamins A and E; it is also packed with antioxidants, omega-6 fatty acids and linoleic acid. When it is applied topically, it eases inflammation, moisturizes skin and boosts cell production.

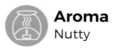 **Aroma**
Nutty

 Key Benefits
» Exfoliates skin and helps fight acne
» May reduce the appearance of stretch marks
» Relieves razor bumps and burns
» Conditions hair and nourishes nails
» Improves cracked or chapped lips

AVOCADO

Avocado oil has actually received prescription drug status in France because of its proven ability to counter the negative effects of arthritis. This oil is produced from the fruit of the avocado tree. Because it is extracted from the fleshy pulp of the fruit, it is one of the few edible oils not derived from a seed. The pulp produces oil full of healthy fats, including oleic acid and essential fatty acids. Avocado oil can be used topically to hydrate dry hair and improve its texture, as well as improve skin health. It also reduces inflammation and boosts nutrient absorption.

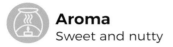 **Aroma**
Sweet and nutty

 Key Benefits
» Reduces inflammation
» May improve arthritis symptoms
» Soothes psoriasis and other skin problems
» Hydrates skin and hair
» Improves hair texture

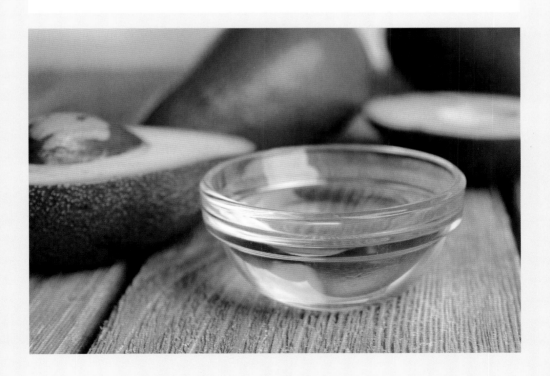

COCONUT

The coconut tree is considered the "tree of life" in much of Southeast Asia, India, the Philippines and other tropical locations. Today, there are over 1,500 articles demonstrating the health benefits of coconut oil. The uses are numerous thanks to its natural healing properties and tremendous use as a product for natural beauty treatments and so much more.

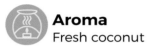 **Aroma**
Fresh coconut

 Key Benefits
» Attacks bacteria and fungi
» Helps reduce cellulite
» Protects the skin and hair
» Improves mental clarity

EVENING PRIMROSE

Primrose is a wild flower that grows in eastern and central North America. The seeds of the flower are cold-pressed for the extraction of their oil, which is high in essential fatty acids. Evening primrose oil has a range of therapeutic properties; it is known to help reduce the pain associated with PMS and relieve skin irritations and conditions. The oil could also be used as an anti-inflammatory agent, and it is commonly used to relieve problems with autoimmune diseases.

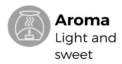 **Aroma**
Light and sweet

 Key Benefits
» Treats skin conditions
» Hydrates skin and hair
» Helps relieve PMS symptoms
» Promotes hormone balance
» May boost fertility

HEMP

Hemp seed is an all-natural way to jumpstart better skin with a wave of incredible vitamins. Hemp seed oil does not contain THC (tetrahydrocannabinol) or the other psychoactive constituents that are present in the dried leaves of Cannabis sativa. With generous amounts of omega fatty acids and proteins, this oil wonderfully reinvigorates the skin as it helps to clear away acne and eczema. Extremely emollient and absorbent, hemp seed oil is packed with vitamins A, B1, B2, B3, B6, C, D and E. It also has abundant levels of anti-inflammatory and antioxidant properties. Hemp seed oil also reduces toxins while alleviating sore muscles and joints.

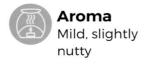 **Aroma**
Mild, slightly nutty

 Key Benefits
» Contains numerous vitamins
» Contains anti-inflammatory and antioxidant properties
» Encourages toxin removal
» Alleviates sore muscles and joints

JOJOBA

Jojoba oil (pronounced ho-ho-ba) is the liquid that comes from the seed of the Simmondsia chinensis plant. It is labeled as an oil, but is actually a liquid plant wax that has been used in folk medicine for a number of ailments. Because jojoba is an emollient, it soothes the skin and unclogs hair follicles. It can be combined with essential oils such as lavender or peppermint to boost skin and hair health.

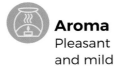 **Aroma**
Pleasant and mild

 Key Benefits
» Moisturizes skin
» Fights bacteria and fungi
» Boosts skin and hair health
» Speeds up wound closures
» Stimulates collagen synthesis

OLIVE

Olive trees have been around for many thousands of years. With a long history dating back to ancient civilizations, olive oil is even considered to be one of the most important Bible foods. High-quality olive oil has well-researched anti-inflammatory compounds and antioxidants. It is made from the fruit of the olive tree, which is naturally high in healthy fatty acids. When used topically, olive oil reduces oxidative damage and works as an anti-microbial agent. It should be used in small amounts, as the olive fragrance could overpower the aroma of essential oils when used in high doses.

Aroma
Slight olive fragrance

Key Benefits
» Helps reduce inflammation
» Protects skin against UV damage
» Can speed up wound healing
» Helps balance hormones

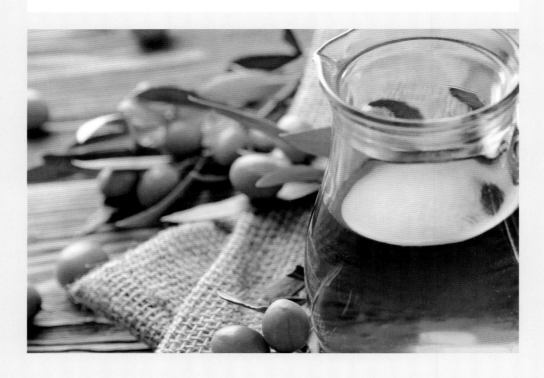

POMEGRANATE

Pomegranate seed oil is considered one of the Bible's powerful foods because of its powerful anti-aging benefits. The dark red color in pomegranate seed oil comes from the bioflavonoids, which protect the skin from sun damage. It has a natural sun protection factor (SPF) and can be used as a sunblock and sunscreen.

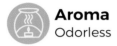 **Aroma**
Odorless

 Key Benefits
» Contains powerful antioxidants
» Helps reduce inflammation
» Works as a natural sunblock
» Nourishes skin
» Boosts skin cell regeneration

ROSEHIP

Rosehip oil is harvested from the seeds of rose bushes predominately grown in Chile. It contains powerful antioxidants, vitamins and essential fatty acids—making it an effective carrier oil for hydrating the skin, relieving itchiness and minimizing the appearances of dark spots, scars and fine lines. Rosehip absorbs easily, and it is non-greasy and light when applied topically.

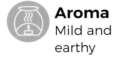 **Aroma**
Mild and earthy

 Key Benefits
» Stimulates collagen production
» Moisturizes skin and hair
» Can reduce the appearance of wrinkles and fine lines
» Protects skin from UV rays and sun damage
» Has anti-aging properties

SEA BUCKTHORN

Sea buckthorn berries and seeds are cold-pressed and CO2 extracted for their oils, which are rich in essential fatty acids and contain vitamins, minerals and nutritive compounds. Sea buckthorn oil is used on the skin to reduce the signs of aging. Because of its intense color that can stain skin when used in high doses, a 1:3 dilution is recommended.

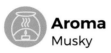 **Aroma**
Musky

 Key Benefits
» Promotes skin regeneration
» Boosts skin elasticity
» Helps treat and prevent acne
» May reduce inflammation
» Soothes the digestive tract

SHEA BUTTER

Shea butter is not a carrier oil, but its natural, beneficial properties make it a lipid suitable for aromatherapy work. It is highly moisturizing, has a smooth, creamy texture and can be included in massage blends, lotions, creams and other natural skin care products. Shea butter can become gritty if not melted and then cooled properly. Once it has cooled, it does not need to be kept in the refrigerator.

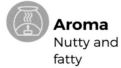 **Aroma**
Nutty and
fatty

 Key Benefits
» Moisturizes skin
» Helps reduce inflammation
» Can improve skin elasticity
» Contains mild SPF properties
» Serves as an under eye wrinkle
   and bag reducer

When shopping for carrier oils, quality matters just as much as it does when it comes to essential oils. For example, you should use only raw, unrefined, grade A shea butter. There are many refined shea butters that are odor-free and bleached to be completely white, but the refining process removes some of the beneficial properties. Similarly, the only coconut oil recommended for use as a carrier oil is raw, unrefined, virgin, organic coconut oil.

WHAT ABOUT MINERAL OIL?

Mineral oil and petroleum jelly are byproducts of petroleum production. They are not of natural, botanical origin and are not used within the scope of holistic therapy. Mineral oil is used in baby oils and many commercially available moisturizers because it is an inexpensive oil to manufacture. It can, however, clog pores, prevent the skin from breathing naturally, prevent essential oil absorption, prevent toxins from leaving the body through the natural process of sweating and may even block vitamins from properly being utilized.

As you continue growing your collection of essential oils, experiment with different carrier oils; they have so many uses as both carriers and in DIY recipes. Find the ones that work best for you to get the most out of your essential oils' therapeutic qualities.

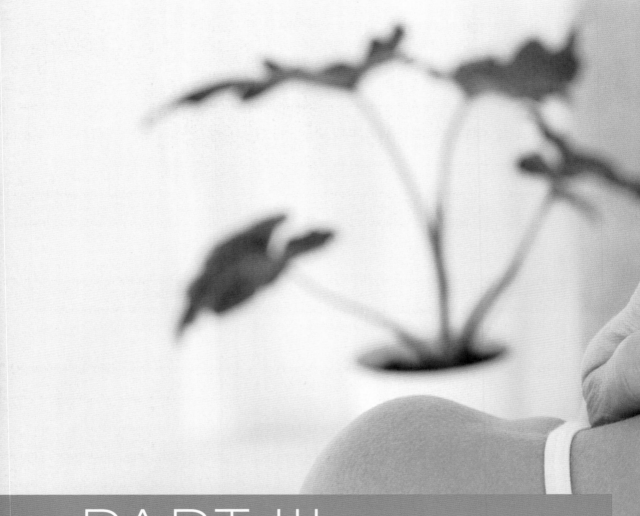

PART III

CONDITIONS

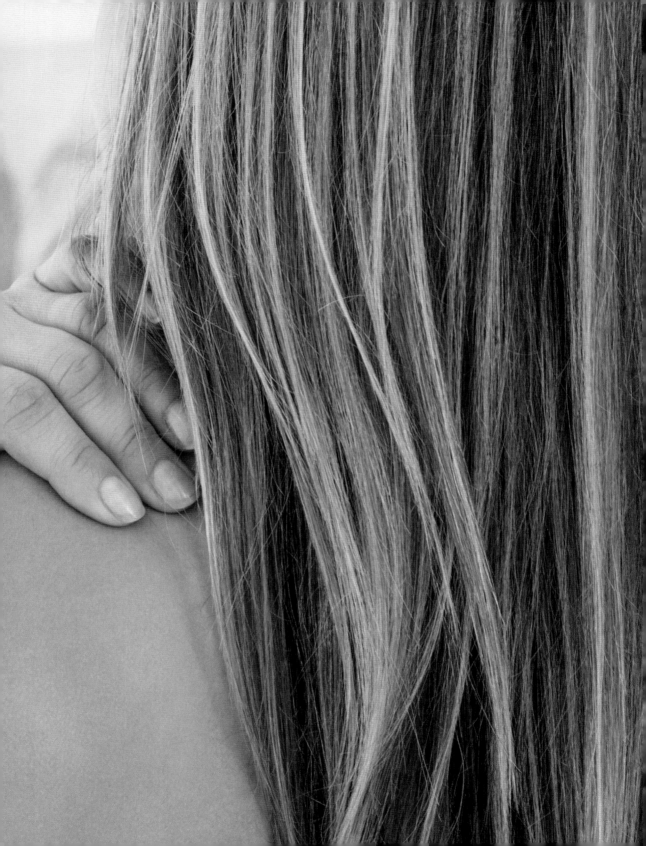

We believe essential oils have the power to change the way you feel. While they are not cure-alls, the use of essential oils through aromatherapy, topical application and internal consumption has a variety of health benefits, providing you with non-invasive home remedies for a multitude of conditions. Even better, they can be used safely in combination with many other therapies.

Some traditional hospitals are catching on to the benefits of essential oils and are using them to aid patients who are being treated for conditions such as anxiety, depression and infections. A 2009 study found that pre-operative patients who received aromatherapy with lavandin oil were significantly less anxious about their surgery than those in the control group. Other oils such as sandalwood, neroli oil and lavender oil have also been used in traditional medicine to help patients better manage anxiety.[1]

Additionally, essential oils have been shown to help patients better manage pain. A 2007 study in the *Journal of Alternative and Complementary Medicine* found that women who used aromatherapy during labor reported less pain overall and were able to use fewer pain medications.[2]

Essential oils can also have anti-bacterial and anti-fungal benefits. When key oils are massaged into the skin, they can promote healing and fight harmful bacteria. Others may help boost the immune system, reduce symptoms of insomnia and aid with digestion.

The power of essential oils rests in their chemical compounds—and in this section, we have detailed the most common conditions from which Americans suffer. For each, we provide you with:

Background: A brief summary of the condition.
Essential Oils: The most effective essential oils for that condition.
Research: Documented research and clinical studies for key uses.
Home Remedy: A DIY remedy to help improve symptoms and promote natural healing.
Suggested Supplements: Two to three recommended supplements to help round out a wellness protocol.

For each oil, we recommend referring to its single oil page in Part II for recommended applications and safety guidelines. If you are taking any prescription medications, please consult with your healthcare practitioner before use.

We hope you will use this section often as a reference guide in your quest for better health and a cleaner lifestyle that most closely resembles the way God intended for us to nourish our bodies inside and out.

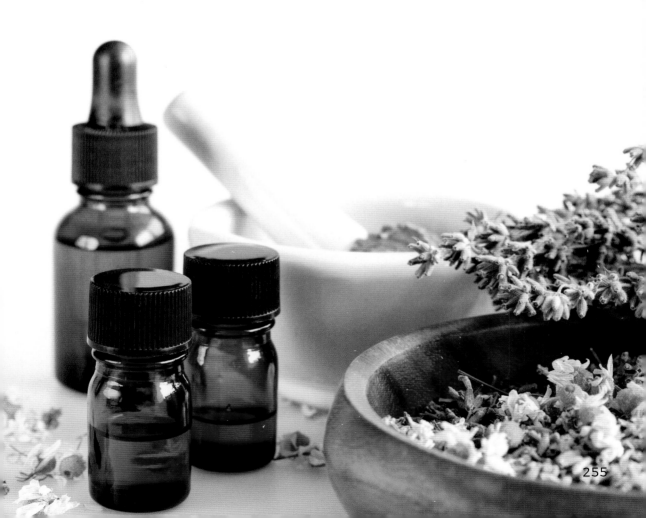

ACID REFLUX

ESSENTIAL OILS

Peppermint. Helps relax the gastrointestinal muscles, allowing painful gas to pass.

Ginger. Can soothe the stomach and help it release its contents into the small intestines.

Fennel. Balances the pH level within the body, especially within the stomach.

Lemon. D-limonene (compound in lemon peels) helps to calm stomach pains and relieve nausea.[3]

Research

A 2015 study evaluated the gastro-protective activity of ginger essential oil in laboratory animals. The ginger essential oil treatment reduced ulcers by 85 percent.[4]

Home Remedy

Reflux ease. Add 1 drop each of peppermint, ginger, fennel and lemon essential oils to a beverage, or mix the oil blend with 1 tablespoon of coconut oil and honey to taste and consume internally.

Background

Between 25 percent and 40 percent of Americans suffer from acid reflux, and an estimated 20 percent of adults experience a more severe form of acid reflux known as gastroesophageal reflux disease (GERD). Despite what we've been told for years, too much stomach acid is not the cause of acid reflux. The primary trigger of heartburn and GERD is acid entering the esophagus because of a leaky valve. Causes of acid reflux include pregnancy, hiatal hernias and an unhealthy diet. Unfortunately, the prescription and OTC drugs that are given for acid reflux do not target the root cause and can have major side effects. Natural acid reflux remedies may help to balance stomach acid and relieve symptoms such as heartburn, gas, bloating, bad breath and sore throat.

Suggested Supplements

» **Digestive enzymes.** Take at the start of each meal to help foods fully digest and nutrients absorb properly.

» **Probiotics.** Reduce levels of bad bacteria and can improve indigestion, leaky gut and acid reflux. Take 25 to 50 billion CFU daily.

ACNE

ESSENTIAL OILS

Melaleuca (Tea Tree). Helps destroy the skin-dwelling bacteria that cause acne.

Holy Basil and Manuka. Ideal for skin care due to their anti-bacterial and anti-microbial properties.

Juniper Berry. A powerful anti-bacterial agent; fights acne yet gentle on the skin.[5]

Lavender. Helps prevent infections, combatting bacteria and fungi. Helps minimize the look of scars.[6]

Research

A 2007 study suggests that tea tree oil is an effective treatment for mild to moderate acne. In regard to overall acne improvement, tea tree oil was 5.8 times more effective than the placebo.[7]

Home Remedy

Acne face wash. Mix 1 tablespoon coconut oil, 3 tablespoons honey, 1 tablespoon apple cider vinegar, 20 drops melaleuca and 2 capsules of probiotics. Pour into a convenient bottle and store in cool, dry place.

Background

Acne is a condition that plagues millions of American children and adults. The main cause of acne is clogged pores that lead to bacteria and yeast overgrowth on the skin. Poor diet, stress and medications such as oral contraceptives and corticosteroids can worsen acne. Other factors such as systemic inflammation, hormone fluctuations and increased cortisol levels can also exacerbate acne. Many patients are unaware that drugs such as tretinoin (the active ingredient in Retin-A) can cause serious side effects, including conjunctivitis, permanently thinned skin, extreme burning and dark circles. We believe it's well worth implementing natural home remedies for acne that tackle the root of the problem and are gentle on the skin.

Suggested Supplements

» **Probiotics.** Support digestion and the immune system, plus improve skin health by fighting acne. Take 25 to 50 billion CFU daily.

» **Zinc.** Promotes immune function and helps balance hormones to improve skin healing.

ADD/ADHD

ESSENTIAL OILS

Vetiver. Inspires a harmonious state while promoting deep concentration.

Cedarwood. May improve focus and clear thinking.

Rosemary. Has been correlated with both improved memory and brain function.

Lavender. May create a calmer mind and more relaxed state.

Research

In 2001, a study found that vetiver oil is effective in helping children with ADHD. After 30 days, vetiver oil was able to double the children's performance levels, helping them to combat ADD and ADHD symptoms such as difficulty concentrating and diminished focus.[9]

Home Remedy

Focus Blend. Combine 1 to 2 drops vetiver with a carrier oil and apply to the wrists or behind the ears. Include ylang ylang and lavender for added calmness and focus.

Background

Everyone can have difficulty sitting still, paying attention or controlling behavior from time to time. For some people, however, the problems are so pervasive that they interfere with every aspect of their life. Attention-deficit/hyperactivity disorder (ADHD) is a behavioral condition affecting 11 percent of school-age children, and symptoms continue into adulthood in more than three-quarters of all cases.[8] It is characterized by difficulty concentrating, impulsiveness and hyperactivity. In ADD, the symptom of hyperactivity is absent. Scientists have discovered genetics may contribute to ADHD. Other contributing factors may include leaky gut syndrome, a high sugar diet, food sensitivities and exposure to toxins such as pesticides or lead.

Suggested Supplements

» **Omega-3.** Significant improvements in reading, spelling and behavior were all noted over the three-month trial using omega-3 fatty acids.[10]

» **B-Complex + Probiotics.** May improve attention and the gut-brain connection.

» **Zinc.** Low levels are associated with poor neurological function, poor attention and a variety of motor disorders.

ADDICTION

ESSENTIAL OILS

Rosemary. Contains mood elevating qualities; helps to reduce stress and anxiety.

Lavender. Shown to have the ability to enhance mood and calm the mind.[12]

Lemon and Bergamot. Enhance mood and increase energy.

Black Pepper and Peppermint. Help relieve discomfort associated with headache, pain and nausea.

Research

A 2006 study found that lemon essential oil had strong anti-stress effects. In the study, laboratory animals were exposed to three stress-inducing behavioral tasks. The results suggested that lemon oil possesses notable antidepressant-like effects.[13]

Home Remedy

Soothing Bath Soak. To help ease the symptoms of withdrawal and curb cravings, add 3 to 5 drops of lavender and rosemary to warm bath water.

Background

People with an addiction have little to no control over what they are doing, taking or using. Addictions can include not only things we consume, such as food, drugs or alcohol, but may include virtually anything, from gambling to psychological dependencies. Recent estimates suggest that as many as 23.5 million Americans are addicted to alcohol or drugs, and one in 20 people have been found to have a food addiction.[11] The causes of addiction vary considerably and are generally caused by a combination of physical, mental, circumstantial and emotional factors. People who are fighting an addiction may often respond well to natural remedies, behavioral modifications, intervention and support from family and friends.

Suggested Supplements

» **GABA.** Helps normalize and restore deficiencies that spur cravings.[14]

» **Probiotics.** Boost your body's ability to extract nutrients from your food, fortify your immune system and manage anxiety, depression and mood.

» **Adaptogenic Herbs.** Ashwagandha, Rhodiola rosea, Reishi and additional adpatogenic herbs help to elevate mood and improve addictive behavior.

ADRENAL FATIGUE

ESSENTIAL OILS

Holy Basil. Helps reduce anxiety; helps regulate serumcortisol levels, which can have systemic impact.[15]

Rosemary. Helps lower cortisol levels. Boosts mood and improves memory.

Clove. A powerful anti-inflammatory agent that can boost energy.

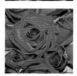

Rose. Shown to promote calm, relaxation and a decrease in blood pressure.

Research

In a 2009 study, the test group receiving rose essential oil rather than a placebo through their skin felt greater feelings of calm and relaxation, as well as a decrease in blood pressure and breathing rate.[16]

 Home Remedy

Warm Adrenal Compress. Dilute 3 to 5 drops of holy basil or rosemary essential oil in a carrier oil and apply it directly to your skin over the kidney area. Then add a warm compress. The oil mixture can also be applied to the reflex points on your feet.

Background

When your brain registers a threat, the body releases adrenaline hormones to help you react (known as the "fight or flight" response). The adrenal cortex then releases corticosteroids to inhibit processes such as digestion, immune system response and other functions not necessary for immediate survival. Adrenal fatigue occurs when the body and adrenal glands can't keep up with the amount of daily stress many people experience, and those "unnecessary functions" become largely neglected for extended periods of time. Most people struggle with adrenal fatigue at some point in their lives. Common symptoms include weight gain, insomnia, reduced sex drive, body aches, trouble concentrating, racing thoughts, irritability, constantly feeling tired, hormone imbalance and food cravings.

Suggested Supplements

» **Ashwagandha.** An adaptogen; especially good at reducing cortisol levels and helping the adrenals adjust to stress.

» **B-Complex.** Vitamin B12 and other B vitamins reduce stress and improve cellular energy.

AGING SKIN

ESSENTIAL OILS

Ylang Ylang. Effective at fighting the development of skin cancer cells and melanoma.[17]

Frankincense. Helps reduce acne blemishes and the appearance of pores, prevent wrinkles and tighten skin.

Lavender. Can help prevent oxidative stress that leads to early aging.

Sandalwood. Helps to soothe, tighten and cleanse the skin. Can reduce inflammation.

Research

Recent studies have shown that frankincense helps tone and lift skin, reduce the appearance of scars and acne and heal wounds. It can also aid in fading stretch marks and surgery scars and in healing dry or cracked skin.[18]

Home Remedy

Anti-Aging Serum. Mix ¼-ounce of jojoba oil, ¼-ounce of evening primrose oil, ¼-ounce of pomegranate oil, 15 drops of vitamin E, 20 drops of lavender or frankincense and 10 drops of carrot seed oil. Place the mixture in a dark glass bottle. Use in the morning and at night on your face and neck.

Background

Many factors cause our skin to age. Some we can influence; others we cannot. Over time, we all get visible lines on our face and notice our skin becoming thinner and drier. Genetics is understood to play a major role in the timing of this process. However, we can have influence over another type of aging, and that is the premature aging caused by environmental factors and lifestyle choices. For example, excessive sugar consumption, stress, toxicity and smoking can lead to an acceleration of the aging process. Even people who already have signs of premature skin aging can benefit from making lifestyle changes and adding certain supplements, including essential oils, to their daily regimen.

Suggested Supplements

» **Green Superfood.** Contains foods high in antioxidant compounds such as chlorella, grass juices, wild berries and herbs that slow aging. Take one scoop daily.

» **Resveratrol.** Shown to reduce cellular damage and slow aging. Take 250 to 500 milligrams daily.

ALLERGIES

ESSENTIAL OILS

Eucalyptus. Aids in clearing the lungs and sinuses.

Peppermint. Unclogs sinuses and soothes scratchy throats.

Ginger. Contains anti-inflammatory properties that may improve symptoms of allergies.

Lemon. Supports lymphatic drainage and rids the body of impurities.

Research

A survey from NYU Medical School discovered that using eucalyptus helped deal with sinusitis. Patients experienced faster improvement whenever supplementing along with eucalyptus oil for allergies and sinus issues.[19]

Home Remedy

Vapor Rub. Pour ¼ cup of olive oil, ½ cup of coconut oil and ¼ cup of grated beeswax into a glass jar. Place a saucepan with 2 inches of water over medium-low heat. Put the jar in the saucepan and allow the oils to melt. Allow it to cool slightly before adding 20 drops each of peppermint and eucalyptus. Pour the mixture into a metal tin and cool before use.

Background

Today, 40 to 60 million Americans are affected by allergies—and the numbers continue to rise, especially in children. Allergies can cause a blocked and runny nose, sneezing, watery eyes, headaches and an impaired sense of smell. For some people, allergies can be life threatening, leading to acute inflammation and shortness of breath. People who suffer from allergies are often told to avoid triggers, but that is nearly impossible when the seasons are changing and our immune systems are impaired by improper diets and environmental toxins. Thankfully, key essential oils serve as a natural and safe way to address the symptoms of allergies and boost our immune systems.

Suggested Supplements

» **Stinging Nettle.** A powerful herb with antihistamine properties.

» **Quercetin.** Shown to reduce symptoms of hay fever and seasonal allergies.

» **Spirulina.** Proven to significantly improve allergy symptoms, including nasal discharge, sneezing, nasal congestion and itching.[20]

ALZHEIMER'S DISEASE

ESSENTIAL OILS

Rosemary. Boosts brain function; promotes the regeneration of neurological tissue.[21]

Frankincense. Helps boost immune function and prevent illness by dangerous pathogens.

Bergamot. Acts as a mood elevating and calming agent.

Lemon. Helps prevent premature aging; improves cellular function.

Research

A recent study found that aromatherapy, particularly the use of rosemary, lavender and citrus, works as an effective non-pharmacological method of therapy for patients with dementia. Patients showed improvement in cognitive function after regular inhalation.[22]

Home Remedy

Daily Brain Boost. Add 1 to 2 drops of lemon essential oil to a glass of water and consume daily. Also, a blend of rosemary and lemon can be diffused or applied topically to your neck.

Background

Alzheimer's disease is an irreversible, progressive brain disorder that slowly destroys memory and other important mental functions. Experts suggest that more than 5 million Americans may have Alzheimer's, with two-thirds of those being women. As this type of dementia progresses, more serious symptoms are experienced, such as mood swings, long-term memory loss, confusion, irritability and aggression. There are several theories to explain the formation of this disease, including free radical damage, an inability to use glucose properly, vitamin deficiencies and environmental toxins. Studies have shown that essential oils may help manage dementia symptoms by supporting brain function and neurological development.

Suggested Supplements

» **Omega-3 Formula High in EPA/DHA.** EPA and DHA are critical for brain function and reducing systemic inflammation.

» **Vitamin D3.** Required for brain function; many of us (especially the elderly) are deficient because of the amount of time spent indoors (5,000 IU recommended daily).

ANXIETY

ESSENTIAL OILS

Lavender. Aids neurological issues such as anxiety, migraines and depression.

Roman Chamomile. May ease feelings of paranoia and aggression.

Vetiver. Used for relaxation; helps to alleviate anxiety, insomnia and depression.

Frankincense. Shown to help reduce heart rate and high blood pressure.

Research

A recent study found that supplementing with lavender essential oil alleviated anxiety, sleep disturbance and depression in participants; lavender oil treatment had no adverse side effects.[23]

Home Remedy

Healing Bath Salts. Combine 3 cups of Epsom salt and 1 cup of baking soda. At bath time, add 1 cup of the dry ingredients and 20 to 30 drops of lavender to warm bath water. Soak for 20 to 30 minutes.

Background

In today's fast-paced, high-pressure society, it's almost impossible not to feel anxious at some point in life. That is why an estimated 40 million American adults are affected by anxiety. For a person with an anxiety disorder, the anxiety does not go away and can get worse over time. These feelings can interfere with daily activities involving his or her job, schoolwork and relationships. Constant anxiety can lead to high blood pressure, insomnia, digestive problems and panic attacks. Some causes include stress, thyroid problems and hormone imbalance, as well as excessive alcohol, caffeine or sugar intake.

Suggested Supplements

» **Ashwagandha.** An adaptogenic herb; shown to improve anxiety symptoms by reducing the effects of stress on the body.[24]

» **Magnesium.** Known as the "relaxation mineral;" reduces tension and calms the nervous system. Take 500 milligrams daily or use magnesium oil topically.

ARTHRITIS

ESSENTIAL OILS

Wintergreen. Acts as a natural analgesic to relieve pain and swelling.

Peppermint. Natural analgesic and muscle relaxant; helps soothe joint discomfort.

Frankincense and Turmeric. Reduce inflammation; help improve circulation.

Ginger. Reduces prostaglandins in the body (compounds associated with pain).[25]

Research
A 2013 study concluded that ginger oil possesses antioxidant activity as well as significant anti-inflammatory and pain-reducing properties.[26]

Home Remedy
Detoxifying Arthritis Bath. Run a warm-water bath and add 2 cups of Epsom salt, plus 20 drops of lavender with 20 drops of peppermint and soak for as long as desired. For added benefit, diffuse frankincense while you are soaking.

Background
It is estimated that more than 52 million people in the U.S. suffer from arthritis symptoms. Arthritis can be defined as inflammation of one or more joints; the types of arthritis range from those related to wear and tear of cartilage (such as osteoarthritis) to those associated with inflammation resulting from an overactive immune system (such as rheumatoid arthritis). Symptoms vary greatly in intensity and include pain and limited function of joints. Essential oils may not only relieve pain but also improve your mood and overall health at the same time.

Suggested Supplements
» **Fish Oil.** An 18-month study showed that taking fish oil "exhibited significant reductions" in arthritis activity.[27] Take 1,000 milligrams of high-quality fish oil daily.

» **Turmeric.** A powerful anti-inflammatory herb; supplement with 1,000 milligrams per day.

ASTHMA

ESSENTIAL OILS

Eucalyptus. Helps open up airways, improving bronchial restriction.

Peppermint. Cleanses the lungs and opens up the bronchial passages.

Thyme. Helps clean lungs for healthier respiratory function.

Ginger. Reduces mucus and inflammation of the respiratory system.

Research

A 2016 study tested one of the main constituents in eucalyptus oil for its anti-inflammatory effects on airway inflammation. The researchers concluded that 1,8-cineole significantly decreases eosinophilic airway inflammation (a main feature of asthma) in laboratory animals.[28]

Home Remedy

Asthma Remedy. Mix 2 drops each of eucalyptus, peppermint, thyme and ginger oil with 1 teaspoon of coconut oil and rub it onto your chest. Take deep, diaphragmatic breaths.

Background

Asthma is a respiratory illness that causes bronchial muscle spasms, swelling of the lung lining, chest tightness, wheezing and increased mucus production, all of which can make it difficult to breathe. Asthma affects more than 22 million people in the U.S. It most often starts in childhood, currently affecting more than 6 million American children. Asthma attacks can be triggered by allergens such as pollen, dust, molds and animal dander. Chemicals, weather changes, exercise, stress and certain medications can also trigger an attack. Asthma medications have a host of side effects—they affect the endocrine system and the immune system and contribute to yeast growth and osteoporosis. For asthma sufferers, essential oils may provide some much-needed relief.

Suggested Supplements

» **Quercetin.** A natural antihistamine and anti-allergenic found in citrus fruits; shown to reduce the severity of exercise-induced asthma.[29]

» **NAC (N-acetyl cysteine).** Helps decrease the severity and frequency of asthma attacks by increasing glutathione and thinning bronchial mucus. Take 200-500 milligrams, two to three times daily.

ATHLETE'S FOOT

ESSENTIAL OILS

Tea Tree. Most effective natural remedy for athlete's foot; fights parasites and fungus.[30]

Oregano. Shows significant anti-bacterial and anti-fungal properties.

Patchouli. Protects cuts or sores on the skin from becoming infected; fights fungus.

Geranium. Helps fight bacterial infections.

Research

A 2013 study found that oregano oil has anti-microbial activity and can be used for the treatment of bacteria, viruses and fungal infections.[31]

Home Remedy

Athlete's Foot Bath. Add 30 drops of tea tree oil to a footbath and soak your feet for 10 minutes. After soaking and thoroughly drying your feet, massage a few drops of the oil directly onto the affected area.

Background

Athlete's foot is a fungal infection that usually begins between the toes. It often occurs in people whose feet have become sweaty while wearing tight-fitting shoes. The infection is contagious and can be spread by contaminated towels, floors or clothing; it can also spread to the toenails, hands, groin and other parts of the body. Some common symptoms of athlete's foot include a scaly rash that can cause itching; burning and stinging; thickened, yellowing toenails; cracking, open flesh; and foot odor. The best way to treat athlete's foot is with an anti-fungal essential oil blend.

Suggested Supplements

» **Garlic.** A compound in garlic known as ajoene is especially effective against the fungus that causes athlete's foot.[32]

» **Grapefruit Seed Oil.** A common remedy for athlete's foot. Spray or apply to your feet and let it fully dry. Can be left on overnight.

AUTISM

ESSENTIAL OILS

Vetiver. Contains relaxing and calming properties; helps with concentration and focus.

Lavender. Calms the mind and body. Can help with neurological issues.

Frankincense. Shown to reduce stress. Helps reduce heart rate and high blood pressure.[33]

Rosemary. Stimulates the senses and supports memory retention.

Research

A recent study found that inhaling rosemary essential oil produced a significant enhancement of performance for overall quality of memory. In addition, inhaling a combination of rosemary and lemon in the morning showed significant improvement in personal orientation.[34]

Home Remedy

Calming and Relaxing Blend. Mix equal parts of vetiver, frankincense, lavender and rosemary. Each morning and evening, inhale for as long as the child is willing. These oils can also be diluted in coconut oil and massaged into the skin.

Background

Autism spectrum disorder (ASD) encompasses a group of complex disorders of brain development. Autism appears to have its roots in very early brain development. However, the most obvious signs of autism and symptoms of autism tend to emerge between two and three years of age. Autism is associated with intellectual disability, motor coordination difficulty, attention issues and physical health issues such as sleep and gastrointestinal disturbances. Most cases of autism appear to be caused by a combination of genetics and environmental factors influencing early brain development.

Suggested Supplements

» **Omega-3.** EPA/DHA found in fish oil are critical for brain function; possesses anti-inflammatory benefits. Supplementation has been shown to reduce symptoms of autism and improve learning.[35]

» **Probiotics.** Can improve leaky gut and nutrient absorption, which may help children who have digestive issues that are affecting the brain.

BACK PAIN

ESSENTIAL OILS

Peppermint and Wintergreen. Cool inflamed joints andreduce back pain.

Frankincense. Improves circulation; helps reduce inflammation associated with back pain.

Cypress. Helps to improve circulation and tissue repair.

Turmeric. Contains anti-inflammatory compounds, which may reduce inflammation.

Research

As a primary source of methyl salicylate, a compound used as an analgesic in over-the-counter dermatological products, wintergreen has the most researched benefits in regard to pain management (for skin and sore muscles).

Home Remedy

Muscle Rub. Pour ½ cup of coconut oil and ¼ cup of grated beeswax into a glass jar. Place the jar in a saucepan with 2 inches of water over medium-low heat. Allow the contents to melt. Add 2 teaspoons of either cayenne powder or turmeric powder. Once combined, allow it to cool slightly and add 15 drops each of peppermint oil and lavender oil. Mix well and allow it to set.

Background

Back pain can range from a dull, constant ache to a sudden, sharp pain. While anyone can have back pain, factors that increase your risk are age, poor physical fitness, being overweight, heredity, your job, pregnancy and chronic conditions such as arthritis. Low back pain can also be a warning sign of spinal abnormalities or a result of poor posture. The most common treatments for back pain are NSAIDS, such as aspirin and acetaminophen, along with more potent prescription pain medications. These drugs can have adverse side effects and have been linked to liver damage and intestinal bleeding.[36]

Suggested Supplements

» **Fish Oil.** Contains omega-3 fats, which help reduce inflammation in the body.

» **Bone Broth Protein Powder and Collagen.** Contain amino acids, including proline and glycine, as well as glucosamine and chondroitin, which support joint and tissue repair.

BLOATING

ESSENTIAL OILS

Peppermint. Can reduce gas in the GI tract and improve digestion.

Juniper Berry. A natural diuretic that helps the body to flush out excess fluids.

Ginger and Fennel. Help relieve bloating, gassiness and indigestion.

Roman Chamomile. Has a relaxing effect on the gut; acts as an anti-inflammatory agent.

Research

A 2007 study demonstrated the benefits of juniper berry essential oil to digestive health. Researchers found that cows given daily juniper and garlic experienced general improved digestion, possibly due to changes in the way protein was broken down.[39]

 Home Remedy

Bloat-Busting Pre-Meal Routine. Add 1 drop of peppermint oil to a glass of water before meals. You may also add 1 to 2 drops each of peppermint oil and ginger oil to a spoonful of coconut oil and consume before meals.

Background

Abdominal bloating, which is the feeling of increased pressure within the gut, is so common these days that it's been called an "epidemic." Causes of bloating are extensive and include overeating, eating too quickly, allergies, hormonal imbalances, thyroid dysfunction, gut troubles and more.[38] Because so many different factors can contribute to bloating—including some that seem totally unrelated, such as a lack of sleep or excessive stress—it's possible to become bloated any time of the day or month.

Suggested Supplements

» **Probiotics.** Good bacteria act like friendly gut bugs in your digestive tract, reducing gas and promoting proper digestion.

» **Digestive Enzymes.** Help break down hard-to-digest proteins and starches that cause gas and bloating.

BODY ODOR

ESSENTIAL OILS

Tea Tree. Has properties that destroy odor-causing bacteria on skin.

Lemongrass. Acts as a safe, natural deodorizer.

Patchouli. Can be used to naturally mask body odor.

Bergamot. Prevents the growth of germs that cause body odor.

Research

A 2006 report stated that tea tree oil contains active ingredients that significantly reduce harmful bacteria that grow on skin.[41]

Home Remedy

DIY Deodorant. Mix ½ cup of coconut oil and ½ cup of baking soda in a bowl. Add in 40 to 60 drops of essential oils and store in a deodorant container. Recommendations for women: lavender, jasmine, lemon and sage. Recommendations for men: sandalwood, cypress, bergamot and rosemary.

Background

Although sweat itself is fairly odorless when skin is clean, once the bacteria that live on skin mixes with sweat, they multiply and begin to leave an unpleasant odor. The sweatiest areas are usually the smelliest, including armpits, back, chest, feet and between the legs. That's because these areas tend to have more sweat-producing follicles and are also dark, warm, moist environments that nurture bacteria. Human body odors change throughout the life cycle, as does someone's ability to detoxify through their pores. So, unless you are part of the lucky 2 percent of people who carry an unusual form of a specific gene that means their underarms never smell, you need the help of natural remedies to keep odor at bay.[40]

Suggested Supplements

» **Super Greens.** Take one scoop of an organic greens formula with sea vegetables, grass juices, vegetables and herbs, all of which help alkalize the body.

» **Soil-Based Probiotics.** Good bacteria such as bacillus subtilis may help clear the digestive tract of odor-causing yeasts (candida) and pathogenic bacteria from the body.

BRONCHITIS

ESSENTIAL OILS

Oregano. Helps fight inflammation, viruses and respiratory infections.[42]

Eucalyptus. Works as an expectorant; helps cleanse the body of toxins and harmful microorganisms.

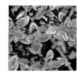

Peppermint. Clears the respiratory tract, unclogs the sinuses and offers relief for a scratchy throat.

Thyme. Supports draining and cleansing of the respiratory and lymphatic systems.

Research

A 2009 study reported that the cineole commonly found in eucalyptus essential oil reduces respiratory exacerbations and improves lung function and health status. This study further suggests cineole to be an active controller of airway inflammation in COPD.[43]

 ### Home Remedy

Respiratory Ease. Make a steam bath by adding 4 drops each of eucalyptus, peppermint and thyme oils to boiling water, placing a towel over your head and inhaling deeply for 5 to 10 minutes.

Background

Bronchitis is an inflammation of the mucous membrane in the bronchial tubes that typically causes bronchospasms and coughing. It often develops after another type of upper respiratory infection such as a cold or flu and can affect any age group. Antibiotics are the most common form of treatment, but conventional medications can lead to damaging side effects such as digestive issues. In cases of acute bronchitis, conventional antibiotics are of little value, as the root cause is viral.

Some people develop chronic bronchitis—a form of chronic obstructive pulmonary disease, or COPD—which is primarily caused by cigarette smoking or environmental irritants. More than 8 million people are diagnosed with chronic bronchitis each year.

Suggested Supplements

» **Echinacea.** Boosts immune system function. Also try a formulation that includes goldenseal.

» **Vitamin C + NAC (N-Acetyl-Cysteine).** A combo that naturally supports the immune system and can help improve respiratory pathways.

CONDITIONS

BRUISING

 ## ESSENTIAL OILS

 Geranium. Helps increase blood circulation below the surface of the skin.

 Helichrysum. A skin soother, dark-spot remover and pain reducer.

 Frankincense and Cypress. Contain compounds that can reduce the appearance of bruising.[44]

 Lavender. Helps cells repair themselves and supports tissue health.

 ## Research

A 2016 study demonstrated that topical application of lavender oil promoted collagen synthesis and has the potential to promote external wound healing.[45]

 ## Home Remedy

Bruise Balm. Combine 10 drops of geranium and 10 drops of helichrysum with ¼ cup of coconut oil, and apply it directly to the bruise to encourage circulation and promote healing.

Background

A bruise is an injury appearing as an area of discolored skin on the body, caused by a blow or impact rupturing underlying blood vessels. Bruises can also be caused by nutrient deficiencies, insufficient blood clotting factors and serious illnesses such as leukemia. They can occur at any age. Symptoms of the bruise vary depending on the cause. Discoloration of the skin is often the first sign. Some bruises appear with very little pain, and you might not notice them. You may also experience pain and tenderness in the area of bruising. These symptoms generally improve as the bruise heals.

Suggested Supplements

» **Bromelain.** An enzyme found in pineapple that reduces swelling. Take 500 milligrams three times daily.

» **Vitamin C.** An antioxidant that helps manufacture collagen, which is critical for healing damaged blood vessels. Take 500 to 1,000 milligrams daily.

BUG BITES

ESSENTIAL OILS

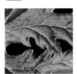
Citronella. Acts as an all-natural bug repellant.

Lemongrass. Repels bugs such as mosquitoes because of its high citral and geraniol content.

Lavender. Feels soothing when applied directly to the skin; can help speed up the healing process.

Holy Basil. Has wound healing abilities, largely due to the presence of eugenol.[46]

Research

A 2016 study tested the effects of the oils of certain plants against mosquito bites. The oils of citrus leaves, citrus fruit peel and Alpinia galanga (rhizome) were used to create a lotion and compared against commercial repellants. The essential oil-based lotions revealed an impressive 90 percent protection against mosquito bites for four hours.[47]

Home Remedy

Bug Spray. Mix ½ cup of witch hazel, ½ cup of apple cider vinegar and 40 drops of essential oils (a mix of citronella, eucalyptus, lemongrass and tea tree) in a spray bottle. Spray your body, avoiding your eyes and mouth.

Background

Many insects and spiders bite or sting, and while the bites of common bugs such as mosquitoes, mites and fleas are itchy and uncomfortable, they're usually harmless. But some bites and stings, such as those from fire ants, wasps, hornets and bees, may cause intense pain or even an allergic reaction. Others, such as poisonous spider bites, may require immediate emergency medical care. Certain oils have the power to soothe the skin and fight possible infections from insects. Essential oils can also ward off bugs; use them to make a homemade bug spray—they will help to fight bacteria and nourish the skin, too.

Suggested Supplements

» **Witch Hazel.** Can help reduce the pain, annoying itching and swelling associated with bug bites; may speed up the healing process.

» **Colloidal Silver + Oatmeal Bath.** Soothes the itching caused by mosquito bites; reduces swelling from bites.

BURNS

ESSENTIAL OILS

Lavender. Naturally soothes burns; helps to calm and disinfect an inflamed injury site.[48]

Tea Tree and Manuka. Help reduce the risk of infection and soothe skin.

Peppermint. Helps reduce pain and improve burns by soothing inflammation.

Frankincense. Helps reduce scarring and inflammation.[49]

Research
A 2015 study reported that the inclusion of tea tree oil in burn treatment reduced the edema resulting from UVB exposure. This represents a promising approach to topical treatment of inflammatory disorders and wound healing.[50]

Home Remedy
Burn Salve. Mix 2 ounces of raw honey, 2 tablespoons of extra-virgin olive oil and 20 drops of lavender oil in a glass jar, and spread the mixture over the burn or wound generously. Cover the injury site with a dressing or adhesive bandage.

Background
Burns occur from exposure to heat, steam, hot liquids, chemicals or the sun. The correct treatment depends on the severity of the burn. Severe burns can destroy all layers of skin and even damage muscles and underlying fat; these kinds of burns need immediate medical attention. Natural therapies can help with healing wounds and decreasing pain associated with burns. Certain natural remedies may also reduce the risk of infection and help areas heal without scarring.

Suggested Supplements
» **Aloe Vera.** Look for a gel that is at least 99 percent pure, or better yet, use fresh aloe from a plant to stimulate healing. Apply it to your skin twice daily.

» **Vitamin E.** An important antioxidant for repairing tissue and healing burns. Take 400 IU daily or use it as a topical gel.

CANCER

ESSENTIAL OILS

Frankincense. Able to cross the blood-brain barrier, unlike chemotherapy chemicals.[51]

Myrrh. Exhibits inhibitory effects on cancer cell growth.[52]

Orange. Primary compound limonene shown to display chemo-preventive properties.[53]

Turmeric. Contains turmerone, which may help fight breast cancer, colon cancer and leukemia. [54] [55]

Research

Researchers from Oxford University discovered turmerone, the active principle of turmeric oil, might help fight colon cancer. In the study, it was found that taking curcumin and turmerone together was more effective at fighting cancer than taking curcumin alone.[56]

Home Remedy

Triple Cancer Threat. Take 2 drops of frankincense, 1 drop of myrrh and 1 drop of turmeric oil internally three times daily, and use these oils topically or diffuse them as a beneficial support to a cancer protocol.

Background

Cancer refers to uncontrolled cell division or abnormal cell growth. Each year 12.7 million people discover they have cancer, and 7.6 million people die from the disease, making it the second most prevalent cause of death in America. There are many possible causes for cancer, including environmental toxins, poor diet, genetics, viruses, infections, stress, poor digestion and lack of exercise. Today, most people turn to conventional treatments such as surgery, chemotherapy, radiation or other drugs that can have serious side effects. There is a large body of evidence that certain foods, herbs and remedies can effectively support cancer treatment without adverse reactions.

Suggested Supplements

» **Greens Powder.** Green superfood powders containing chlorella, spirulina, juiced grasses, vegetables and berries can help provide critical nutrients and antioxidants for healing.

» **Proteolytic Enzymes.** Bromelain and papain have been shown to have a powerful anti-cancer effect.

CANDIDA

ESSENTIAL OILS

Clove. Proven as effective as nystatin, a drug prescribed to manage yeast infections.[57]

Oregano. Acts quickly to combat fungi, bacteria and viruses within the body.[58]

Cinnamon. One of the top oils for fighting harmful fungi and bacteria.[59]

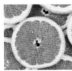

Grapefruit. Contains d-limonene, which can help dry up excess dampness in the body.

Research
A 2005 study observed that clove was as effective as nystatin, which is a drug commonly prescribed to manage yeast infections of the mouth (thrush) that includes a slew of harmful side effects.[60]

Home Remedy
Candida Cleanse. Add 1 drop of clove oil to a smoothie for two weeks under the care of a physician or nutritionist; also, eliminate all sugar and grains during this time and consume a diet consisting of probiotic fermented foods, bone broth, cooked vegetables and organic meat.

Background
Candida is a yeast that aids with nutrient absorption and digestion when produced in proper levels in the body; however, if the body's natural pH balance is upset, candida can quickly grow out of control. With approximately 460,000 cases each year, candida (or candidiasis) is a common yeast infection that can lead to many health problems, from a sore throat to serious stomach conditions. Common causes of candida overgrowth include taking antibiotics, birth control pills and oral corticosteroids; excess sugar consumption; and experiencing too much internal dampness. Candida can cause a white coating on the tongue, headaches, an inability to concentrate, chronic fatigue, sugar cravings and stomach issues. Oral thrush is a yeast infection caused by the same strain of candida that affects other mucous membranes, including the vagina.

Suggested Supplements

» **Pau D'arco.** An herb traditionally used to eliminate candida from the body. Consume 1 cup of tea or supplement two to three times daily.

» **Probiotics.** Help clear candida and bad bacteria from the body. Take 50 billion CFU twice daily.

CARPAL TUNNEL SYNDROME

 ## ESSENTIAL OILS

Wintergreen and Peppermint. Can reduce inflammation and pain.

Cypress. Improves circulation and reduces swelling.

Helichrysum. May decrease pain; supports nerve tissue repair.

Frankincense. Known to reduce inflammation, which may help ease pain.[61]

 ### Research

According to a 2015 study, the anti-inflammatory response of methyl salicylate (active ingredient in wintergreen oil) is comparable to that of a commonly prescribed NSAID (anti-inflammatory) drug known as fenoprofen.[62]

 ### Home Remedy

Apply a mixture of 1 to 2 drops each of wintergreen, cypress and helichrysum topically to the affected area three times daily. You can also add the oils to a warm-water bath.

Background

Carpal tunnel syndrome is a painful progressive condition caused by compression of the median nerve in the wrist. It is extremely common, affecting up to 6 percent of adults in the U.S. The carpal tunnel, which houses the median nerve, can become thickened and cause the nerve to be compressed. The result may be pain, weakness or numbness in the hand and wrist, radiating up the arm. Women are three times more likely than men to develop carpal tunnel syndrome, perhaps because the carpal tunnel itself may be smaller in women. Other contributing factors include trauma or injury to the wrist that cause swelling, such as sprain or fracture, hypothyroidism, arthritis, work stress, repeated use of vibrating hand tools or fluid retention during pregnancy or menopause.

Suggested Supplements

» **Vitamin B6.** Reduces nerve inflammation. Take 100 milligrams three times daily.

» **Bromelain.** An enzyme found in pineapple; has a natural anti-inflammatory effect. Take 500 milligrams three times between meals.

CHICKENPOX

ESSENTIAL OILS

Lavender. Speeds healing of blisters and scabs; soothes skin and relieves itchiness and irritation.

Manuka. Soothes the skin and has anti-viral benefits to fight off infections of all kinds.

Tea Tree. Helps to relieve skin inflammation. Fights bad bacteria and infections.

Roman Chamomile. Promotes healthy skin and relieves irritations. Can penetrate below the skin surface.[63]

Research
A 2016 study indicated that a topical application of lavender oil promoted collagen synthesis and encouraged skin healing. It concluded that the beneficial effect of lavender oil on wound healing raises the possibility of new approaches to wound treatment.[64]

Home Remedy
Pox Ease. Mix equal parts of lavender, tea tree, lemon and oregano oils (diluted with coconut oil). Soak a cotton swab with the mixture and apply it three times per day. Use an immune-building blend with these oils and apply along your spine and the soles of your feet.

Background
Chickenpox is a viral infection that causes an itchy, blister-like rash. It can be contagious to people who haven't had the disease or haven't been vaccinated against it. For most people, chickenpox is a mild disease; the infection usually lasts about five to seven days. Common signs and symptoms of chickenpox include a rash, fever, loss of appetite, headache and tiredness. Once the chickenpox rash appears, it will go through three phases: raised pink or red bumps, fluid-filled blisters that will break and leak after a day and finally, crusts and scabs that take several days to heal.

Suggested Supplements

» **Elderberry.** Promotes the production of cytokines, which are the body's cellular messengers that keep the immune system healthy.

» **Probiotics.** Boosts the immune system (80 percent of your immune system function is located in your digestive tract).

CHOLESTEROL

ESSENTIAL OILS

Lavender. Shown to decrease emotional stress, which can lower cholesterol levels.

Lemongrass. Shown to sustain healthy levels of triglycerides and reduce LDL cholesterol.[65]

Rosemary. Helps reduce cholesterol due to antioxidant properties.

Cypress. Boosts circulatory function.

Research

According to a recent study, lavender oil treatment exerted hypolipidemic (lipid or fat lowering) effects by balancing LDL/HDL levels.[66]

 ### Home Remedy

Cholesterol Protocol. Take 1 drop of lemongrass oil and 1 drop of rosemary oil in a teaspoon of honey. Follow up by applying 1 to 2 drops each of cypress oil and lavender oil mixed with a carrier oil to the liver area and the soles of your feet.

Background

Cholesterol is a naturally occurring substance made by the liver and required by the body for the proper function of cells, nerves and hormones. Normally, cholesterol is kept in balance, but the standard western diet contains a large amount of hydrogenated fats and refined carbohydrates, which leads to an upset in this balance. This is manifested in elevated LDL levels and low HDL levels, an imbalance that affects 102 million Americans. Over time, LDL cholesterol can oxidize and build up in the arteries and lead to serious health problems, such as heart attack or stroke. To address this, millions of cholesterol-lowering prescriptions are written each year (statins are the most common), many of which can cause cramping, constipation, liver problems and more.

Suggested Supplements

» **CoQ10.** Take 200-300 milligrams of CoQ10 daily if you're on cholesterol-lowering medications, because these medications decrease levels of this important co-enzyme.

» **Omega-3.** Take 1,000 milligrams of an omega-3 fish oil supplement once or twice daily to support healthy cholesterol levels.

CHRONIC FATIGUE SYNDROME

ESSENTIAL OILS

Holy Basil. An adaptogen that improves energy and reduces stress.

Roman Chamomile. Ideal for fighting stress and insomnia.

Lavender and Ylang Ylang. Relax the mind and body; increase circulation.

Rosemary. May improve energy by decreasing inflammation and supporting brain health.

Research

A study conducted on college students found that using lavender oil improved overall quality of sleep by 60 percent. This included length of sleep, time it took to fall asleep and restfulness.[67]

Home Remedy

Healing Bath Salts. Mix 3 cups of Epsom salt and 1 cup of baking soda. At bath time, add 1 cup of the dry ingredients and 40 drops of the essential oil of your choice to your bath (as warm as you can stand). Soak for 20 to 40 minutes.

Background

Chronic fatigue syndrome (CFS) is an illness characterized by extreme fatigue that lasts for more than six months. One of the disease's challenges is that it's impossible to diagnose with lab tests alone. However, some experts believe it is closely related to adrenal fatigue or system-wide inflammation of the body. Over a million Americans are suffering from this debilitating illness that manifests with a lack of energy and motivation, and women are two to four times more likely than men to be diagnosed. When left untreated, it decreases stamina, memory, concentration and overall quality of life. People who suffer from CFS must do their best to manage stress and get plenty of rest—and essential oils can help with that.

Suggested Supplements

» **B-Complex Vitamins.** B-vitamins, especially B12, boost energy and improve mood.

» **Magnesium and Potassium.** Symptoms of a potassium deficiency include the common CFS symptoms; CFS patients commonly have low magnesium levels.[68]

COLIC

ESSENTIAL OILS

Fennel. Contains mild laxative-like effects.[69]

Peppermint. Gives a cooling sensation and has a calming effect on the body.

Chamomile (German or Roman). Slight muscle relaxant with mild sedative properties.[70]

Ginger. Known to help ease stomach and digestive issues.

Research

Researchers found that fennel seed oil can reduce pain and increase motility in the small intestine, making it an excellent natural remedy for colic.[71]

Home Remedy

Colic Tummy Rub. Mix 1 to 2 drops of fennel, peppermint and chamomile with a carrier oil, and apply the mixture to the infant's stomach with gentle circular rubbing.

Background

Colic is not a disease but a combination of baffling behaviors in an otherwise healthy baby. Occurring in one out of five infants, the true definition of colic follows the "rule of three:" The baby's crying starts at around three weeks old, lasts more than three hours at a stretch, occurs at least three days a week and persists for at least three weeks in a row. It usually starts a few weeks after birth and often improves by the age of three months. Underlying causes of colic are not fully understood, but some experts believe colic manifests due to an immature digestive system, infant acid reflux, food allergies or sensitivity or tobacco exposure. It is generally less common in breastfed babies.

Suggested Supplements

» **Infant Probiotic.** Can help the baby break down hard-to-digest food.

» **Natural Formula.** If you use formula, switch to a goat- or coconut-based blend, or try a predigested organic milk protein formula.

COMMON COLD

ESSENTIAL OILS

Thyme. Helps drain congestion; proven to fight infections and rid the body of toxins.[73]

Lemon. Can support lymphatic drainage and help to overcome a cold quickly.

Ginger. Relieves discomfort caused by congestion and infections.

Eucalyptus and Peppermint. Work as expectorants and help cleanse the body.

Research

According to a 2002 study, d-limonene (a primary compound found in lemon oil) directly activates the immune response of alveolar phagocytes. Phagocytes are cells that protect the body by ingesting harmful foreign particles, bacteria and dead or dying cells.[74]

Home Remedy

Steam Bath. Make a steam bath by mixing 10 drops each of eucalyptus oil and peppermint oil, placing a towel over your head and inhaling deeply for 5 to 10 minutes.

Background

According to estimates, adults and children in the U.S. get 1 billion colds each year. There are over 200 viruses that can cause a cold. Cold viruses take up residence in the lining of the nose and grow, eventually attempting to infect the body. If the body is weak or unable to resist the germs, it will get sick. Despite what some people think, there's no evidence that cold weather, large tonsils or other such wives' tales can make you "catch" a cold.[72] Evidence does suggest that stress and allergies can increase your chances of getting a cold. Colds generally last from about two days to two weeks. Some common symptoms of a cold include runny or stuffy nose, low-grade fever, sore throat, cough and body aches.

Suggested Supplements

» **Echinacea and Elderberry.** Act as anti-inflammatories, helping reduce symptoms of cold and flu.

» **Garlic.** Some studies suggest supplementing with garlic will lead to fewer colds and faster recovery.[75]

CONSTIPATION

ESSENTIAL OILS

Peppermint. Proven to reduce symptoms of IBS, including constipation.

Fennel. Soothes the digestive tract and reduces stress, which can support the colon.

Ginger. Relaxes the smooth muscles in the gut lining and helps food move along.[77]

Marjoram. Relaxes the digestive system with its sedative properties.

Research
A 2007 study used peppermint oil to treat irritable bowel syndrome. After four weeks of peppermint oil therapy, patients reported a 50 percent reduction in symptoms, including abdominal bloating, abdominal discomfort, diarrhea, constipation and pain during elimination.[78]

Home Remedy
Constipation Ease Blend. Take 1 to 2 drops each of fennel oil, peppermint oil and ginger oil in a spoonful of honey or applesauce just before meals.

Background
Constipation is slower than normal movement of food waste through the digestive tract. This slow movement leads to difficulty in emptying the bowels, usually associated with hardened feces. Estimates suggest that as many as 63 million people suffer from constipation in the U.S.[76] It is often accompanied by symptoms such as bloating, gas, back pain, hemorrhoids or fatigue. The main cause stems from a lack of water, healthy fats, probiotics and fiber in the diet. Stress, inactivity, certain medications, an imbalance in intestinal flora, thyroid problems and a magnesium deficiency can also cause constipation. For some people, being constipated is just the prelude to other major health problems. Lifestyle choices are key—move more, drink more, eat clean and take the right supplements, including essential oils.

Suggested Supplements
» **Magnesium.** Improves gut motility.

» **Chia and Flax Seeds.** High in fiber and healthy fats; help to lubricate the colon.

» **Probiotics.** Support normal levels of flora that may improve constipation.

COUGH

ESSENTIAL OILS

Peppermint. Helps open the airways. Can relieve pain associated with a sore throat.

Eucalyptus. Shown to cleanse the body of toxins and harmful microorganisms.[79]

Lemon and Orange. Encourage lymphatic drainage and boost the immune system.

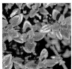
Thyme. Thins mucus and naturally supports the immune system.

Research

According to studies, menthol, the primary constituent in peppermint oil, suppresses a cough evoked in the lower airways primarily through a reflex initiated from the nose.[80]

Home Remedy

Cough Syrup. Add 1 drop each of lemon oil, frankincense oil, peppermint oil and Roman chamomile oil to a spoonful of honey and take as needed.

Background

Coughing is a common reaction of the respiratory system trying to expel harmful microbes, dust or irritants. As mucus or other substances accumulate in the airways, this reflexive action attempts to facilitate unobstructed breathing. A cough can be nothing more than the body's natural reaction to an irritant, or it can be a symptom of an underlying illness or even lung cancer. Coughing is generally caused by an infection (such as upper respiratory infections, sinus infections and pneumonia) but may also have noninfectious causes (such as asthma, allergies, GERD and chronic bronchitis). Essential oils are widely known to provide relief for stubborn coughs.

Suggested Supplements

» **Vitamin C.** Helps with immune system function and boosts white blood cells.

» **Echinacea.** Can help fight off colds; best taken at the first sign of illness.

CUTS AND SCRAPES

 ## ESSENTIAL OILS

 Oregano. Has proven and powerful anti-microbial capabilities.[81]

 Cedarwood. Defends the body against bacteria.

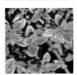 **Tea Tree and Manuka.** Destroys parasites and fungi.

 Thyme. Controls infections on the skin and within the body.[82]

Research

In clinical studies, plant-derived active biomolecules found in thyme and tea tree oil exhibit powerful antioxidant, anti-microbial and anti-inflammatory attributes that can be useful for wound care.[83]

 ## Home Remedy

Cut and Scrape Care. Clean out the damaged area with water and a clean towel. If dirt is present, use hydrogen peroxide. Once it's clean and dry, apply 2 to 3 drops of anti-bacterial essential oils and cover with a bandage. Apply a new covering and additional oils daily to keep the area from getting infected until it's completely healed.

Background

Cuts and scrapes can be caused by various types of injuries. Most cuts or scrapes are harmless and improve after a few days, but sometimes they can become infected, which is why it's important to take immediate and decisive steps to promote natural healing. Minor cuts and scrapes usually don't require a trip to the emergency room, but it's important to follow some basic guidelines for caring for minor skin wounds, such as washing your hands, stopping the bleeding if necessary with gentle pressure, cleaning the wound and then applying essential oils with natural anti-bacterial properties.

Suggested Supplements

» **Bromelain.** An enzyme found in pineapple that reduces swelling; take 500 milligrams, three times daily.

» **Vitamin C.** A powerful antioxidant that helps manufacture collagen, critical for healing damaged blood vessels; take 500-1000 milligrams daily.

DENTAL HEALTH

ESSENTIAL OILS

Thyme. Helps destroy oral germs; can be a remedy for gum disease.

Clove. Helps relieve oral pain and discomfort.

Peppermint. Has performed better than mouthwash for reducing cavities.[84]

Myrrh. Has properties that may improve gum disease.

Research

A study found that clove essential oil had the same numbing effect as benzocaine, a topical agent commonly used before needle insertion. Use with teething infants by mixing it with coconut oil and rubbing it on the gums.[85]

Home Remedy

Homemade Mouthwash. Add 5 drops each of peppermint oil and tea tree oil to 2 cups of spring water. Mix it together in a BPA-free plastic dispenser bottle. Sip and swish around in your mouth, gargle for 30 seconds and spit out. Do not swallow.

Background

Oral health touches every aspect of our lives but is often taken for granted. One common oral concern is tooth decay, which occurs when foods containing carbohydrates such as milk, soda, cakes and candy are frequently left on the teeth. Bacteria that live in the mouth thrive on these foods and produce acids as a result. Over time, these acids destroy tooth enamel, resulting in tooth decay and other dental concerns. Over 90 percent of adults ages 20 to 64 have had tooth decay. Some common causes of dental issues include lack of good oral hygiene habits, consumption of processed sugar, a lack of fat-soluble vitamins (A, D, E, K) and a deficiency in minerals such as calcium, magnesium and phosphorus. Essential oils can present some safe, effective options for great oral care.

Suggested Supplements

» **Coconut Oil.** Try a technique called oil pulling for oral detoxification. Swish a tablespoon of coconut oil in your mouth for 20 minutes and then spit out, rinse and brush your teeth.

» **Vitamins D3 and K2, and Magnesium.** Consider taking these vitamins and minerals essential for building strong teeth and bones.

DEPRESSION

ESSENTIAL OILS

Bergamot. Can create feelings of joy and energy by improving circulation of the blood.[86]

Ylang Ylang. Acts as a mild sedative and can lower stress responses.

Lavender. Known to aid neurological conditions, including depression and anxiety.

Roman Chamomile. Inhaling it may help lessen anxiety and general depression.

Research

A 2012 study took 28 high-risk postpartum women and found that after a four-week treatment plan of lavender aromatherapy, they had a significant reduction of postnatal depression and reduced anxiety disorder.[87]

Home Remedy

Invigorating Inhalation. Rub 1 drop each of bergamot oil, lavender oil and ylang ylang oil into your hands and cup your mouth and nose. Breathe in the oil slowly. Also try rubbing the oils on your feet and stomach.

Background

Depression is a common but serious mood disorder caused by changes in brain chemistry. It affects approximately 14.8 million American adults. Depression causes severe symptoms that affect how you feel, think and handle daily activities. Symptoms include fatigue, sadness, low sex drive, lack of appetite, feelings of helplessness and disinterest in common activities. Research indicates that other factors contribute to the onset of depression, including genetics, changes in hormone levels, certain medical conditions, stress, grief or difficult life circumstances. Antidepressant medications have serious side effects that can include suicidal thoughts, weight gain and personality changes; what's worse, studies have shown that antidepressants fail to cure the symptoms of major depression in half of all treated patients.

Suggested Supplements

» **Fish Oil.** High in EPA, which is critical for neurotransmitter function—an important component in emotional and physiological brain balance.

» **Vitamin D3.** Helps improve seasonal affective disorder (may manifest as depression).

DIABETES

ESSENTIAL OILS

Cinnamon. Helps lower blood sugar levels; can improve sensitivity to insulin.

Coriander. Works with your liver to help balance blood sugar levels.

Ginger. Contains compounds that may help support insulin response.

Lavender. Reduces stress and supports cortisol levels.

Research

A 2009 study concluded that cinnamon is a viable anti-diabetic therapy, as it possesses anti-hyperglycaemic properties and the potential to reduce postprandial blood glucose levels.[88]

Home Remedy

Diabetes Foot Rub. Take 2 drops of both coriander oil and cinnamon oil with one teaspoon of coconut oil. Vigorously rub the mixture on the soles of your feet to support healthy blood glucose levels. Alternatively, add 1 drop of cinnamon oil to a smoothie or coconut oil and take with meals.

Background

Diabetes has grown to "epidemic" proportions since the latest statistics state that 25.8 million Americans are diabetic or pre-diabetic. It is also the seventh leading cause of death in America. Type 1 diabetes is an autoimmune disease where the immune system attacks the insulin-producing cells in the pancreas. Some of the causes that trigger this response may include exposure to a virus, genetically modified organisms (GMOs), heavy metals, vaccines or foods such as wheat, milk and soy. Type 2 diabetes is the most common form of diabetes and is caused by insulin resistance; it is generally caused by genetics and unhealthy lifestyle habits. The most common complications from diabetes include high blood pressure, blindness, kidney disease, neuropathy, Alzheimer's disease and in extreme cases, amputations. With the right diet and supplementation, type 2 diabetes is reversible; and essential oils can support the fight to reverse this terrible disease.

Suggested Supplements

» **Chromium.** Can decrease cholesterol levels in individuals being treated for type 2 diabetes. Take 200 micrograms, one to three times daily with meals.[89]

» **Fish Oil.** Omega-3 fatty acids from fish oil can help lower triglycerides and apoproteins (markers of diabetes) as well as raise HDL.[90]

DIARRHEA

ESSENTIAL OILS

Peppermint. Can help soothe the digestive tract.

Ginger. Contains compounds that may improve digestive function.[91]

Roman Chamomile. Soothes digestive distress and calms emotional stress.

Turmeric. Reduces inflammation and supports a healthy digestive system.

Research

Peppermint oil taken internally has been proven to be effective at naturally relieving symptoms of IBS that can include diarrhea. One study found a 50 percent reduction of IBS symptoms in 75 percent of patients who used it.[92]

 ### Home Remedy

Stomach Ease. Mix 2 to 3 drops each of ginger oil, Roman chamomile oil and peppermint oil with equal parts carrier oil and rub the mixture onto your abdomen. Additionally, take 1 to 2 drops of peppermint oil with honey internally to improve diarrhea.

Background

Diarrhea is a natural reaction to toxins that need to be expelled from the digestive system. When you have diarrhea, your bowel movements (stools) are loose and watery. It's incredibly common and although it feels bad, it's usually not serious. For many people, diarrhea strikes once or twice each year. If you have certain conditions, such as irritable bowel syndrome (IBS), it can happen more often. Diarrhea can have a variety of causes, including food allergies, infections, emotional stress or autoimmune diseases such as Crohn's. Symptoms of diarrhea include an urgent feeling that you need to go to the bathroom, bloating, cramps and thin, loose or watery stools. Chronic diarrhea is problematic and can lead to dehydration and nutrient deficiencies.

Suggested Supplements

» **Probiotics.** Help fight infection and can help re-colonize the gut with healthy bacteria.

» **Bentonite Clay.** Helps to absorb toxins and bind water within the intestines to slow down bowel movements.

EAR INFECTION

ESSENTIAL OILS

Basil. Fights infections and bacteria; traditionally used for ear infections.

Frankincense. Relieves pain and inflammation associated with an ear infection.[93]

Manuka. Has anti-viral properties and supports immunity, which may target the cause of ear infections.

Tea tree. Effective for ear infections due to its anti-bacterial and anti-viral compounds.

Research

In a 2005 study, researchers examined the middle ear cultures of laboratory animals that were given basil oil and found that basil's chemical components were highly effective against two types of bacteria that cause middle ear infections.[94]

Home Remedy

Ear Ease. Rub 1 drop each of frankincense oil and basil oil behind your ears and on the soles of your feet to speed up recovery time from ear infections while also reducing pain and swelling. For children, dilute the oil with a carrier oil.

Background

An ear infection is an inflammation of the inner, middle or outer ear caused by a bacterial or viral infection. Children between the ages of 6 months and 2 years are more susceptible to ear infections because of the size and shape of their ear tubes, and because of their immature immune systems. Symptoms may include earaches and thick, yellow fluid coming from the ears. A middle ear infection is generally related to an allergy or upper respiratory infection and is caused by fluid buildup in the ear. Swimmer's ear is caused by water getting trapped in the ear canal due to the buildup of wax; this causes bacteria to grow and an infection to occur. Ear infections can either be viral or bacterial, but viral infections are much more common; therefore, treatment with conventional antibiotics typically is ineffective and may include adverse side effects.

Suggested Supplements

» **Garlic and Mullein Oil Ear Drops.** Anti-bacterial and anti-inflammatory. Place 2 warm drops in the ear daily.

» **Zinc.** Boosts immune function, promotes healing. For ages 2 and older, take 10 milligrams twice daily.

ECZEMA

ESSENTIAL OILS

Lavender. Brings circulation to skin cells.

Geranium. Contains anti-bacterial properties; soothes allergic reactions.[96]

Manuka. Soothes and helps heal damaged skin.

Myrrh. Treats skin irritations; soothes chapped or cracked skin.

Research

A 2010 study reported that myrrh essential oil helped maintain elevated white blood cell count throughout the healing period after dermal injury; this implied it was also able to induce activation of the immune responses involved in wound healing.[97]

 ### Home Remedy

Eczema Ease. Mix a teaspoon of coconut oil with 5 drops of geranium oil, and then rub the mixture onto the infected area twice daily until results are noticeable.

Background

Eczema is an itchy, red rash that can appear all over the body and, in particular, occurs among people who have very dry, sensitive skin. The skin can blister and crack in some cases. There are 31.6 million people in the U.S. with eczema.[95] It is usually diagnosed at a very young age. Babies with eczema typically have it on the face, especially the cheeks and chin, but they can also have it on the scalp, chest, back and outer arms and legs. Children and adults typically have the telltale rash on their necks, wrists, ankles and in areas that bend. The specific cause of eczema remains unknown, but it is believed to develop due to a combination of hereditary and environmental factors. Symptoms can worsen with exposure to common food allergens or other substances such as perfumes or soaps.

Suggested Supplements

» **Omega-3 + Vitamin D3.** Essential fats and vitamin D are critical for wound healing and reduce inflammation.

» **Probiotics.** Provide friendly bacteria that help support gut health and immunity.

EDEMA

ESSENTIAL OILS

Roman Chamomile. Contains anti-inflammatory properties; acts as a disinfectant due to the presence of azulene.

Juniper. Shown to regulate hormone levels and reduce bloating and inflammation.[98]

Lavender. Can lessen swelling in the feet, ankles and legs.

Cypress. Improves circulation, thereby helping reduce edema more quickly.

 Research
A 2015 study reported that an inflammatory response in laboratory animals was reduced through the pre-treatment of the animals with lavender oil. The results reveal lavender's analgesic and anti-inflammatory activities, as well as demonstrate its therapeutic potential.[99]

 Home Remedy
Edema Massage. Mix 2 drops each of cypress oil and juniper oil with equal parts of coconut oil, and massage the mixture onto inflamed areas twice daily. It can also be added to a warm-water bath or applied with a warm compress.

Background
Edema is swelling caused by excess fluid that is trapped in the body's tissues. It is estimated that approximately 4.4 million people in the U.S. regularly experience edema. Common symptoms include swelling or puffiness of the tissue directly under the skin, skin that retains a dimple or mark after being pressed for several seconds, increased abdominal size and stretched or shiny skin. It can appear suddenly, but usually develops subtly—the patient may first gain weight, or wake up with puffy eyes. Edema can be the result of medication, pregnancy, physical inactivity, sitting or standing for long periods, surgery, heat, birth control pills, excessive salt intake, poor diet or an underlying disease.

Suggested Supplements

» **Omega-3.** EPA/DHA found in fish oil is beneficial for lowering inflammation, which may improve edema.

» **Turmeric + Black Pepper.** This combination helps improve blood flow and reduces inflammation.

ERECTILE DYSFUNCTION

 ESSENTIAL OILS

 Sandalwood. Can balance testosterone levels; acts as a natural aphrodisiac.

 Patchouli. Stimulates hormones and helps increase libido or sex drive.[100]

 Ylang Ylang. Widely used as a natural impotence remedy to help increase libido.

 Jasmine and Rose. Natural aphrodisiacs; increase arousal and elevate mood.

Research

Compared with a placebo, jasmine oil caused significant increases of physical signs of arousal in a study conducted in healthy adult women. Subjects in the jasmine oil group also rated themselves as more alert and more vigorous than subjects in the control group.[101]

 ## Home Remedy

Invigorating Men's Cologne. Mix 5 drops of sandalwood oil, 5 drops of bergamot oil, 2 drops of cedarwood oil and ½ pint (300 milliliters) of 70 percent alcohol or vodka in a glass roll-on tube or glass cologne spray bottle and apply it to smell great and boost libido.

Background

Erectile dysfunction (ED), also known as impotence, occurs when a man can't get or keep an erection firm enough for sexual intercourse. Recent studies suggest that approximately 10 percent of men aged 40 to 70 have severe or complete erectile dysfunction, defined as the total inability to achieve or maintain erections sufficient for sexual performance. An additional 25 percent of men in this age category have moderate or intermittent erectile difficulties, meaning they are able to achieve an erection but cannot maintain it. Causes of erectile dysfunction may be physiological or psychological. Common causes include low levels of testosterone, certain medications, poor diet, underlying illnesses, fatigue, stress, depression or heavy metal poisoning.

Suggested Supplements

» **L-arginine.** Helps with blood vessel dilation and improves blood flow. Take 1,000 milligrams twice daily.

» **Vitamin D3.** Supports hormone and testosterone production. Take 5,000 milligrams once or twice daily.

FIBROMYALGIA

ESSENTIAL OILS

Frankincense. Shown to decrease muscle pain and support the healing of nerve tissue.[102]

Turmeric. Contains compounds that reduce inflammation and support healthy muscles and nerves.

Lavender. Contains properties that help relieve tension and pain.

Peppermint. Acts as an effective natural pain reliever and muscle relaxant.

Research
A study shows that peppermint oil applied topically has pain relief benefits associated with fibromyalgia and myofascial pain syndrome.[103]

Home Remedy

Muscle Rub. Mix ½ cup of coconut oil and ¼ cup of grated beeswax in a glass jar. Place the jar in a saucepan with 2 inches of water and allow the contents to melt over medium-high heat. Stir and then add 2 teaspoons of cayenne and 2 teaspoons of ginger or turmeric. Allow it to cool slightly before adding 15 drops each of peppermint oil and lavender oil. Mix well. Pour the mixture into metal tins and let it cool.

Background
Fibromyalgia is a syndrome that includes long-term, body-wide pain in the muscles and connective tissues as well as general weakness, fatigue and intermittent depression. For a diagnosis to be made, the pain must be present in at least 11 of 18 specific trigger points. This characteristic pain may be accompanied by fatigue and headaches, along with experiencing difficulty with sleep, anxiety and depression. Females in the age group 20 to 50 are the most likely to suffer from fibromyalgia. The specific cause of fibromyalgia is yet to be determined, but some potential causes include allergies to chemicals or foods, viruses, hormonal problems, poor digestion, candidiasis, spinal misalignments, stress or neurotransmitter deficiency.

Suggested Supplements
» **Magnesium.** Magnesium deficiency is often linked to fibromyalgia. Take 500 milligrams daily.

» **Bone Broth Protein Powder.** Contains type 2 collagen that supports healthy muscles, joints and connective tissue.

FLU

ESSENTIAL OILS

Tea Tree and Manuka. Help with congestion andrespiratory tract infections.[104]

Lemon. A natural disinfectant that can fight bacteria and viruses in the home and on the body.

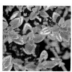

Thyme. Shown to drain congestion and help with infections in the chest andthroat.[105]

Eucalyptus and Peppermint. Expectorants that help to cleanse the body of toxins and harmful microorganisms.

Research

A 2009 study reported that tea tree oil showed anti-viral activity against influenza virus subtype H1N1; the anti-viral activity is principally attributed to terpinen-4-ol, the main active component. They concluded that tea tree is a promising treatment for influenza.[106]

Home Remedy

Steam Bath. Make a steam bath by pouring a cup of boiling water into a bowl, and then mix 10 drops of eucalyptus or peppermint essential oil, place a towel over your head and inhale deeply for 5 to 10 minutes.

Background

The flu is a common viral infection that attacks the lungs, nose and throat. The flu is similar to the common cold, but generally the symptoms are more severe. It is incredibly common, with more than 10 percent of the U.S. population affected each year. Symptoms include a temperature of 100 degrees or higher, cough or sore throat, runny or stuffy nose, headaches, body aches, chills, fatigue, nausea, vomiting and diarrhea. Young children, adults, pregnant women and people with chronic disease or weak immune systems are at high risk. Essential oils can provide immune support and may ease some of the flu's most bothersome symptoms.

Suggested Supplements

» **Elderberry.** Helps with immune system function; boosts white blood cells.

» **Echinacea.** Helps your body fight off infections; best taken at the first sign of illness (1,000 milligrams, two to three times daily).

GINGIVITIS (GUM DISEASE)

ESSENTIAL OILS

Clove. Contains eugenol, which may support healthy gums and the remineralization of teeth.

Cinnamon. Highly potent against bacteria responsible for gum disease.[107]

Myrrh. Contains anti-inflammatory compounds that may aid in healing gum disease.

Tea Tree and Manuka. Have anti-bacterial properties that can prevent gingivitis.

Research

A recent study evaluated clove's ability to slow dental erosion compared to eugenol, eugenyl-acetate, fluoride and a control group. Not only did clove oil lead the pack by significantly decreasing decalcification, it was observed that it actually remineralized teeth.[108]

Home Remedy

Oil Pulling. Take 1 teaspoon of coconut oil and 2 drops of an anti-bacterial essential oil, such as clove, and gently swish the mixture in your mouth for 5 to 20 minutes to help fight gingivitis.

Background

Gingivitis is a common form of gum disease (periodontal disease) that causes irritation, redness and swelling (inflammation) of your gums. There are more than 200,000 reported cases each year. Because gingivitis can be mild, you may not be aware that you have the condition, but it's important to take it seriously and treat it promptly. Gingivitis can lead to much more serious gum disease and eventual tooth loss. Common symptoms of gingivitis are red gums that are swollen and bleed easily. This can be due to poor dental hygiene, smoking, immune-related illnesses, emotional stress, poor nutrition or excess consumption of sugar.

Suggested Supplements

» **Coenzyme Q10.** Can have a healing effect on gingivitis; take 100 milligrams daily.

» **Vitamin C + Collagen Protein.** Help strengthen gums and aid with healthy tissue formation.

HAIR LOSS (ALOPECIA)

ESSENTIAL OILS

Rosemary. Stimulates hair growth and helps prevent baldness, slow graying and treat dandruff.

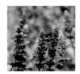

Lavender. Shown to promote hair growth and reduce emotional stress.

Clary Sage. Helps to strengthen and tone hair follicles.[109]

Cedarwood. Helps naturally thicken hair and improves emotional well-being.

Research

Researchers evaluated 86 people who were experiencing hair loss and had them massage their scalps with essential oils including lavender oil. They did this daily for seven months and at the end, those who used the essential oils daily noticed significant hair regrowth.[110]

Home Remedy

Rosemary Mint Shampoo. Mix 6 ounces of aloe vera gel, 3 tablespoons of olive oil, 10 tablespoons of baking soda, 20 drops of rosemary oil and 10 drops of peppermint oil. Store in an 8-ounce glass or plastic bottle.

Background

Anyone—men, women and children—can experience hair loss. Hair loss can affect just your scalp, or it can affect your entire body. Although hair loss may seem like a more prominent problem in men (two-thirds of men face hair loss by age 35), women are nearly as likely to lose, or have thinning, hair. Male-pattern baldness is an inherited sensitivity to DHT, a by-product of testosterone, which leads to finer hair, a receding hairline and finally a deserted scalp. Female pattern baldness is characterized by thinning on the top or center of the head. Female hair loss is generally due to high levels of stress, hormone imbalance, thyroid conditions or toxic exposure. The good news is that lifestyle changes to reduce stress, dietary improvements and taking certain hair loss remedies can often improve hair growth.

Suggested Supplements

» **Saw Palmetto.** A natural DHT blocker that can improve hair growth. Take 320 milligrams daily.

» **Zinc.** Addresses the cause of hair loss by blocking DHT binding sites and improving prostate health. Take 30 milligrams twice daily.

HEADACHES

ESSENTIAL OILS

Peppermint. Improves circulation and reduces pain.[111]

Lavender. Reduces muscle tension; used as a mood stabilizer, sedative and effective migraine remedy.

Eucalyptus. Opens nasal airways; eliminates sinus pressure that can lead to headaches.

Rosemary. Stimulating, anti-inflammatory and analgesic.

Research

A 2012 study measured the results of inhaling lavender oil for 15 minutes. The 47 participants were asked to record the effects every half hour, for two hours. Out of 129 headache attacks, 92 responded positively to the lavender oil remedy.[112]

Home Remedy

Headache Ease. Rub a mixture of peppermint oil, lavender oil and a carrier oil on your temples, chest and the back of your neck. Before washing your hands after application, cup your hands and breathe in deeply for several minutes.

Background

Headaches are an extremely common ailment that affects millions of people across the globe. It has been estimated that up to three-quarters of adults have had a headache at least once within the last year. A headache is a good indicator that the body is missing something—it may be the result of dehydration, nutrient deficiency or a food sensitivity that is causing this built-up tension. A multitude of headache triggers exist, including stress, fatigue, allergies, eyestrain, poor posture, alcohol or drugs, low blood sugar, hormones, constipation and nutritional deficiencies. The most severe form of a headache is known as a migraine, which can cause vision disturbance and vomiting.

Suggested Supplements

» **Magnesium.** Migraine sufferers have lower levels of magnesium both during and between attacks compared with healthy individuals.[113]

» **Feverfew.** Reduces the frequency of migraine headaches and headache symptoms, including pain, nausea, vomiting and sensitivity to light and noise.[114]

HEARTBURN

ESSENTIAL OILS

Ginger. Blocks the production of acid and helps prevent ulcers.

Peppermint. Relaxes the muscles, allowing painful digestive gas to pass.[115]

Fennel. Balances the pH level within the body, especially within the stomach.

Lemon. Helps temporarily excrete digestive acids.

Research

A 2015 study reported that ginger essential oil treatment inhibited ulcers in laboratory animals by 85 percent, suggesting the promising gastro-protective activity of ginger.[116]

Home Remedy

Heartburn Quick Fix. Add 1 drop each of peppermint and lemon essential oils to a tablespoon of apple cider vinegar plus a spoonful of honey for a soothing way to combat digestive issues.

Background

Heartburn is a form of indigestion caused by acid regurgitation into the esophagus. Often considered a symptom of acid reflux, the most common times to experience heartburn occur in the evening after a heavy meal, during movement such as bending or lifting or when lying down. Symptoms include burning or pain in the chest, stomachaches after eating, a bitter taste in the mouth, belching and nausea. Roughly 20 percent of American adults endure painful heartburn on a weekly basis—and yet many are unaware of simple and natural remedies that work quickly to correct the underlying digestive problem, as diet and lifestyle habits are the biggest contributors to heartburn.

Suggested Supplements

» **Raw Apple Cider Vinegar.** Naturally acidic; lowers the pH in your stomach. Take 1 tablespoon before meals.

» **HCL with Pepsin.** Increases the level of acid in the stomach necessary for proper digestion. (Only take with meals that contain protein; do NOT use if you take corticosteroids or anti-inflammatory medications such as NSAIDs.)

» **Digestive Enzymes.** Help break down hard-to-digest starches and proteins.

HEMORRHOIDS

ESSENTIAL OILS

Cypress. Contains anti-inflammatory properties; helps shrink swollen blood vessels.

Helichrysum. Reduces inflammation and improves the condition of blood vessels.[117]

Manuka. Contains cooling, anti-viral and anti-bacterial properties.

Frankincense. Contracts and tones tissues, which helps to speed regeneration.

 ### Research

Tea tree oil's anti-inflammatory properties have been widely researched and studied in recent years and show tremendous promise as a topical treatment for conditions such as hemorrhoids.[118]

 ### Home Remedy

Hemorrhoid Salve. Mix 2 to 4 drops each of cypress oil and helichrysum oil with a carrier oil and apply it to hemorrhoids with a cotton ball. Repeat every few hours as needed to ease pain, inflammation and swelling.

Background

Hemorrhoids are swollen and inflamed veins in the rectum and anus that cause discomfort and bleeding. About half of adults will have experienced the symptoms of hemorrhoids by age 50. They can be either internal or external and are also known as piles. They may occur with constipation, lifting heavy objects, obesity, pregnancy and childbirth. Hemorrhoids cause pain, severe itching and difficulty sitting, but luckily, they are treatable. Natural remedies for hemorrhoids (such as essential oils) can effectively prevent and help heal the condition quickly.

Suggested Supplements

» **Butcher's Broom.** Can help reduce swelling and inflammation of hemorrhoids. Take 200 to 300 milligrams daily.

» **Diosmin.** Bioflavanoid that helps improve venous and capillary health, including hemorrhoidal tissue.

HERPES

ESSENTIAL OILS

Thyme. Shows excellent promise as a treatment for drug-resistant strains of herpes.[119]

Manuka. Balances inflammation; soothes irritated skin.

Myrrh. Acts as an antiseptic and is used to clean and heal cuts or wounds.

Lavender. Provides nourishment and hydration to dry or cracked skin.

Research

In a 2014 study, thyme essential oil demonstrated excellent activity against an antibiotic-resistant strain of bacteria, making it a promising alternative treatment for herpes.[120]

 ### Home Remedy

Lavender Mint Lip Balm. Mix 1 tablespoon of beeswax, 1 tablespoon of coconut oil and 2 tablespoons of shea butter in a pot over medium heat. Remove from the heat and add 7 drops each of lavender oil and peppermint oil. Whisk well. Pour it quickly into tins or tubes and let it cool.

Background

Herpes is a virus causing sores, typically around the mouth or on the genitals. The most common types of herpes are cold sores (herpes type 1), which appear around the lips, and genital herpes (herpes type 2). Both are highly contagious and both can occur in either area of the body. More than 50 percent of Americans have type 1, and one out of every six people in the U.S. has type 2. Most people do not have apparent symptoms for many months, or even years, after becoming infected. Those who do have symptoms during the initial period will usually notice them about four to seven days after being infected. Causes include sexual contact, immune system suppression and nutritional deficiencies. Stress can trigger a recurrence of symptoms.

Suggested Supplements

» **L-lysine.** Can help prevent outbreaks. Take 1,000 milligrams, three times daily.

» **Zinc and Vitamin C.** Improve immunity, which may provide broad anti-viral support.

HYPERTENSION (HIGH BLOOD PRESSURE)

 ESSENTIAL OILS

 Clary Sage. Relaxes the arteries; may help decrease your risk of heart problems.

 Ylang Ylang. Known to improve blood flow and fight inflammation.

 Frankincense. Has sedative properties; promotes relaxation.[121]

 Lavender. Helps to reduce stress, which is a cause of high blood pressure.

 Research

A 2009 study found that clary sage oil can bring about a significant decrease in systolic blood pressure.[122]

 Home Remedy

BP-Lowering Inhalation. Add 1 drop each of frankincense, lavender, clary sage and ylang ylang oils into a bowl containing steaming water. Cover your head with a soft towel and inhale for a minimum of 3 minutes before going to bed.

Background

Hypertension, more commonly known as high blood pressure, is a condition in which the force of the blood against the artery walls is too high and the arterial wall becomes distorted. About 70 million American adults have high blood pressure—that's 1 in every 3 adults. Anyone, including children, can develop high blood pressure. It greatly increases the risk for heart disease and stroke, the first and third leading causes of death in the U.S. Causes of high blood pressure include a diet high in salt, stress, alcohol, caffeine, smoking, obesity, inactivity, birth control pills and heavy metal poisoning. Frequently, there are no symptoms as blood pressure increases, but warning signs for dangerously high blood pressure can include chest pains, confusion, headaches, ear noise or buzzing, irregular heartbeat, nose bleeds, tiredness or vision changes.

Suggested Supplements

» **Omega-3.** EPA/DHA found in fish oil reduces blood pressure and inflammation when taken long-term; take 1,000 to 2,000 milligrams daily.

» **Magnesium.** Helps with relaxation of smooth muscle and reduces blood pressure. Take 500 milligrams before bed daily, or as needed.

HYPOTHYROIDISM

ESSENTIAL OILS

Holy Basil. Works as an adaptogen to naturally balance cortisol levels.

Myrrh. Has hormone balancing properties and reduces systemic inflammation.

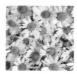

Lemongrass. Reduces inflammation and balances insulin.[123]

Roman Chamomile. Improves thyroid health while helping to reduce stress.

Research

In a study to determine holy basil's efficacy against breast cancer cells, the essential oil was found to positively impact hormone levels in the body.[124]

 ### Home Remedy

Thyroid Support. Rub 2 to 4 drops each of lemongrass oil and myrrh oil directly to the thyroid area along with the reflexology points on your feet (big toes) and on your wrists multiple times per day.

Background

Hypothyroidism is a condition related to having an underactive thyroid gland that doesn't properly make or release thyroid hormones. The thyroid gland normally releases many crucial hormones that travel throughout the bloodstream and reach receptors that are found throughout the body, so a disturbance in thyroid function can cause widespread, noticeable health problems. According to some estimates, 40 percent of the population suffers with some form of low thyroid function. Women (especially older women) are the most susceptible group for developing hypothyroidism. Common symptoms of hypothyroidism include a slow metabolism, poor digestion, low energy levels, increased carbohydrate cravings, trouble sleeping, depression, thinning hair and signs of accelerated aging.

Suggested Supplements

» **Ashwagandha.** Helps hypothyroidism patients significantly increase thyroxine hormone levels, which can reduces the severity of the disorder.[125]

» **Iodine + Selenium.** Promote healthy thyroid function. If you have an autoimmune disease such as Hashimoto's, consult with a doctor before taking iodine.

IMMUNE DEFENSE

 ESSENTIAL OILS

 Frankincense. Has superior immune-boosting ability; multiplies white blood cells.[126]

 Thyme. Has anti-viral and immune-boosting compounds that protect the body.

 Orange. Contains limonene, which is a powerful defender against oxidative stress.

 Myrrh. Contains anti-inflammatory properties.

 Research

In a clinical study on chickens, thyme essential oil was found to reduce the incidence of disease.[127]

 Home Remedy

Immune-Boosting Juice. Extract the juice of 1 bell pepper, 1 head/stem of broccoli and 1 cucumber. Mix the juice in a blender with 1 to 2 drops of lemon oil or orange oil, 1 to 2 drops of ginger oil and 1 tablespoon of apple cider vinegar.

Background

The immune system is a network of cells, tissues and organs that work together to protect the body from infection. Your immune system does a remarkable job of defending against disease-causing microorganisms, but it isn't perfect—some germs invade successfully and make you sick. However, it is possible to intervene in this process and make your immune system stronger. Some essential oils have the power to target invading microbes, infected cells and even tumors—protecting the body from disease and other health conditions.

Suggested Supplements

» **Probiotics.** Line your digestive tract and support your body's ability to absorb nutrients and fight infection.

» **Bone Broth Protein Powder.** Contains type 2 collagen, which helps repair gut lining and improves immunity.

305

INFICTION

 ## ESSENTIAL OILS

Oregano. Has proven and powerful antibiotic capabilities.[128]

Cedarwood. Defends the body against toxins; fights off bacteria in the body.

Tea Tree and Manuka. Destroys parasites and fungi.

Thyme. An antiseptic; controls infections on the skin and within the body; antibacterial.[129]

Research

A study conducted at the Department of Oral Medicine and Radiology found that cedarwood is effective in controlling both bacteria and yeasts responsible for oral infections.[130]

 ### Home Remedy

Infection-Fighting Lotion. Mix 1 to 2 drops each of tea tree, cedarwood, manuka and thyme oils into a squirt of natural lotion and apply it to areas of infection or to your lymph nodes to fight internal infection. Additionally, take oregano oil internally for up to two weeks.

Background

An infection is the invasion of body tissues by disease-causing agents. These agents are able to multiply, cause a reaction in bodily tissues and produce toxins within the body. An infection can lead to countless symptoms, from a sore throat and fever to far more serious and sometimes fatal complications. Worldwide, infectious diseases are the leading cause of death of children and adolescents, and one of the leading causes in adults. Infections are caused by germs such as viruses, bacteria, parasites and fungi. Many of the constituents in essential oils have been proven to fight these germs and help you recover from or possibly evade infection.

Suggested Supplements

» **Elderberry.** Fights infections, including influenza, herpes, viral infections and bacterial infections.

» **Echinacea.** Evidence suggests that phytochemicals in echinacea have the capacity to reduce viral infections.[131]

INFERTILITY

ESSENTIAL OILS

Roman Chamomile. Acts as a mild sedative that calms the nerves and reduces anxiety.

Thyme. Provides progesterone-balancing effects.[132]

Ylang Ylang. Serves as a mood enhancer and natural energizer.

Sandalwood. Works as a natural aphrodisiac and can help increase libido, especially for men.

Research

Recent research noted that of 150 herbs tested for progesterone production that inhibit the growth of human breast cancer cells, thyme oil is one of the top six to have the highest estradiol and progesterone binding.[133]

Home Remedy

Revitalizing Inhalation. Place 1 to 2 drops each of thyme oil and ylang ylang oil in your palms and inhale deeply for several minutes. Also diffuse it, or apply it topically.

Background

Infertility is defined as the inability to become pregnant for at least 12 consecutive months. According to the Center for Disease Control and Prevention, millions of women in America are suffering from infertility, with some 7.3 million between the ages of 15 and 44 reporting infertility. Many blame the rising infertility rate on the toxins in our environment polluting the body and compromising precious functions. Infertility can stem from either the male or female and causes may include poor nutrition, emotional stress, sexually transmitted diseases, thyroid disorders, candida, medical conditions, eating disorders, excessive exercise, obesity, polycystic ovary syndrome (PCOS) and hormonal problems. The best ways to boost fertility are to decrease stress, exercise regularly, balance hormones and minimize exposure to toxins.

Suggested Supplements

» **Vitex (Chasteberry).** Helps balance estrogen/progesterone ratios and stimulates the ovaries. Take 160 to 240 milligrams daily.

» **Stinging Nettle.** An herb used in Chinese medicine to remedy fertility because it supports the kidneys, adrenals and reproductive organs.[134]

INFLAMMATION

ESSENTIAL OILS

Frankincense. Encourages circulation and helps decrease symptoms of joint or muscle pain.

Turmeric. Helps relieve inflammation in the entire body, including joints and gut.

Patchouli. Can address internal inflammation and conditions such as arthritis and gout.

Ginger. Contains zingiberene and gingerols, which have potent anti-inflammatory properties.

Research

Frankincense has been shown to be a potent inhibitor of 5-lipoxygenase, an enzyme responsible for inflammation in the body.[136]

 ### Home Remedy

Anti-Inflammatory Pain Relieving Rub. Mix ½ cup of coconut or jojoba oil, 10 drops of helichrysum oil and 10 drops of lavender oil in a bottle and massage it into inflamed areas.

Background

Inflammation is your body's response to stress—whether from your diet, lifestyle or environment—that results in an inflamed or heated area. When you catch a cold, you may have inflammation in the form of a fever as your body heats up to eradicate the effects of the invading virus. This kind of inflammation is acute and beneficial, but the modern epidemic of chronic, low-grade inflammation destroys the balance in your body. When your body's systems experience a constant inflammatory response, you become more susceptible to aging and disease.[135] Over time, dietary and environmental toxins build up in the body, turning on the immune system and keeping it highly reactive and in an inflamed state. Other causes of inflammation include stress, leaky gut and chronic food allergies or food sensitivities. Essential oils can work together with healthy diet and lifestyle choices to reduce inflammation and help prevent disease.

Suggested Supplements

» **Omega-3.** EPA/DHA found in fish is nature's anti-inflammation prescription.

» **Proteolytic Enzymes.** Enzymes (bromelain, papain and actinidin) help our bodies respond to inflammation by breaking down inflammatory proteins and toxins.

INSOMNIA

ESSENTIAL OILS

Lavender. Helps relax the body; able to reduce feelings of uneasiness, stress and anxiety.

Roman Chamomile. Inhalation is a natural remedy for anxiety and general depression.[137]

Clary Sage. Reduces inflammation and has a calming effect.[138]

Ylang Ylang. May improve mood and help put the body into a more relaxed state.

 Research

Researchers have discovered that one constituent of Roman chamomile works on the brain in a way similar to that of benzodiazepines, a group of anxiolytic (anxiety-reducing) drugs that include Xanax and Valium[139]

 Home Remedy

Sleepy Time Blend. Diffuse clary sage, Roman chamomile and lavender oils by the bed at night, or rub them onto the back of your neck. These oils can also be added to a warm bath with Epsom salt, which contains magnesium and helps to calm the body and reduce muscle pain.

Background

Insomnia is the inability to fall asleep or stay asleep. As much as 15 percent of the U.S. population suffers from insomnia, with even higher percentages among older people and women. Insomnia can negatively affect energy levels, mood, work performance, quality of life and overall health. Causes of insomnia include stress and anxiety, overuse of stimulants, sugar, indigestion, pain, alcohol, lack of physical activity, restless leg syndrome, hormonal changes, sleep apnea or other medical conditions. While it may be the primary problem, insomnia could also be due to an underlying disease or side effect of a prescription medication. These essential oils are well known to promote relaxation and feelings of calm.

Suggested Supplements

» **Melatonin.** Helps promote sleep, best used for short periods of time. Take 1 to 3 milligrams 30 minutes before bed.

» **Passionflower.** Helps relax the nervous system; take 500 milligrams before bed.

IRRITABLE BOWEL SYNDROME

ESSENTIAL OILS

Ginger. Shown to have gastro-protective properties that aid intestinal issues.[140]

Peppermint. Proven to ease symptoms of IBS and provide relief.

Fennel. May have a relaxing effect on the body.

Roman Chamomile. Promotes relaxation and may reduce intestinal gas and bloating.

Research

Peppermint oil taken internally in capsule form has been proven to be effective at naturally addressing IBS. One study found a 50 percent reduction in IBS symptoms with 75 percent of patients who took peppermint capsules.[141]

Home Remedy

IBS Ease. Add 1 drop each of fennel, ginger and peppermint oils to water three times daily, or rub the mixture over your abdomen twice daily.

Background

Irritable bowel syndrome (IBS) is an intestinal disorder causing pain and bloating in the gut, gas, diarrhea and constipation. The amount of people who now struggle with some form of IBS is a shocking 60 million people— that's 20 percent of Americans. IBS affects about twice as many women as men and most often occurs in people younger than age 45. Some of the primary causes of IBS include a low fiber diet, food allergies, gluten, dairy, nutritional deficiencies, emotional stress, leaky gut and poor lifestyle choices such as the use of drugs or alcohol. Non-GI conditions that people with IBS often have include chronic fatigue syndrome, depression, anxiety and chronic pelvic pain. The good news is you can help IBS symptoms naturally through diet, lifestyle changes and natural remedies.

Suggested Supplements

» **Probiotics.** Can help re-colonize the gut with healthy bacteria. Take 50 to 100 billion CFU daily.

» **Digestive Enzymes.** Help with nutrient absorption. Take two before each meal.

» **Bone Broth Protein and Collagen Powder.** Contain collagen, which helps repair the gut lining and supports digestion.

LEAKY GUT SYNDROME

 ## ESSENTIAL OILS

Ginger. Helps relieve nausea, bloating and digestive distress.

Peppermint. Known as a premier digestive remedy.[146]

Turmeric and Roman Chamomile. Reduce inflammation, which may support the gut.

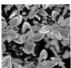
Thyme. May support healthy microbial levels and gut-related immune response.

 ### Research
A 2015 study reported that thymol, the active compound in thyme oil, is effective in suppressing pathogens in the small intestine, with no harm to beneficial commensal colonic bacteria in the distal gut.[147]

 ### Home Remedy
Stomach Ease. Take 1 drop each of ginger oil and peppermint oil internally in a glass of water. Also, mix 2 drops each of these oils with coconut oil and rub it over your abdomen twice daily.

Background
Leaky gut syndrome is a condition also referred to as increased intestinal permeability where the "net" in your digestive tract gets damaged, which allows proteins (such as gluten), bad bacteria and undigested particles to pass into your bloodstream. These particles cause systemic inflammation and an immune reaction over time. A growing body of research has linked leaky gut to a number of seemingly unrelated health concerns and diseases, such as chronic sinusitis, fibromyalgia, migraines, chronic fatigue syndrome, Parkinson's and rheumatoid arthritis.[142-145] Some of the initial symptoms of leaky gut can include food allergies, skin issues such as acne and eczema, and digestive issues such as bloating and gas. In order to repair leaky gut, you must make specific diet changes and look to natural remedies for improvement.

Suggested Supplements
» **Probiotics.** Can help re-colonize the gut with healthy bacteria. Take 50 to 100 billion CFU daily.

» **Bone Broth Protein Powder.** Contains amino acids glutamine and proline, which may help repair the digestive tract.

LUPUS

ESSENTIAL OILS

Frankincense. Reduces inflammation and immune reactions.

Helichrysum. Supports the nervous system.[148]

Lavender and Geranium. Used to lessen skin inflammation.

Ginger and Turmeric. Support gut-immune response—a cause of autoimmune disease.

Research

In clinical studies, an active constituent in frankincense has been shown to be potent against 5-lipoxygenase, an enzyme responsible for inflammation in the body.[149]

 ### Home Remedy

Take 3 drops of frankincense with water, three times daily. Sweeten the mixture with honey if desired. You can also apply 1 to 2 drops of helichrysum, lavender, turmeric and frankincense to your neck area to help ease some of the symptoms associated with lupus.

Background

Lupus is an inflammatory disease caused when the immune system attacks its own tissues. This attack leads to inflammation and chronic pain in the skin, joints and muscles. Lupus can also cause sun sensitivity, weight loss, hair loss and digestive problems. In 50 percent of cases, lupus causes a rash on the face known as a butterfly rash, which can get worse with sunlight and also appear on other parts of the body. Research indicates that at least 1.5 million Americans have lupus. Potential causes include allergic reactions, viruses, emotional stress, estrogen disruption due to pregnancy or birth control, hormonal imbalances, poor digestion and metal toxicity. Natural remedies for lupus—including an anti-inflammatory diet, exercise and essential oils for pain and stress reduction—can help manage symptoms and prevent further complications.

Suggested Supplements

» **Omega-3.** EPA/DHA in fish is critical for reducing systemic inflammation. Take 1,000 to 12,000 milligrams daily.

» **Bone Broth Protein Powder.** Contains type 2 collagen, along with the amino acids proline, glycine and glutamine, which support the gut and immune system.

LYME DISEASE

 ESSENTIAL OILS

 Frankincense. Can help modulate immune reactions and reduce inflammation.

 Roman Chamomile. Helps relieve stress, supports immunity and fights off parasites.

 Helichrysum. Helps protect from infections and reduce pain.

 Lemongrass. Wards off insects, fights bacteria and helps relieve muscle pain.

 Research

A 2014 study reported that both citronella and clove were effective at repelling ticks. While citronella was reasonably effective, clove outperformed it substantially with over 90 percent efficacy.[151]

 Home Remedy

Lyme Disease Bath. Add 10 drops each of Roman chamomile, frankincense and lemongrass oils along with 1 cup of Epsom salt to a warm bath. Soak for 20 to 30 minutes at least three times a week in the evening.

Background

Lyme disease is a bacterial infection primarily transmitted by deer ticks and black-legged ticks. According to estimates, more than 300,000 Americans are diagnosed with the tick-borne disease each year.[150] Because diagnosing Lyme can be difficult, many people who have Lyme disease may be misdiagnosed with other conditions. Thus, many experts believe the true number of cases is much higher. Symptoms can start with flu-like symptoms, including headaches and muscle and joint pain. A "bulls eye" rash may occur at the spot of the bite. It can also cause arthritis that persists months or years after the tick bite. Over time, the symptoms can continue to worsen and turn into a chronic inflammatory condition.

Suggested Supplements

» **Probiotics.** Improving digestive and immune system health with the use of probiotics can aid in reducing symptoms of Lyme disease.

» **Bone Broth Protein Powder.** Contains type 2 collagen and amino acids proline, glycine and glutamine that can help support healthy levels of inflammation.

MENOPAUSE

ESSENTIAL OILS

 Clary Sage. Offers relief from symptoms such as hot flashes.

 Roman Chamomile. Acts as a mild sedative that calms nerves and reduces anxiety.

 Peppermint. Helps cool the body during hot flashes.

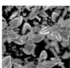 **Thyme.** May delay menopause by stimulating hormones.[152]

Research

Inhalation of clary sage oil was found to reduce cortisol levels by 36 percent and improve thyroid hormone levels in 22 post-menopausal women in their 50s. Clary sage also had an antidepressant effect.[153]

 ### Home Remedy

Hot Flash Massage. Dilute 5 drops each of clary sage, Roman chamomile and peppermint oils with 1 tablespoon of a carrier oil and massage it onto your body. Also add these oils to a bath.

Background

Menopause is a natural decline in reproductive hormones that begins when a woman reaches her 40s or 50s. The duration of menopause is very hard to predict, as each woman's situation is vastly different. Women typically begin experiencing hot flashes, mood swings, vaginal dryness and other menopause symptoms when they are going through perimenopause. This stage is generally considered part of the menopause period and can last anywhere from 10 months to four years, as the ovaries gradually decrease estrogen production. However, menopause is not considered to have officially begun until a woman misses her period for 12 straight months. Menopause is a natural biological process; although it ends fertility, women can stay healthy and vital.

Suggested Supplements

» **Black Cohosh.** Can help prevent menopausal symptoms; helps improve sleep quality and reduce hormonal imbalances tied to diabetes or fibroids.[154]

» **Natural Progesterone Cream.** A natural way to reduce menopausal symptoms such as loss of bone density, vaginal dryness and fibroids. Best used under the guidance of a physician specializing in anti-aging medicine.

MULTIPLE SCLEROSIS

 ## ESSENTIAL OILS

 Frankincense. Shown to provide neurological support.

 Helichrysum. Helps detoxify the body and relieve pain and swelling.[155]

 Rosemary and Basil. May support nerve tissue and reduce inflammation.

 Turmeric. Contains anti-inflammatory and immune-supportive compounds.

 ## Research

Research studies suggest that essential oils high in linalool (such as basil) are highly useful in the control of MS symptoms and other inflammatory diseases.[156]

 ## Home Remedy

Soothing Bath Soak. Add 5 to 10 drops each of helichrysum, basil and rosemary oils to a warm bath and soak for at least 20 minutes. To fight inflammation, take 2 drops of frankincense oil internally, three times a day for three weeks.

Background

Multiple sclerosis (MS) is an autoimmune disease in which the immune system eats away at the protective covering of nerves, causing nerve damage. MS affects 2.5 million people worldwide and around 400,000 people in the U.S. MS affects women more than men, and while the disorder is most commonly diagnosed between ages 20 and 40, it can be seen at any age. Although no specific cause is known, some possible suspects include infections, mold toxicity, emotional stress, hormonal imbalances, toxic exposure, vitamin D deficiency, food allergies and immunizations. Common symptoms of MS include blurred or double vision, trouble thinking, loss of coordination, loss of balance, numbness, tingling and limb weakness.

Suggested Supplements

» **Omega-3.** EPH/DHA found in fish can reduce inflammation and promote better nerve functioning. Take 1,000 to 12,000 milligrams daily.

» **Lion's Mane Mushroom.** Promotes neurological function and helps restore nerve cells.

MUSCLE ACHES

ESSENTIAL OILS

Peppermint and Wintergreen. Effective natural pain relievers and muscle relaxants.

Cypress. A sedative with a calming and relaxing effect on the body.

Marjoram and Lemongrass. May reduce muscle spasms and muscle pain.

Lavender. Indicated for muscular spasms, cramps, sprains and rheumatism.[157]

Research

A study shows that peppermint oil applied topically has pain relief benefits associated with fibromyalgia and myofascial pain syndrome. The study found that peppermint, eucalyptus, menthol, capsaicin and other herbal preparations may be helpful.[158]

 ### Home Remedy

Muscle Compress. Put 3 drops of peppermint oil, 3 drops of cypress oil and 1 teaspoon of coconut oil on the area of concern, and then cover it with a hot compress for 3 to 5 minutes.

Background

A muscle cramp is an involuntarily and forcibly contracted muscle that does not relax. Most people experience a muscle cramp at some time in their life. There is a variety of types and causes of muscle cramps. One of the most common causes of muscle cramps is dehydration, but other causes include increased physical activity or a lack of activity, stress, nutritional deficiencies and hormonal changes. The body may not be getting enough electrolytes, such as potassium or magnesium. Some other medical explanations include fibromyalgia, statin drugs, flu symptoms, hormonal changes and Lyme disease. Essential oils such as peppermint and cypress are ideal home remedies for muscle aches and pains.

Suggested Supplements

» **Magnesium.** Can help with muscle relaxation. Take 250 milligrams twice daily.

» **Bone Broth Protein Powder.** Supports healthy joints and muscles and promotes tissue repair.

NAUSEA

ESSENTIAL OILS

Peppermint. Can reduce nausea, as well as bloating and gas.

Ginger. Known to reduce nausea and upset stomach.[159]

Basil. An anti-spasmodic that can lessen cramps associated with motion sickness.[160]

Lavender. Works as a mild sedative; helps to relax the body during times of stress.

Research
A medical study found that peppermint oil use reduced chemotherapy-induced nausea better than standard medical treatments.[161]

Home Remedy
Nausea Ease. Rub peppermint, ginger and lavender oils behind your ears or on your stomach, or take it internally to help relieve nausea.

Background
Almost everyone at some point in life has experienced symptoms of nausea, that sick feeling in your stomach that often comes just before vomiting. There are many causes of nausea, but some of the most common include pregnancy, food poisoning, motion sickness, flu symptoms, gallbladder distress, medications, migraine headaches and emotional stress. Morning sickness is nausea and/or vomiting that occurs during pregnancy. The timing of the nausea or vomiting can sometimes indicate the cause. For example, when it appears shortly after a meal, nausea or vomiting may be caused by food poisoning, gastritis (inflammation of the stomach lining) or an ulcer. If nausea leads to severe vomiting, dehydration becomes a concern. The next time your stomach is uneasy, use essential oils for natural relief.

Suggested Supplements
» **Vitamin B6.** Helps reduce nausea. Take 25 milligrams, three times daily.

» **Digestive Enzymes.** Help the body digest macronutrients and can reduce symptoms of nausea when consumed consistently. Take 1 to 3 capsules daily with meals.

NECK PAIN

ESSENTIAL OILS

Wintergreen. Acts as a natural analgesic to relieve pain and swelling.[162]

Peppermint. Provides a cooling sensation; effectively relieves sore muscles.

Lavender. Soothing and calming to the body and mind.

Black Pepper and Ginger. Warming; promote circulation.

Research

In one study, it was determined that a cream containing a 3 percent concentration of essential oils including black pepper, peppermint and lavender improved range of motion and decreased neck pain compared to those using an unscented cream.[163]

Home Remedy

Neck Relief. Apply 2 to 3 drops of wintergreen, diluted with a carrier oil, onto your neck to relieve pain. A warm compress can be added to intensify wintergreen's benefits.

Background

Neck pain, soreness and stiffness are some of the most common types of muscle aches that children and adults experience. Triggers include poor posture, exercise-induced strains and repetitive work movements— even strenuous housework and landscaping can bring on a stiff neck. Sometimes, neck pain is caused by injury from a fall, contact sports or whiplash. Neck pain can also be a symptom of a heart attack, but it often presents with other symptoms of a heart attack. Neck pain or stiffness is sometimes accompanied by numbness or loss of strength in the arms or hands; shooting pain into the shoulder or down the arm often occurs with more serious cases. Chances are your stiff neck can be resolved without the need for drugs or serious intervention.

Suggested Supplements

» **Omega-3.** EPA/DHA fats found in fish help reduce inflammation in the body.

» **Turmeric Extract.** An anti-inflammatory supplement high in antioxidants that helps relieve pain and stiffness.

OSTEOPOROSIS

ESSENTIAL OILS

Cypress and Helichrysum. Can strengthen bones and reduce discomfort.[164]

Fir Needle. Can assist in bone repair.[165]

Clary Sage. Helps maintain healthy estrogen levels.

Myrrh. Contains compounds that support hormones.

Research

A scientific review concluded that conifer oils such as cypress and fir needle oils may be able to assist in bone repair.[166]

Home Remedy

Bone Aid. Apply a few drops of fir needle oil to the problematic area three times per day; dilute it with a carrier oil before applying it to your skin.

Background

Bone is living tissue that is constantly being broken down and replaced. Osteoporosis occurs when the creation of new bone doesn't keep up with the removal of old bone, which causes bones to become weak, brittle and easily fractured. Today, 44 million Americans have osteoporosis. It affects men and women of all races, but white and Asian women—especially older women—are at highest risk. The main causes of osteoporosis include inactivity, aging, hormonal imbalances, long-term use of certain medications, steroid use, low vitamin D levels, emotional stress and nutritional deficiencies. There typically are no symptoms in the early stages of bone loss. Over time, symptoms include fractures in the hip, wrist or spine; gradual loss of height; stooped posture and back pain. Certain essential oils may increase bone density and speed fracture healing.

Suggested Supplements

» **Magnesium + Calcium.** Required for proper calcium metabolism. Take 500 to 1000 milligrams daily.

» **Vitamin D3 + K2.** Fat-soluble vitamins necessary for healthy bone formation.

PARKINSON'S DISEASE

 ESSENTIAL OILS

 Lavender. Shown to reduce oxidative toxicity caused by certain Parkinson's treatments.[167]

 Helichrysum. Helps reduce swelling in the brain; boosts immunity.[168]

 Frankincense and Rosemary. Can destroy toxins that may lead to neurological damage.

 Vetiver. Acts as an anxiolytic (inhibits anxiety), which may help with tremors.[169]

Research

A nine-month long study found that people with Parkinson's who either used a blend of essential oils (clary sage, marjoram and lavender) in aromatherapy or received massages with them experienced more symptom relief than those who did not.[170]

 ### Home Remedy

Nervous System Support. To help relieve symptoms, rub 2 drops of frankincense, helichrysum, lavender and vetiver oil on your temples and neck twice daily. Additionally, put 2 drops of frankincense on the roof of your mouth.

Background

Parkinson's disease is a degenerative illness of the nervous system that affects the smooth natural movements of the body and results in extreme dysfunction, loss of motor skills and dementia. Parkinson's affects up to 1 million people in the U.S., and 60,000 new cases occur each year. Parkinson's strikes 50 percent more men than women, and the average age of onset is 60. Generally, those with Parkinson's lose the ability to speak properly, have difficulty walking and may also experience tremors. This happens because people with Parkinson's do not produce enough dopamine, which is an important chemical necessary for proper body movements and function. There is no specific known cause, but some aggravating factors include exposure to toxicity, inflammatory brain disorders, free radicals, poor nutrition and food allergies.

Suggested Supplements

» **Coenzyme Q10.** A powerful antioxidant that can help slow the progression of Parkinson's disease. Take 1,200 milligrams daily.

» **Turmeric Extract.** An antioxidant that supports healthy inflammation in the body and brain.

PLANTAR FASCIITIS

ESSENTIAL OILS

Rosemary. Reduces cortisol levels, which helps to relieve pain and oxidative stress.[171]

Marjoram and Lemongrass. May reduce muscle spasms and muscle pain.

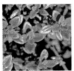

Thyme and Turmeric. Help relieve pain. Increase circulation; may speed healing.

Wintergreen and Peppermint. May help temporarily relieve pain.

Research

Researchers found that thyme oil can suppress the inflammatory COX-2 enzyme in a manner similar to resveratrol (protects the body against damage). The chemical carvacrol found in thyme and oregano oil was primarily responsible for this suppressive activity.[172]

Home Remedy

Warming Heel Rub. Warm up a tablespoon of coconut oil and add 2 drops each of rosemary, thyme and turmeric oils. Deeply massage the mixture into your heel.

Background

Plantar fasciitis is an inflammation of a thick band of tissue (called the plantar fascia) that connects the heel bone to the toes. If you strain your plantar fascia, it gets weak, swollen and irritated or inflamed. As a result, your heel or the bottom of your foot hurts when you stand or walk. This inflammation is the most common cause of heel pain. Around one in 10 people will develop plantar fasciitis at some time in their life, and it is seen regularly among middle-aged people, athletes or people who are on their feet a lot. It is twice as common in women as it is in men. You are also more likely to develop plantar fasciitis if you have pronated feet, high arches, are overweight or wear ill fitting or worn out shoes. Pain is the main symptom, and it is often at its worst when you take your first steps after getting up in the morning, or after long periods of rest where no weight is placed on your foot.

Suggested Supplements

» **Magnesium.** An essential mineral for bone formation and the utilization of calcium. Muscle and tissue relaxer. Required for protein synthesis, nerve function and the production of the antioxidant glutathione.

» **Vitamin B5.** Helps the body avoid nerve damage and impairment. Also known to accelerate the healing process.[173]

PNEUMONIA

ESSENTIAL OILS

Eucalyptus and Peppermint. Cooling and soothing; help with symptoms of pneumonia.

Thyme. Shown to be an effective alternative to antibiotics for superbugs.[174]

Lavender and Clove. Effective in fighting common infection causes.

Ginger. May reduce inflammation of the respiratory tract and fight infections.

Research

Studies suggest that clove has strong anti-microbial agents and exerts considerable control over Pseudomonas aeruginosa, which causes pneumonia.[175]

Home Remedy

Bedtime Chest Rub. Mix 10 drops each of eucalyptus oil and peppermint oil with 1 tablespoon of coconut oil. Before bed, rub the mixture on your neck and chest. Leave it on overnight, then rinse it off in the morning. Repeat nightly until symptoms improve.

Background

Pneumonia is an infection caused by bacteria or viruses that inflame the air sacs in one or both lungs, which may fill with fluid. For most people, pneumonia can be treated at home; it often clears up in two to three weeks. But older adults, infants and people with other diseases or a weakened immune system can become very ill. In the U.S., about 3 million cases of pneumonia are reported each year, and about 60,000 people die as a result of the condition. About one-third of cases occur in people over age 65. You may be more likely to present symptoms of the disease after having a cold or the flu; these illnesses make it hard for your lungs to fight infection, so it is easier to get pneumonia. Having a long-term, or chronic disease also makes you more likely to contract pneumonia. Symptoms of pneumonia include cough, fever, fast or labored breathing, chills, nausea, diarrhea, chest pain and extreme fatigue.

Suggested Supplements

» **Elderberry.** Supports healthy immune system response and fights viral invaders.

» **Echinacea.** Boosts the immune system; best taken at the first sign of illness (1,000 milligrams, two to three times daily).

POLYCYSTIC OVARY SYNDROME

 ## ESSENTIAL OILS

Holy Basil. May improve cortisol and insulin levels that support overall hormone balance.

Clary Sage. Stimulates the uterus and aids in regulating reproductive hormones.[176]

Geranium. Promotes hormone balance and supports detoxification of the liver and kidneys.

Roman Chamomile. May help lower stress and improve fertility.

 ### Research

A study found that using clary sage oil on humans caused improvements in overall hormone levels, as 22 post-menopausal women saw a reduction in depression (by 36 percent) and cortisol, and increases in 5-HTP and better levels of thyroid hormones.[177]

 ### Home Remedy

Hormone Balancing Blend.
Combine 2 drops each of clary sage, holy basil, geranium and Roman chamomile oils and mix with 1 teaspoon of coconut oil. Rub it on your lower abdomen and the front of your neck 2 to 3 times a day.

Background

Polycystic ovary syndrome (PCOS) is one of the most common hormonal disorders affecting nearly 20 percent of women of reproductive age. Women with PCOS develop enlarged ovaries with multiple cysts on them, which then start producing higher than normal levels of androgen hormones, such as testosterone. This reaction can also cause imbalanced levels of estrogen and low levels of progesterone and may be responsible for as much as 70 percent of infertility in women. Symptoms of PCOS may include irregular periods, trouble conceiving, acne, stubborn weight loss, insulin resistance, fatigue and low sex drive. In severe cases, PCOS can cause severe hair thinning and masculine characteristics (like hair growth on the face). Major improvements can occur with a good diet (less sugar and more vegetables, healthy fats and bone broth), managing stress and using natural compounds.

Suggested Supplements

» **Vitex (Chasteberry).** Helps balance estrogen/progesterone ratios and stimulates the ovaries. Take 160 to 240 milligrams daily.

» **Chinese Herbs (Rehmannia, White Peony and Astragalus).** These herbs remove dampness from the body, which improves organ function and hormone levels.

PREMENSTRUAL SYNDROME

 ## ESSENTIAL OILS

 Clary Sage. Helps to balance hormones naturally.

 Holy Basil. Shown to balance hormones and reduce PMS symptoms.[178]

 Cypress. Improves circulation and relieves cramps and aches.

 Ylang Ylang. Helps reduce tension, stress and cramping.

Research

A study concluded that aromatherapy massage using clary sage oil was more highly associated with reduction in the level of menstrual pain than acetaminophen.[179]

 ### Home Remedy

PMS Ease. To reduce symptoms of PMS, rub 2 to 3 drops of clary sage on your lower abdomen and apply a warm compress for 5 minutes.

Background

Premenstrual syndrome (PMS) is a group of symptoms linked to the menstrual cycle. These symptoms include mood swings, bloating, acne, tender breasts, food cravings, fatigue, headache, irritability and depression. It's estimated that as many as three of every four menstruating women have experienced some form of PMS. Symptoms may start a week or two before the period and can be mild to severe. Changes in hormones during the menstrual cycle seem to be an important cause; chemical changes in the brain may also be involved. Stress and emotional problems do not seem to cause PMS, but they may make it worse. About 3 to 8 percent of women have a more severe form of PMS, called premenstrual dysphoric disorder (PMDD), which can be debilitating. The good news is that if you improve your diet, manage stress and implement natural remedies, you can experience significant improvements in the symptoms associated with PMS.

Suggested Supplements

» **Vitex (Chasteberry).** Helps balance estrogen/progesterone ratios. Take 240 milligrams daily.

» **Vitamin B-Complex.** Vitamin B6 and other B vitamins are involved in estrogen metabolism.

PROSTATITIS

ESSENTIAL OILS

Rosemary. Helps promote hair growth and prostate health.[180]

Frankincense. Shown to reduce inflammation that is associated with prostatitis.

Thyme and Oregano. Effective against one of the known bacterial causes of prostatitis.

Turmeric. Contains powerful anti-inflammatory compounds.

Research

A constituent in oregano and thyme, carvacrol, has been found to be particularly effective against some drug-resistant strains of bacteria. Carvacrol is a strong inhibitor against E. coli, which is the cause of 80 percent of all cases of prostatitis.[181]

Home Remedy

Prostate Blend. Take 2 drops each of rosemary, frankincense and oregano oils and mix with 1 teaspoon of coconut oil. Rub the mixture on the areas below the genitals twice daily. These oils can also be taken internally, using 1- to 2-drop doses for up to six weeks.

Background

Prostatitis is often described as an infection of the prostate; it can also be inflammation with no infection. According to the National Institutes of Health, prostatitis may account for up to 25 percent of all office visits for complaints involving the genital and urinary systems from young and middle-aged men—and chronic (long-term) prostatitis is the number-one reason men under age 50 visit a urologist. How the prostate becomes infected is not fully clear; the bacteria that cause prostatitis may get into the prostate from the urethra by backflow of infected urine or stool from the rectum. Common symptoms include the frequent urge to urinate, difficulty urinating, chills, fever and pain or burning during urination.

Suggested Supplements

» **Saw Palmetto.** Can improve symptoms of non-infective prostate enlargement. Start with 320 milligrams, three times daily for 4 months, and then drop down to 320 milligrams once daily.

» **Zinc.** Necessary for prostate health; take 50 milligrams daily.

PSORIASIS

ESSENTIAL OILS

Geranium. Known to revitalize body tissues.

Myrrh. May relieve red, dry and flaking skin by reducing inflammation.

Tea Tree and Manuka. Soothe irritated and infected skin; relieve dry, flaky skin.

Lavender and Frankincense. Soothing to the skin; helps reduce inflammation.[182]

Research

In laboratory studies, geraniin (an active compound in geranium) protected against nephrotoxicity (kidney toxicity) by inhibiting oxidative stress and inflammatory response.[183]

 Home Remedy

Revitalizing Salve. Mix 5 drops of geranium oil and 3 drops of myrrh oil with 1 teaspoon of shea butter; rub the mixture onto any areas of concern twice daily. Oils can also be added to your body wash and lotion.

Background

Psoriasis is a chronic inflammatory disease of the immune system. It mostly affects the skin and joints, but it also may affect the fingernails, toenails, genitals and inside of the mouth. Approximately 7.5 million people in the U.S. have psoriasis. It occurs in all age groups but is primarily seen in adults. With plaque psoriasis (the most common form), skin cells build up and form scales and itchy, dry patches. The scaly patches, also known as psoriatic plaques, take on a silvery-white appearance. Up to 40 percent of people with psoriasis experience joint inflammation that produces symptoms of arthritis; this is called psoriatic arthritis. Patients with psoriasis have an increased incidence of low self-esteem, heart disease and type 2 diabetes.

Suggested Supplements

» **Hydrochloric Acid.** Helps with protein digestion and may help decrease psoriasis flare-ups. Take 1 to 3 capsules per meal.

» **Omega-3 + Vitamin D3.** Reduce inflammation and have been shown to improve psoriasis symptoms. Recommended dose is 1,000 to 12,000 milligrams of omegas and 5,000 IU of vitamin D daily.

RASH

ESSENTIAL OILS

Geranium. Helps to speed up the healing process of rashes, cuts and wounds.

Rose. May help prevent or slow the spread of harmful cells.[184]

Lavender. Shown to heal skin irritations and restore skin complexion.

Myrrh and Manuka. Reduce skin irritation and inflammation.

Research

Results from a comparison study suggest that lavender oil may improve skin healing through increasing growth factors in the dermis and epidermis more than other topical applications.[185]

Home Remedy

Rash Balm. Rub 3 drops each of lavender oil and geranium oil on the affected area three times daily; for sensitive skin, mix 3 drops with ½ teaspoon of coconut oil.

Background

Rashes are small, often-red bumps that appear on the skin; hives are raised white or yellow bumps surrounded by red, inflamed skin. Both rashes and hives usually start as a burning sensation followed by itching. They can be caused by an allergen or irritant from food, clothing or household chemicals. Medications, poor digestion or illness may also cause rashes or hives. One of the most common forms of a rash is contact dermatitis, which is caused when a substance of some sort irritates the skin. A more severe reaction may cause swelling, redness and larger blisters. Rashes can be caused by many things, including poison ivy, poison oak, soaps, detergents, shampoos, perfumes, lotions, a latex allergy and a food allergy. They may also occur from viral infections such as shingles, fungal infections, acne, eczema, psoriasis, rosacea, Lyme disease, bug bites or heat exposure.

Suggested Supplements

» **Vitamin C.** A powerful antioxidant with antihistamine properties. Take 2,000 milligrams daily.

» **Nettle Leaf.** Shown to be effective in reducing hives because it reduces overall histamine production. Take 300 milligrams, three times daily.

RESTLESS LEGS SYNDROME

 ## ESSENTIAL OILS

Roman Chamomile. Helps reduce muscle spasms; fights anxiety and depression; helps fight insomnia.

Cedarwood and Cypress. Contain antispasmodic properties; work as calming and soothing agents.

Helichrysum. Supports the neurological system; antispasmodic.[186]

Marjoram. May assist in relieving muscle aches and spasm.

Research

Roman chamomile contains coumarin, which has been shown to reverse inflammatory pain and shows promise for pharmaceutical and medicinal applications such as pain therapy.[187]

 ### Home Remedy

RLS Bath Soak. Add 5 to 10 drops each of cedarwood, Roman chamomile and helichrysum oils to a warm-water bath. For additional relief, rub 2 to 3 drops each of these oils mixed with a carrier oil onto your legs and cover with a warm compress for 10 minutes before bed.

Background

Restless legs syndrome (RLS) is a neurological condition characterized by a nearly irresistible urge to move the legs. The most distinctive aspect of the condition is that lying down and trying to relax activates the symptoms, which include throbbing, pulling, creeping or other unpleasant sensations in the legs. The sensations can be irritating and painful, and moving the legs helps to relieve the discomfort. Most people with RLS have difficulty falling asleep and staying asleep. When left untreated, RLS can lead to sleep deprivation and affect a person's ability to concentrate and complete daily tasks. This may also lead to depression and impaired memory. As many as 10 percent of the U.S. population may have RLS, and childhood RLS is estimated to affect almost 1 million children. The most common treatments for RLS are dopamine-related medications, even though long-term use can actually worsen symptoms in many individuals.

Suggested Supplements

» **Magnesium.** Relaxes muscles and nerves and is scientifically linked with improved sleep.[188]

» **Multivitamin.** Several deficiencies (iron, vitamin D and B-vitamins) can contribute to restless legs syndrome.

ROSACEA

ESSENTIAL OILS

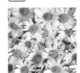
Roman Chamomile. Helps cell re-growth and encourages healing of damaged skin.

Geranium and Rose. Contain properties that cause contraction of skin cells.

Tea Tree. Helps with dermatologic infections and inflammatory conditions.[190]

Lavender. Has calming and anti-inflammatory effects on the skin.

Research

Tea tree oil exhibited a dose-dependent extermination effect on demodex mites, the most common ectoparasite found in the human skin.[191]

Home Remedy

Cooling Toner. Mix 1 ounce of apple cider vinegar and 1 ounce of natural aloe vera gel. Then add 5 drops of geranium oil and 5 drops of Roman chamomile oil and shake. Put the mixture into a spray bottle and use directly on your face, avoiding your eyes.

Background

Rosacea is a skin condition that causes redness and tiny, red bumps on the face. It is estimated to affect at least 16 million people in the U.S, most of whom are Caucasian with fair skin. The condition commonly affects the central third of the face, especially the nose, and has periodic ups and downs (flares and remissions). People typically equate rosacea with having a red, flushed face, but for most sufferers, the symptoms go beyond this and can include "spider veins" (visible broken blood vessels); swollen and painful skin; bloodshot eyes; sensitive skin that easily reacts to the sun, skin care products, heat or sweat; stinging or burning skin; and rough, itchy or scaling skin. The underlying causes of rosacea are still relatively unknown, but some experts now believe that rosacea is caused by demodex mites.[189] Common rosacea triggers can include alcohol, hot or spicy foods, emotional stress and heat.

Suggested Supplements

» **Bone Broth or Collagen Protein Powder.** Fights inflammation and promotes healthy skin, nails and hair.

» **Evening Primrose Oil.** High in gamma-linolenic acid, which improves the health of the skin. Take 500 milligrams twice a day.

SHINGLES

ESSENTIAL OILS

Tea Tree. Strengthens the immune system and helps fight against viruses.

Peppermint. Has cooling and soothing effects on the skin.

Helichrysum. Fights infections and supports healthy immune response.[192]

Oregano. Contains anti-viral properties; acts as a natural anti-bacterial agent.

Research

Research shows that oregano and its major component, carvacrol, are highly effective against various human and animal viruses.[193]

Home Remedy

Shingles Salve. Mix 2 to 4 drops each of tea tree, peppermint and helichrysum oils and mix with ¼ teaspoon of coconut oil; rub the mixture on the affected areas at least three times daily. Repeat until your symptoms improve and the rash fades.

Background

Shingles is a painful skin rash caused by the chickenpox virus. Once you contract chickenpox, the virus "sleeps" in your nerve roots. In some people, it stays dormant forever; in others, the virus "wakes up" when disease, stress or aging weakens the immune system, which is why shingles (closely associated with chickenpox) is most common in older adults and in people who have compromised immune systems. Shingles symptoms happen in stages: At first, you may have a headache, light sensitivity and flu symptoms. Next, you may feel itching, tingling or pain in an area before a rash appears in a band or strip on one side of the face or body. The rash later turns into clusters of blisters that fill with fluid and crust over, taking up to four weeks to heal. About one out of every three people will develop shingles in their lifetime—so boost your immune system with natural remedies, including essential oils.

Suggested Supplements

» **Vitamin B12 and Zinc.** Support immune function and may improve shingles symptoms.

» **Echinacea and Elderberry.** Can help your body fight off infections, including viruses. Take 500 milligrams, three times daily.

CONDITIONS

SINUSITIS

ESSENTIAL OILS

Eucalyptus. Helps to open the sinus pathways, clearing out mucus.

Peppermint. Helps reduce the swelling associated with sinusitis.

Thyme. Contains carvacrol, which reduces inflammation.[195]

Lemon. Supports mucus clearing in nasal and sinus regions.

 ### Research

An active ingredient in thyme oil, thymol, has been shown to be effective against multidrug-resistant bacteria strains, showing promise as a therapy for highly drug-resistant infections.[196]

 ### Home Remedy

Vapor Rub. Pour ¼ cup of olive oil, ½ cup of coconut oil and ¼ cup of grated beeswax into a jar; place the jar in a pan with water over medium heat. Once melted, stir. Allow it to cool slightly. Add 10 drops each of peppermint oil and eucalyptus oil. Allow it to set. Rub the mixture onto your chest multiple times each day.

Background

Sinusitis is an inflammation of the tissue lining the sinuses that often causes an infection and can result in mucus build-up and pain. It's an incredibly common condition, with almost 40 million Americans suffering from sinusitis each year. Causes include respiratory infection, allergies, nasal polyps and a weakened immune system. Symptoms of sinusitis may include fever, weakness, fatigue, cough, congestion and mucus drainage in the back of the throat, called postnasal drip. About 90 percent of adults seen in the U.S. by a general practice physician for sinusitis are prescribed an antibiotic, even though antibiotics may not always be the best remedy, according to recent research and physician experts.[194] Your body should be able to naturally overcome mild or moderate sinusitis without medication that can cause antibiotic resistance. Essential oils can greatly help with sinusitis symptoms, allowing your immune system to do its job.

Suggested Supplements

» **Xylitol-Based Nasal Spray.** Has been shown to be an effective disruptor of biofilms, which are protective measures used by germs that have invaded your sinuses.[197]

» **Colloidal Silver.** Supports the immune system's ability to fight infections. Can be consumed orally or in a nasal spray.

STREP THROAT

ESSENTIAL OILS

Eucalyptus. Stimulates immunity; improves respiratory circulation.[198]

Peppermint. Contains menthol, which helps to soothe a sore throat and thin mucus.

Thyme. Contains anti-bacterial properties that boost immunity and fight infections.

Oregano. Proven to fight infections and promote healing.

Research

Oregano has been shown to destroy the superbug MRSA both as a liquid and as a vapor. Researchers concluded that oregano oil shows tremendous promise as a natural anti-microbial.[199]

Home Remedy

Sore Throat Gargle. Gargle with 2 to 3 drops of oregano oil, 1 to 2 drops of peppermint oil and 1 teaspoon of salt in warm water for up to 1 minute, and then spit it out. Repeat three times daily.

Background

Strep throat is a bacterial infection that causes inflammation and pain in the throat and is caused by group A *Streptococcus* bacteria. Strep throat can affect children and adults of all ages. However, it's especially common in children between the ages of 5 and 15. Sneezing and coughing can spread the infection from one person to another. The common symptoms of strep throat include sudden fever; sore, red throat with white patches; headache; chills; swollen lymph nodes and trouble swallowing. If a child has six or more severe throat infections in one year, his or her doctor might suggest surgery to remove the tonsils. However, many children tend to stop having recurring instances of strep throat as they get older. The decision to remove a child's tonsils must be weighed against the risks of anesthesia and bleeding, as well as the missed school days to recover from the procedure.

Suggested Supplements

» **Garlic.** Fights germs and boosts the immune system.

» **Echinacea.** Can help your body fight off infections; it is best to take it at the first sign of illness (1,000 milligrams, two to three times daily).

TEETHING

ESSENTIAL OILS

 Clove. A natural analgesic with a long history of safe use in dentistry.[200]

 Peppermint. Soothes painful areas. Dilute before use.

 Lavender. Can be used diluted and applied to the jawline.

 Roman Chamomile. Helps promote calmness and relaxation.

 ### Research
A 2006 study showed that clove oil worked just as well as benzocaine at numbing the pain caused by toothache and infection.[201]

 ### Home Remedy

Teething Oil. Mix 1 teaspoon of olive oil and 1 teaspoon of coconut oil with 1 to 2 drops of clove oil. Shake well and apply it sparingly to the gums with your fingertip. Reapply every 2 to 3 hours as needed. Test the mixture on yourself before applying to make sure it is not too strong.

Background
Teething can be very challenging for babies and parents. While teething can begin as early as three months of age, you'll most likely see the first tooth start pushing through your baby's gum line when your little one is between four and seven months old. Researchers note that during teething, there is a notable increase in biting, drooling, gum rubbing, sucking, irritability, wakefulness and ear rubbing. Your baby might also have a facial rash and decreased appetite. These symptoms tend to manifest in the few days before and after a tooth's emergence from the gums. Although tender and swollen gums could cause your baby's temperature to be a little higher than normal, teething doesn't usually cause high fever or diarrhea. Essential oils such as clove can help your baby through the most uncomfortable teething symptoms. Remember to use common sense when it comes to essential oils and babies—as a little bit goes a long way.

Suggested Supplements

» **Pineapple Core.** Allow the baby to suck on a non-ripe (very hard) pineapple core. Bromelain found in the stem and core of a pineapple helps with inflammation and pain.

» **Homeopathic Teething Tablets.** Made with natural ingredients that dissolve easily under your baby's tongue.

TENDONITIS

ESSENTIAL OILS

Frankincense. Works to numb the affected area to provide relief.[202]

Cypress. Helps to reduce inflammation within the body; soothes pain.

Peppermint. A natural analgesic and muscle relaxant.

Turmeric. Contains potent anti-inflammatory compounds.

Research

Menthol (a primary compound found in peppermint oil) has been proven to enhance the dermal penetration of other medicines. This is perhaps what makes it an effective way to bring cooling relief to inflamed tendons.[203]

Home Remedy

Warm Compress. To help reduce pain and speed up blood flow, mix 2 drops each of frankincense, cypress and peppermint oils with ½ teaspoon of coconut oil. Apply the mixture to the painful area three to five times daily with a warm compress.

Background

Tendonitis is an inflammation or irritation of a tendon—a thick cord that attaches bone to muscle. It is most often caused by repetitive, minor impact on the affected area, or from a sudden, more serious injury. Activities that often cause tendonitis are carpentry, gardening, tennis, golf, painting and scrubbing. Anyone can get tendonitis, but it is more common in adults, especially those over 40 years of age. As tendons age, they tolerate less stress, are less elastic and tear easier. Symptoms include pain at the site of the tendon and surrounding area. Shoulder tendonitis involves the loss of motion and flexibility and is often called "adhesive capsulitis," or frozen shoulder. Conventional treatments for tendonitis such as NSAIDs (ibuprofen, aspirin, etc.) and corticosteroid injections can lead to liver problems, stomach pain, high blood pressure and more. Try these essential oils for a safer way to get relief from tendonitis pain.

Suggested Supplements

» **Bromelain.** An enzyme that comes from pineapples that reduces inflammation. Take 250 milligrams twice daily.

» **Bone Broth and Collagen Protein.** Support healthy inflammation response and joint, ligament and tendon health.

TOENAIL FUNGUS

ESSENTIAL OILS

Oregano. Shown to be superior to some prescription medications.[204]

Tea Tree. A natural anti-fungal agent; soothes the skin.

Clove. Effective in treating multiple forms of fungi.

Lemongrass. Helps fight internal and external fungal infections.

Research

Tea tree oil has been shown to have the ability to penetrate the fungal organelle membrane, which ultimately leads to eradication of the fungus at a cellular level.[205]

Home Remedy

Fungus Fighter. Combine 3 drops of oregano oil and 2 drops of tea tree oil, and then apply the mixture directly on the toenail four times a day. This must be done consistently, every day, for maximum benefit.

Background

Nail fungus (or onychomycosis) is a common condition that begins as a white or yellow spot under the tip of your nail. The fungus causes the toenail, particularly on the big toe, to thicken and discolor; the end may separate from the nail bed. Often, the nail is so thick you can't cut it. In severe cases, the nail may detach and fall off. Older people are more likely to suffer from nail fungus, and those with compromised immune systems are even more susceptible. It also affects more men than women. Diabetes and vascular problems are additional risk factors. Few are aware that toenail fungus symptoms can actually be a sign of candida yeast overgrowth within your system. Toenail fungus can cause pain and difficulty walking, not to mention self-consciousness when wearing sandals. Toenail fungus is notoriously difficult to treat, but the essential oils listed below have been shown to be effective against some fungus strains.

Suggested Supplements

» **Probiotics.** A quality probiotic supplement will help reduce levels of the systemic yeast behind the toenail fungus.

» **Olive Leaf Extract.** Has powerful anti-microbial action that can help eliminate yeast within your system.

ULCERS

ESSENTIAL OILS

Roman Chamomile. Reduces stress and aids the digestive system.

Lemon. Calms the stomach and aids digestion.[206]

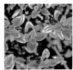

Thyme. Its active compound, thymol, is effective against ulcers.

Peppermint. Reduces stomach acids and has anti-microbial properties.

Research

Thymol, a primary compound in oregano and thyme oil, was found to display promising gastroprotective actions on acute and chronic ulcer models.[207]

Home Remedy

Ulcer Tonic. Add 2 drops each of peppermint oil and Roman chamomile oil to your water twice daily until symptoms subside.

Background

About one in every 10 Americans will suffer from the burning, gnawing abdominal pain of a peptic ulcer (in the stomach) or gastric ulcer (in the small intestine) at some point in life. Ulcers are similar to burns that form in the lining of the upper part of the GI tract. Until the mid-1980s, it was widely believed that ulcers formed as a result of stress, a genetic predisposition to excessive stomach acid secretion and poor lifestyle habits. While excessive stomach acid secretion certainly plays a role in the development of ulcers, a recent theory holds that bacterial infection is the primary cause of peptic ulcers. Other factors that may contribute to ulcer formation include excessive use of over-the-counter painkillers (such as aspirin, ibuprofen and naproxen), heavy alcohol consumption, psychological stress and smoking. With burning pain as the most common symptom, peptic ulcers affect as many as 5 million people in the U.S. alone.

Suggested Supplements

» **Licorice Root.** Can help stimulate regeneration of mucus membranes in the stomach and may help inhibit H. pylori. Take 500 milligrams before meals.

» **Aloe Vera.** Helps heal the intestinal lining. Take ¼ cup, three times daily.

URINARY TRACT INFECTION

ESSENTIAL OILS

Oregano. Prevents bacterial overgrowth in the bladder's interior walls.[208]

Clove. Fights the bacteria that lead to UTIs. Can fight parasites that thrive in the intestines.

Myrrh. Helps soothe the discomfort associated with UTIs and addresses the cause.

Lemongrass. Supports urinary tract health.

Research

Myrrh has been shown to have powerful analgesic properties and anti-inflammatory benefits that support the traditional uses of myrrh as an anti-inflammatory and pain reliever.[209]

Home Remedy

Bladder Soothe. Consume 5 drops of oregano oil diluted with 1 tablespoon of coconut oil or honey three times daily either until symptoms subside or up to 7 days. Also, take daily doses of probiotics.

Background

A urinary tract infection (UTI), or bladder infection, is an infection involving the kidneys, ureters, bladder or urethra that is caused by bacterial overgrowth in the bladder's interior walls. It leads to pain during urination, a frequent need to urinate and fever. The culprit in at least 90 percent of UTIs is a type of bacteria called Escherichia coli, better known as E. coli. If you're a woman, your chance of getting a UTI is high; some experts rank your lifetime risk of getting one as high as one in two—with many women having repeat infections, sometimes for years on end. UTIs are much more common in adults than in children, but about 1 to 2 percent of children do get them. In the U.S., UTIs account for more than 7 million visits to medical offices and hospitals each year. The most common causes of a UTI include sexual intercourse, overconsumption of sugar, pregnancy, antibiotic use, hormone imbalances and injury to the area.

Suggested Supplements

» **D-mannose.** Prevents bacterial buildup in the bladder. Take 500 milligrams, four times daily.

» **Probiotics.** Help increase good bacteria in the bladder and reduce the growth of infection-causing bacteria. Take 50 billion CFU daily.

VARICOSE VEINS

 ## ESSENTIAL OILS

 Cypress. Increases circulation and supports healthy vein walls.

 Thyme. Increases blood circulation and balances hormones.

 Fir Needle. Helps to increase metabolism and blood circulation.

 Geranium. Shown to strengthen the capillary walls of blood vessels.[210]

Research

Thyme oil was shown to improve the fatty acid composition in laboratory animals, which may help improve the appearance of varicose veins.[211]

 ### Home Remedy

Varicose Massage. Combine 10 drops each of geranium oil and fir needle oil, 5 drops of cypress oil and 4 teaspoons of a carrier oil. Use 1 teaspoon of this mixture to massage your legs twice daily. Using one hand and a gentle grip, start at ankles and stroke firmly but gently upward on either side of the varicose veins (never directly over them). Elevate legs after massaging.

Background

Varicose veins are enlarged veins that can be blue, red or flesh-colored. They often look like cords and appear twisted and bulging. Spider veins are similar to varicose veins but are smaller and closer to the surface of the skin. An estimated 30 to 60 percent of adults have varicose veins or spider veins. Varicose veins are typically caused by weak or damaged valves in the veins, while spider veins are most often caused by the backup of blood. They can also be caused by hormone changes, excessive exposure to the sun and injuries. Varicose veins often affect the legs, since they are the farthest from the heart and gravity makes it harder for the blood to flow upward. For many people, varicose veins and spider veins are simply a cosmetic concern. For others, varicose veins can cause aching pain and discomfort. Sometimes varicose veins lead to more serious problems. Some potential causes of varicose veins include obesity, pregnancy, standing for long periods of time, inactivity and hormone imbalance.

Suggested Supplements

» **Horse Chestnut.** Helps strengthen veins and can help reduce swelling. Take 100 milligrams daily.

» **Diosmin.** Can reduce inflammation of the veins and improve circulation.

WARTS

ESSENTIAL OILS

Tea Tree. Loaded with anti-viral ingredients that can fight warts.

Oregano. Its active ingredient, carvacrol, powerfully works to remove warts.

Lemongrass. Shown to effectively fight viruses.

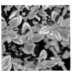
Thyme. Helps destroy viruses that live on the skin.[212]

Research
Studies have shown that lemongrass oil can effectively eliminate the herpes simplex type 1 virus (causes cold sores), both at the onset of a cold sore and even after it's already appeared, which demonstrates its anti-viral capabilities.[213]

Home Remedy
Wart Bomb. Add 20 drops each of oregano, lemongrass and tea tree oils to a 2-ounce glass dropper bottle. Add raw, organic apple cider vinegar (but do not fill to the top). Fill the remainder with fractionated coconut oil. Apply it directly to warts using 1 to 3 drops and a cotton swab. Apply it nightly until the warts have receded.

Background
A wart is a small, hard, benign growth on the skin caused by a virus. In order to target the exact course of action for eliminating warts, it helps to determine exactly what type of warts you have. Types of warts include common warts (which represent 70 percent of non-genital warts), flat warts, plantar warts and genital warts. Since they are caused by a virus, warts generally do not respond to medication. The root cause of every wart is human papillomavirus (HPV), of which there are more than 100 types. Warts are caused by direct contact with HPV, which is contagious and makes skin grow faster than usual. HPV can infect the skin via areas of minimal trauma such as cuts or abrasions. The main symptoms of warts are small, fleshy, grainy bumps. Essential oils provide what antibiotics can't—the ability to fight viruses and help address the root cause of warts.

Suggested Supplements
» **Apple Cider Vinegar.** Promotes skin healing and stimulates the immune system. Also helps to destroy the wart by making the area inhospitable for the virus.

» **Garlic.** A potent anti-viral that aids the immune system. Consume raw garlic or aged garlic supplements to support your immune response, and apply raw garlic directly to your warts.

WEIGHT GAIN/ OBESITY

ESSENTIAL OILS

Cinnamon. Contains cinnamaldehyde, which promotes healthy blood sugar.

Grapefruit. May reduce cravings for sweets and improve metabolism.

Ginger. Helps reduce systemic inflammation and improve digestion.

Black Pepper. Naturally warms the body; stimulates metabolism.[215]

Research

In a study, the scent of grapefruit oil stimulated loss of body fat, strengthened adrenal function and reduced appetite in laboratory animals. Researchers concluded grapefruit oil has tremendous potential as a weight loss aid.[216]

 ### Home Remedy

Weight Loss Boost. Add 1 to 3 drops of grapefruit oil to a glass of water three times daily, or add a blend of cinnamon, grapefruit, ginger and black pepper to a diffuser and take in deep breaths for two minutes, one to three times daily.

Background

"Overweight" and "obesity" are both labels for ranges of weight that are greater than what is generally considered healthy for a given height. The terms also identify ranges of weight that have been shown to increase the likelihood of certain diseases and other health problems. More than 35 percent of U.S. adults are obese, and more than 34 percent are overweight for a combined total of a whopping 69 percent.[214] An adult who has a BMI between 25 and 29.9 is considered overweight. An adult who has a BMI of 30 or higher is considered obese. Excess weight is often caused by an overconsumption of calories and physical inactivity. Some other causes may include hormonal imbalances, stress, medical conditions, genetics, toxins or certain medications. The good news is there are steps to treat weight gain and obesity naturally, which include eating a healthy diet, doing weekly exercise and using natural supplements.

Suggested Supplements

» **Bone Broth Protein Powder.** High in easy-to-digest protein, which may support healthy blood sugar and metabolism.

» **Probiotics.** Studies have shown improved weight loss with probiotic use; helps clear excess yeast, which may contribute to food cravings.

ADDITIONAL CONDITIONS

Here is a list of additional common conditions. For each, you will find the three to four most effective oils to use to ease symptoms and promote healing, as well as suggested supplements to enhance the recovery process. For each oil, we recommend referring to its single oil page in Part II for recommended applications and safety guidelines. If you are taking prescription medication, please consult with your healthcare practitioner before use.

Anemia
Effective Oils: Cinnamon, Grapefruit and Holy Basil
Suggested Supplements: Iron, Probiotics and B-Complex

Autoimmune Disease
Effective Oils: Frankincense, Holy Basil and Roman Chamomile
Suggested Supplements: Bone Broth Powder, Probiotics, Medicinal Mushrooms and Omega-3

Bad Breath
Effective Oils: Peppermint, Cinnamon and Lemon
Suggested Supplements: Probiotics, Pau D'arco and Ginger

Bipolar Disorder
Effective Oils: Vetiver, Holy Basil and Roman Chamomile
Suggested Supplements: Omega-3, Vitamin D and Ashwagandha

Bone Fracture
Effective Oils: Fir, Cypress and Lemongrass
Suggested Supplements: Vitamin D, Magnesium and Bone Broth Protein Powder

Chronic Obstructive Pulmonary Disease (COPD)
Effective Oils: Eucalyptus, Thyme and Ginger
Suggested Supplements: Vitamin C, NAC and Vitamin D

Crohn's Disease
Effective Oils: Peppermint, Ginger and Roman Chamomile
Suggested Supplements: Probiotics, Digestive Enzymes and Bone Broth Protein Powder

Dermatitis
Effective Oils: Geranium, Lavender, Rose Manuka and Myrrh
Suggested Supplements: Omega-3 and Probiotics

Fibroids
Effective Oils: Clary Sage, Frankincense and Thyme
Suggested Supplements: Vitex, Omega-3 and B-Complex

Food Allergies (Sensitivities)
Effective Oils: Ginger, Frankincense and Roman Chamomile
Suggested Supplements: Probiotics, Digestive Enzymes and Bone Broth Protein Powder

Foot Odor
Effective Oils: Tea Tree, Lemongrass, Patchouli and Fir Needle
Suggested Supplements: Zinc and Probiotics

Gallbladder Problems (Gallstones)
Effective Oils: Citrus, Rosemary and Peppermint
Suggested Supplements: Digestive Enzymes, Ox Bile and Milk Thistle

Gout
Effective Oils: Turmeric, Peppermint, Lime and Holy Basil
Suggested Supplements: Celery Seed, Black Cherry and Nettles

Grave's Disease
Effective Oils: Frankincense, Myrrh and Holy Basil
Suggested Supplements: Ashwagandha, Vitamin D and Bone Broth Protein Powder

Hashimoto's Thyroiditis
Effective Oils: Holy Basil, Frankincense and Myrrh
Suggested Supplements: Probiotics, Ashwagandha and Bone

Broth Protein Powder

Heavy Metal Exposure
Effective Oils: Cilantro, Coriander, Turmeric and Grapefruit
Suggested Supplements: Milk Thistle, Probiotics and Chlorella

Heel Spurs (Bone Spurs)
Effective Oils: Rosemary, Thyme, Lavender and Cypress
Suggested Supplements: Magnesium and Vitamin B5

Hypotension (Low Blood Pressure)
Effective Oils: Rosemary, Ginger, Bergamot and Holy Basil
Suggested Supplements: Ginseng, Licorice and Reishi

Jock Itch
Effective Oils: Lavender, Myrrh, Tea Tree, Manuka and Turmeric
Suggested Supplements: Apple Cider Vinegar and Cornstarch

Kidney Stones
Effective Oils: Geranium, Lemon, Juniper and Thyme
Suggested Supplements: Magnesium, B Vitamins and Cranberry Extract

Lice
Effective Oils: Tea Tree, Clove, Eucalyptus and Lavender
Suggested Supplements: Coconut Oil and Omega-3

Low Testosterone
Effective Oils: Sandalwood, Cedarwood and Rosemary
Suggested Supplements: L-Arginine, Vitamin D3, Ashwagandha, Shilajit and Zinc

Migraines
Effective Oils: Peppermint, Lavender and Ginger
Suggested Supplements: Magnesium, Butterbur, Feverfew and Bone Broth Protein Powder

Obsessive Compulsive Disorder (OCD)
Effective Oils: Cypress, Lavender and Frankincense
Suggested Supplements: Omega-3, Magnesium and B-Complex

Pink Eye
Effective Oils: Roman Chamomile, Manuka and Frankincense
Suggested Supplements: Colloidal sliver, Elderberry and Echinacea

Poison Ivy
Effective Oils: Tea Tree, Geranium and Roman Chamomile
Suggested Supplements: Baking Soda, Apple Cider Vinegar and Vitamin C

Postpartum Depression
Effective Oils: Rose and Lavender
Suggested Supplements: Fish Oil or Cod Liver Oil and Bright Light Therapy

Ringworm
Effective Oils: Tea Tree, Oregano, Lemongrass and Myrrh
Suggested Supplements: Garlic and Grapefruit Seed Extract

Sciatica
Effective Oils: Basil, Frankincense, Peppermint and Eucalyptus
Suggested Supplements: Vitamin B Complex, Calcium and Magnesium

Seasonal Affective Disorder (SAD)
Effective Oils: Lavender, Jasmine, Ylang Ylang and Bergamot
Suggested Supplements: B Vitamins and St. John's Wort

Shin Splints
Effective Oils: Frankincense, Lavender, Clove and Peppermint
Suggested Supplements: Fish Oil or Cod Liver Oil and Organic Green Superfood

Small Intestinal Bacterial Overgrowth (SIBO)
Effective Oils: Lemon, Ginger, Oregano, Thyme and Peppermint
Suggested Supplements: Digestive Enzymes, Bone Broth Protein Powder and Probiotics

Sprains/Strains
Effective Oils: Cypress, Lemongrass and Turmeric

Suggested Supplements: Bone Broth Protein Powder + Collagen, Omega-3 and Proteolytic Enzymes

Stress
Effective Oils: Jasmine, Sandalwood, Vetiver and Lavender
Suggested Supplements: Ginseng, Ashwagandha, Rhoidola and Magnesium

Stroke
Effective Oils: Cypress, Helichrysum, Cedarwood and Frankincense
Suggested Supplements: Coenzyme Q10 and Vitamin B3 (Niacin)

Sunburn
Effective Oils: Peppermint, Lavender and Helichrysum
Suggested Supplements: Aloe Vera Gel and Apple Cider Vinegar

Swimmer's Ear
Effective Oils: Tea Tree, Basil and Frankincense
Suggested Supplements: Garlic, Mullein Oil and Colloidal Silver

Temporomandibular Joint Dysfunction (TMD or TMJ)
Effective Oils: Lavender, Peppermint and Marjoram
Suggested Supplements: Magnesium, Omega-3 and Collagen Protein

Thrush (Oral)
Effective Oils: Clove, Thyme, Cinnamon and Oregano
Suggested Supplements: Probiotics and Coconut Oil

Toothaches
Effective Oils: Clove, Peppermint and Tea Tree
Suggested Supplements: Sea Salt and Ginger Root

Ulcerative Colitis
Effective Oils: Ginger, Peppermint and Roman Chamomile
Suggested Supplements: Digestive Enzymes, Probiotics and Bone Broth Protein Powder

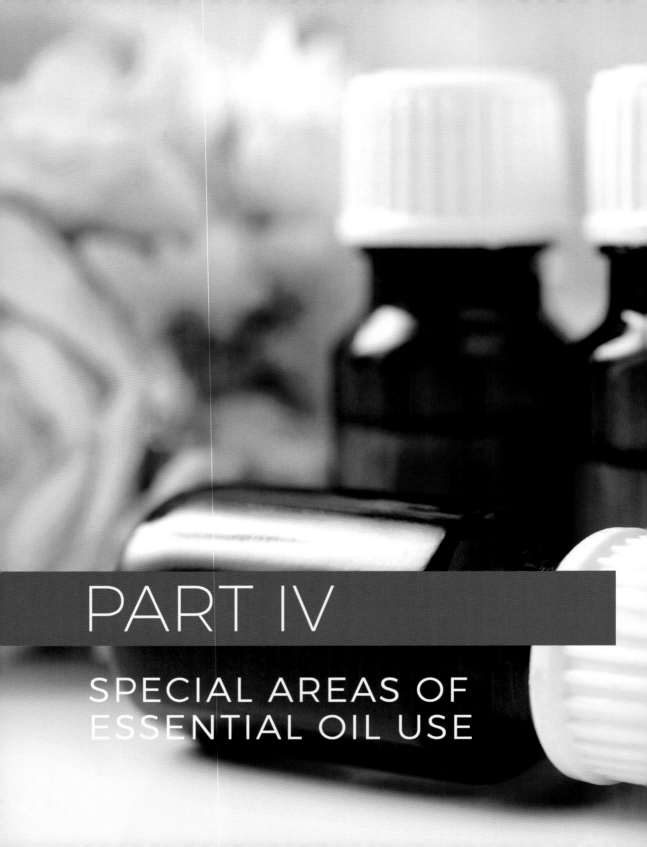

PART IV

SPECIAL AREAS OF ESSENTIAL OIL USE

Thanks to the powerful compounds in essential oils, their uses are enormously broad and varied. There are few supplements that can boast the ability to be used in natural remedies, personal and home care products, therapeutic massage and spiritual practice, and are powerful yet safe enough for use in infant care and during pregnancy. They are even great for our four-legged friends!

In this section, we will detail six special areas of essential oil use as follows:

Chapter 6: Reflexology and Massage
Chapter 7: Healing Touch "By His Wounds" Therapy
Chapter 8: Pregnancy and Baby Care
Chapter 9: Skin and Body Care
Chapter 10: Home Cleaning and Detoxing
Chapter 11: Natural Pet Care

The three of us are so thankful for the gift of essential oils in our lives. We encourage you to utilize these sections that include reference tables as a guide to understanding some of the more specialized areas of essential oil usage.

CHAPTER 6

REFLEXOLOGY AND MASSAGE

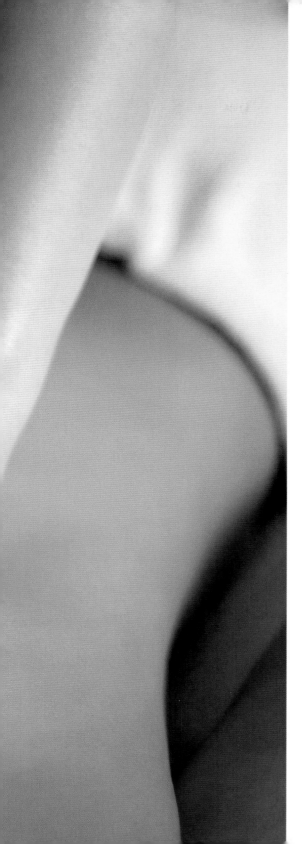

The human body is an amazing, complex and uniquely designed machine. The fact that our bodies turn food into both fuel and living tissue, our hearts pump blood through thousands of miles of blood vessels and our brains send billions of bits of information throughout the body that control every action—right down to the flicker of an eyelid—is a demonstration that we are the work of an intelligent and skillful designer. What's even more amazing is that, according to Genesis 1:27, "...God created man in His own image, in the image of God created He him, male and female created He them."

We truly are "fearfully and wonderfully made." Our bodies have an incredible level of organization from the molecular level to the tissue level. God put such thought into the balance of our bodily functions and systems—so much that one change at the micron level can lead to health issues and even disease.

In this chapter, we are going to examine two forms of body therapy that assist our bodies in doing their intricate, immense and unremitting jobs. The power of touch can move energy and focus to the areas of the body in need of special attention—and in combination with the use of essential oils, body therapies can facilitate healing on all levels and be an effective way to relieve symptoms that occur both internally and externally.

REFLEXOLOGY

"Reflexology" and "foot massage" are often synonymous, but putting these two in the same category does this ancient practice an injustice. Reflexology involves massaging the feet, but more specifically, it is a hands-on complementary therapy that is based on the premise that there are zones and reflex areas in the feet (also the hands and ears) that correspond to all body parts. The physical act of applying specific pressures using thumb, finger and hand techniques results in stress reduction that causes physiological changes in the body.

Reflexology dates back thousands of years to the ancient civilizations of Egypt, India and China. The oldest known documentation of reflexology is a pictograph found in the tomb of an Egyptian physician that depicts patients having treatments done on their hands and feet.

The modern form of reflexology was first brought to light in the early 1900s by a surgeon named Dr. William Fitzgerald. He discovered that exerting pressure on the tips of the toes or fingers caused corresponding parts of the body to become anaesthetized. From this, Dr. Fitzgerald divided the body into 10 equal zones and aptly named it "zone therapy." Amazingly, by using tight elastic bands on the middle sections of the fingers or small clamps on the tips of the fingers, he found it was no longer necessary to use anesthetic agents during minor surgeries!

The subject of zone therapy was a controversial one, although it met with a certain amount of success with osteopaths and dentists in the mid 1900s. A physiotherapist named Eunice Ingram worked in a doctor's office where Dr. Fitzgerald's zone therapy was being used on patients' hands. Ms. Ingham thought, however, that it would be more effective to be practiced on the feet rather than the hands.

She extended the work of Dr. Fitzgerald and painstakingly mapped the feet, where one point on the foot corresponds to a certain part of the body. See figure 6.1 for a map of these corresponding areas on the feet.

Foot Reflexology Chart

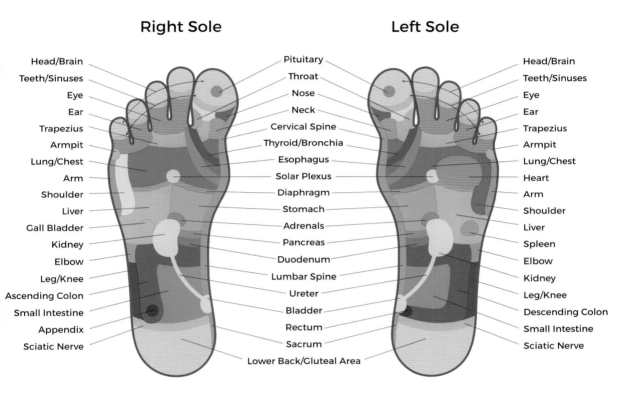

Right Sole

Head/Brain
Teeth/Sinuses
Eye
Ear
Trapezius
Armpit
Lung/Chest
Arm
Shoulder
Liver
Gall Bladder
Kidney
Elbow
Leg/Knee
Ascending Colon
Small Intestine
Appendix
Sciatic Nerve

Left Sole

Pituitary
Throat
Nose
Neck
Cervical Spine
Thyroid/Bronchia
Esophagus
Solar Plexus
Diaphragm
Stomach
Adrenals
Pancreas
Duodenum
Lumbar Spine
Ureter
Bladder
Rectum
Sacrum
Lower Back/Gluteal Area

Head/Brain
Teeth/Sinuses
Eye
Ear
Trapezius
Armpit
Lung/Chest
Heart
Arm
Shoulder
Liver
Spleen
Elbow
Kidney
Leg/Knee
Descending Colon
Small Intestine
Sciatic Nerve

Figure 6.1. Foot Reflexology Chart. By using acupressure or massage techniques on these points in the feet, a positive effect is created in the corresponding body part.

HOW DOES IT WORK?

There are many theories about how reflexology works, but the most commonly held belief is that the practice works to relax reflexes that are connected to various parts of the body, improving lymphatic drainage and circulation as well as relaxing muscles and stimulating nerve connections. Since experts believe that stress causes up to 90 percent of all illness, by relaxing the recipient, reflexology may help to prevent and heal damage from stress.[1]

Reflexology works with zones, and it is believed that by "clearing" the zones, you allow energy to flow in the body and healing can occur. Nerve endings can become calcified and therefore dysfunctional. Through reflexology, you can "break up" this calcification and re-establish communication in the body by stimulating circulation and promoting detoxification.

Reflexology also works through the communication of the nervous system. There are over 7,200 nerve endings in each foot. Stimulating these nerves has a huge impact on the entire body. By applying calm, healing touch, the entire body can relax and be soothed.

WHAT DOES IT DO?

One large review of reflexology summarized 168 research studies and abstracts from journals and meetings from around the world.[2] Many of these studies originated in peer-reviewed journals in China and Korea. All of the studies contained information about the frequency and duration of the reflexology application. Based on the studies reviewed, it was concluded that reflexology may:

» **Have a positive impact on specific organs.** Various reports state that MRI readings have demonstrated an increase in blood flow to kidneys and to the intestines after reflexology massage.

» **Be associated with an improvement of a wide variety of symptoms.** Positive changes were noted in kidney functioning with kidney dialysis patients. In another study, 100 percent of cancer patients reported significant improvement in symptoms after three reflexology sessions.

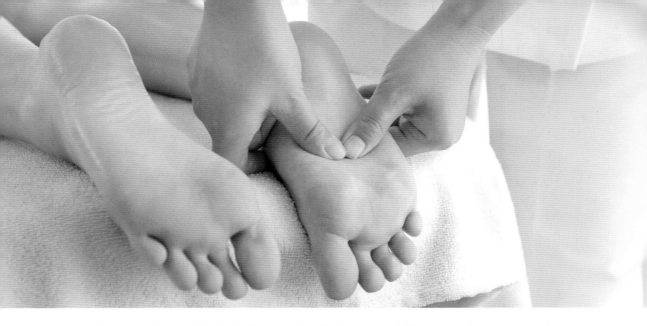

Improved areas included appetite, fatigue, mobility, mood, nausea, pain and sleep.[3]

» **Create a relaxation effect.** In certain studies, blood pressure was decreased and anxiety was lowered after a series of reflexology massages.

» **Aid in pain reduction associated with certain conditions.** Twenty-seven separate studies demonstrated a positive outcome for reduction in pain; e.g., AIDS, chest pain, peripheral neuropathy of diabetes mellitus, kidney stones and osteoarthritis.[4]

» **Help alleviate headache pain.** After three months of reflexology massage, 81 percent of the patients in one study claimed that the therapy either considerably helped or completely eliminated their headaches, and 19 percent who previously took prescription or OTC drugs to manage the pain were able to stop their medication altogether.[5]

» **Boost cardiovascular health.** By reducing baroreceptor reflex sensitivity, reflexology boosts heart health while also relieving stress, anxiety and pain that can put the cardiovascular system at risk.[6]

It is important to note that reflexology does not "heal" any ailments; the body repairs itself. The human body responds to touch, which can facilitate restoration on all levels. This makes reflexology a phenomenal way to supplement other natural and conventional therapies.

DEEP REFLEX FOOT MASSAGE USING ESSENTIAL OILS

The use of essential oils during a reflexology massage can greatly enhance its benefits. The numerous therapeutic properties of essential oils coupled with the proven uses of reflexology form a powerful combination of restorative therapy for a myriad of health challenges and conditions.

If you are interested in receiving a reflexology session, there are likely several practitioners nearby. Ask around or search an online holistic practitioner directory to find one near you.

Alternatively, you can start by practicing some reflexology techniques at home. The following will provide you with a step-by-step guide for using essential oils to perform a basic reflexology foot massage on a friend or a loved one.

» **Step 1:** Use a diluted essential oil or blend to massage one foot, starting clockwise on the center of the arch. Slowly increase the size of the circles and add pressure for a few minutes, and then switch to the other foot—creating a balance between each foot as you go through the massage.

» **Step 2:** Press your knuckle into the center of the foot, activating the liver on the right foot and spleen on the left foot. Massage in small circles on one foot and then switch.

» **Step 3:** Use your thumbs and knuckles to massage the balls of the feet, relieving tension and pressure. Focus on one foot for a few minutes and then switch.

» **Step 4:** Unblock the control areas of the brain by pressing your knuckle or thumb into the big toe, making a downward and circular movement—working the middle, base and neck of the toe. This will help to unblock emotions and relieve stress. Continue to massage each toe the same way before switching to the other foot.

» **Step 5:** Work the heel of the foot, putting pressure on the bottom center and large bones on each side of the foot. This will target the reproductive organs in both men and women and the prostate in men.

» **Step 6:** To end the massage, work the top of the feet and ankles.

If the person being massaged feels pain, reduce the pressure slightly. As the area is massaged over time, the pain will begin to minimize—indicating that the massage is unblocking the area and benefiting the corresponding organ.

Essential Oil Use Guide for Reflexology

The best way to keep the bodily systems working properly is to massage a few major pressure points each day, applying a few drops of essential oils, either neat or diluted, with a carrier oil. Use this table to select the ideal oils to use for your specific areas of concern.

Body Part/Organ	Reflex Point	Essential Oils
Adrenal	Middle of both feet	Holy basil, clove, rosemary
Colon	Lower-outer side, right foot	Ginger, lemon, peppermint
Ears	Fourth and fifth toes	Basil, frankincense, tea tree, lavender
Heart	Upper-middle of left foot	Frankincense, cypress, rose, ylang ylang
Kidney & Bladder	Middle of both feet	Geranium, lemon, grapefruit, thyme
Liver & Gallbladder	Middle-outer side, right foot	Geranium, rosemary, lavender, bergamot
Lungs	Top of foot, center	Eucalyptus, peppermint, rosemary, thyme

Body Part/Organ	Reflex Point	Essential Oils
Ovaries	Inner ankle	Cypress, fennel, frankincense
Sciatic Nerve	Heel	Peppermint, ginger, lavender
Shoulder	Upper-outer side, both feet	Turmeric, lemongrass, peppermint
Spine	Upper-inner side, both feet	Tea tree, peppermint, white fir, lemongrass
Spleen	Middle-outer side, left foot	Lemon, tea tree, basil, orange
Stomach	Upper-inner side, both feet	Ginger, oregano, peppermint
Testes	Outer ankle	Clary sage, rosemary, sandalwood, turmeric
Uterus	Inner ankle	Clary sage, geranium, frankincense, jasmine

TOUCH MASSAGE

The practice of using touch as a healing method derives from customs and techniques rooted in ancient history. Massage therapy began as a sacred system of natural healing; however, cultural shifts rendered it little more than a form of indulgence for extensive periods of history. Thankfully, massage has experienced a resurgence in modern times. Today, massage is used as a form of holistic therapy for its ability to reduce pain, increase alertness, relieve feelings of depression and enhance immune function.

Modern massage therapists practice a multitude of techniques originating from methods that are as old as time. The goal is simple—to help others promote their physical and emotional well-being and experience a higher quality of life. The body of research dedicated to proving massage therapy's benefits continues to grow and has revealed that massage may:

» **Help fight depression.** A 2010 meta-analysis investigated the effects of massage therapy on depression symptoms by reviewing 17 studies containing 786 participants. All trials displayed the positive effects of touch massage when compared to control groups.[7]

» **Aid in reducing stress.** A review published in Sports Medicine states that touch massage therapy produces positive effects on recovery and muscle soreness after physical exertion or injury.[8]

» **Alleviate pain.** In 2014, 404 patients with fibromyalgia were analyzed after receiving massage therapy for at least five weeks. The meta-analyses showed that massage therapy improved pain, anxiety and depression in patients.

» **Promote hormone balance.** A study found that massage was associated with an increase in the hormone oxytocin, as well as reductions in adrenocorticotropin hormone, nitric oxide and beta-endorphin levels.

» **Lessen systemic inflammation.** A 2012 study evaluated the effects of massage on young male participants with muscle damage. Massage reduced the production of the inflammatory compounds and mitigated cellular stress.

There is no shortage of massage therapists, but not all of them utilize essential oils in their therapy. Make sure to ask plenty of questions before you book a session.

TOUCH MASSAGE TECHNIQUE

If you are interested in incorporating massage therapy into your family's health regimen, the technique below is an excellent primer to begin to understand how to give a healing massage. We've also included a brief list of oils that address specific areas of concern.

» **Step 1:** Depending on the desired effect of the massage (overall relaxation, pain relief, inflammation reduction, etc.), choose an appropriate essential oil. Create a blend or use 5 to 10 drops of one oil diluted with a teaspoon of a carrier oil. Use the following chart to determine which oils to use based on the desired benefit.

Benefit	Essential Oils
Alleviate Pain	Peppermint, lavender, eucalyptus, rosemary, turmeric
Boost Immunity	Clove, frankincense, lemon, myrrh, ginger, thyme
Boost Mood	Ylang ylang, lavender, orange, frankincense, rose, vetiver
Reduce Inflammation	Roman chamomile, frankincense, eucalyptus, peppermint, rosemary, turmeric
Reduce Stress	Lavender, bergamot, Roman chamomile, frankincense, rose, ylang ylang

» **Step 2:** Position the recipient's body correctly, resting stomach-down on a flat, comfortable surface. Take pressure off the neck by allowing it to be straight during the massage. It should not be tilted up or pulled to one side. A pillow can also be placed under the feet to take pressure off the lower back.

» **Step 3:** Warm up the oil in your hands before applying it to the back. Start by distributing the oil over the length of the spine. Press your hands, palms down, into the back lightly and make three clockwise circles over the heart area. Then slide one hand to the bottom of the spine and the other hand to the base of the skull—building a connection and sense of balance.

» **Step 4:** The first step of massage is called effleurage; this helps to distribute the oil evenly while warming up the tissues. Standing at the recipient's head, maintain the same pressure throughout this movement and rhythmically move up and down the spine, placing your palms down side by side. Use light but firm, broad strokes, making sure to cover the entire back with oils.

» **Step 5:** Petrissage is a kneading movement that can be used with the palms, knuckles or fingertips that is designed to increase circulation. With one hand, make small circles and move up the side of the back and slide back down the spine. Repeat this three times, and then switch to the other side. The pressure should be slightly firmer than the pressure used during effleurage.

» **Step 6:** To apply more pressure, add one hand on top of the other and continue kneading up the back and back down the spine. This is called reinforced kneading, and it boosts lymphatic circulation.

» **Step 7:** Place both hands on the spine with your fingers pointing away from you. Slide one hand from the spine to the side of the back using mild pressure; repeat using the other hand. Continue this movement, working from the base of the spine up to the base of the skull. Do this three times, and then switch to the other side.

» **Step 8:** Stand at the recipient's head and place your hands, palms down, on the shoulders. Push your hands out to the points of the shoulders. Then rotate your hands and pull them to the neck, moving along the neck from top to bottom.

» **Step 9:** Grip the earlobe between your thumb and forefinger, working your fingers in small circles with gentle pressure. Slide your thumbs along the backs of the ears.

» **Step 10:** End the massage by repeating step 4—moving up and down the spine with gentle pressure.

Reflexology and massage are both excellent therapies that promote vitality and healing. Our lives would certainly not be complete without them, and we believe you will gain even more benefit from massage by incorporating essential oils into your therapy. The oils we recommend in this chapter are just the beginning; there is virtually no end to the combination of oils you can use in conjunction with various forms of massage therapy.

CHAPTER 7

HEALING TOUCH
"BY HIS WOUNDS"
THERAPY

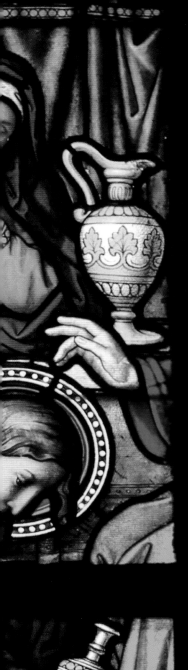
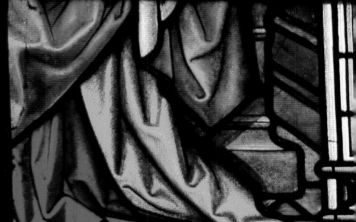
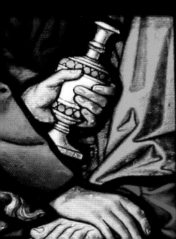
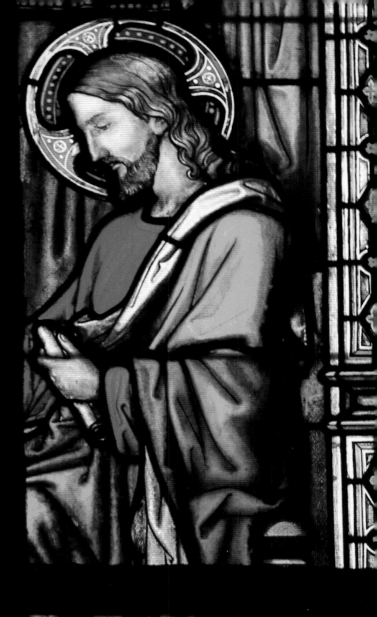

In the last chapter, we discussed the benefits of two forms of massage and the use of essential oils during therapeutic bodywork. Here we introduce a truly holistic therapy that can transform your body, mind and spirit, and create deep connections between the one who provides the therapy and the recipient.

In order to explain this new essential oil healing system and why it is so dear to our hearts, we'll first explain where the idea for this unique form of spiritually-based therapy originated.

Jordan had been aware of essential oils for decades before they ever became an instrumental part of his life in 2008, when he was given a death sentence. Doctors told him there was a 100 percent chance he would be dead within three months from an aggressive form of metastatic cancer if he did not take the traditional cancer treatment route (chemotherapy and surgery).

Jordan felt strongly that this was not the answer he needed if he wanted to survive this prognosis—and that is when he made the life-changing decision to embark upon a dramatic physical, mental, emotional and spiritual healing plan that spanned 40 days. During that period of time, he spent 12 to 14 hours a day focused on diet, detoxification and body therapies, as well as engaging in a major spiritual attack on cancer.

Part of Jordan's daily regimen involved a massage that was a combination of lymphatic drainage and essential oil therapy and included the use of up to a dozen or more oils at a time. The essential oil session alone lasted an hour every single day, seven days a week, for all 40 days of his healing plan. Jordan also diffused essential oils all day long throughout his home, added them to cleansing beverages, poured them on his head and rubbed oils on his feet.

This multi-faceted attack that was a combination of holistic and spiritual therapies resulted in a total healing, and Jordan truly became more than a conqueror. It was a supernatural miracle, made possible by God's direct hand on Jordan and aided by natural therapies.

Essential oils also became a bigger part of Dr. Josh's life after his mother's victorious battle against cancer. As a part of her natural path to cancer treatment, she received two to three lymphatic massages per week using various essential oils.

There was no doubt in our minds how restorative and powerful essential oils could be. And slowly, over the course of the last decade, they have taken on more and more of a primary role in each of our lives.

THE BIBLICAL SIGNIFICANCE OF OILS IN ANOINTING

Beyond simply the healing power of oils, we believe their power also comes from their significance in Scripture. The oils and aromatics mentioned in the Bible were more valuable than gold and silver. Israel's King Hezekiah kept "the spices, and the precious ointment" (2 Kings 20:13) together with silver and gold in the royal treasure chamber.

People and objects were anointed throughout the Bible: Aaron and his sons were anointed priests, the Tabernacle and all of its vessels were anointed before being put into service and Saul and David were anointed to be kings. It has been suggested that the holy anointing oil described in Exodus 30:23-25 is a symbol of being set apart for special purposes in God's kingdom.

The Hebrew word for Messiah, Moshiach, means "Anointed One." Jesus Christ was twice anointed with the oil of spikenard, which was so expensive that Judas was indignant that it wasn't sold to raise money for the poor. Psalm 45 informs us that the garments of the Messiah are fragrant with myrrh, aloes and cassia.

In one translation of Philippians 4:18, Paul described gifts given as "a fragrant aroma, an acceptable sacrifice, well-pleasing to God." In Proverbs 27:9, we are told "ointment and perfume rejoice in the heart." The New Testament also suggests that incense offering represents the prayers of saints rising up to God in Heaven.

There is no doubt that oils play a significant role both spiritually and therapeutically in the Bible. Now, although Jordan never formally studied the existing aromatherapy massage techniques, as he was coaching people who were having some health challenges, he was inspired to create an essential oil system that was healing to the body in a physical and spiritual sense.

He soon felt led to develop a system that is based on the healing properties of essentials oils and serves as a symbolic representation of the areas of Jesus' body that bled (for us) in the hours leading up to and during the crucifixion.

He called it BHW, or By His Wounds.

THE BIBLICAL ESSENTIAL OIL HEALING SYSTEM

By His Wounds (BHW) Therapy is a modern anointing system that allows you to connect to God in a meaningful, deep way. The idea is that you quite literally anoint the areas of the body where Jesus bled with special oils. This system was revealed to Jordan, in part because of the significant role essential oils played in his healing, and also because of the Biblical importance of oils themselves in anointing.

There are seven key areas where the anointing occurs, with each area representing a place on Christ's body from which he bled:

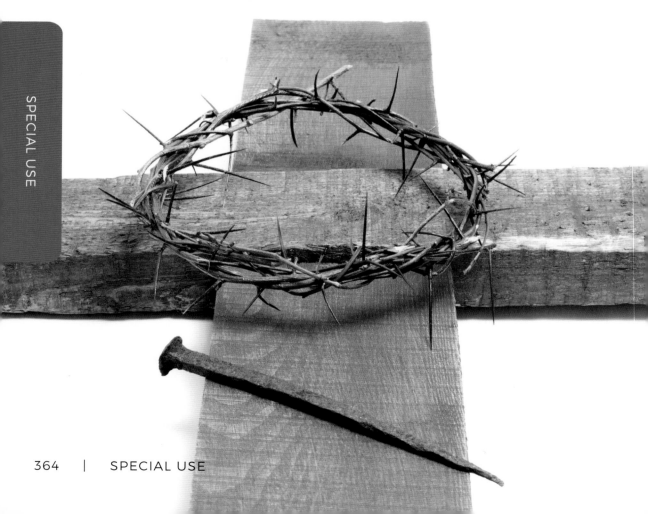

1. **Feet.** Jesus shed blood from his feet when a large nail or spike was driven through skin, tendon, nerve and bone in order to secure his feet to the cross—a heavy price to pay for our peace.

2. **Hands.** In the same manner in which his feet were nailed to the cross, so too were his hands (or perhaps his wrists). Jesus paid for our inheritance, and because of his sacrifice, we have authority in His name.

3. **Head.** Jesus was mocked by Roman soldiers, who placed a crown of thorns upon his head. Matthew 27:29 tells us, "And plaiting a crown of thorns, they put it on His head, and a reed in His right hand. And they bowed the knee before Him and mocked Him, saying, Hail, King of the Jews!" The King of Kings could have silenced them without a word, but he endured the humiliation for us.

4. **Sides.** Jesus shed blood from his side. When it was pierced, it is said that both blood and water came from Him. Some believe this is a physical symbol that his heart burst. He truly paid the price to heal the broken hearted.

5. **Chest.** Jesus was beaten and bruised so severely that internal bleeding was evident under his skin, including on his chest. He bled on the inside for our iniquities.

6. **Neck.** The scourging on Jesus' entire body was brutal. Scourging was a punishment so severe, humiliating and demeaning that it was reserved only for slaves and non-Romans—those who were viewed as the lesser elements in Roman society. The scourging undoubtedly caused our Savior's neck and shoulders to bleed.

7. **Back.** Just before His crucifixion, the Romans viciously flogged Jesus. Deuteronomy 25:3 states that a criminal should not receive more than 40 lashes. In order to avoid possibly breaking this command, the Jews would only give criminals 39 lashes, which is why many infer this is the number of lashes Jesus received. He paid for our healing by His stripes, His wounds. And by His wounds we are healed.

The pure, perfect innocence of Jesus Christ, His wisdom and creative power, were all present in His human body. This flawless Shepherd chose to accept an undeserved, cruel death in order to save us. The Father chose to send His son to the cross, and Jesus chose to take our punishment. They conspired to save all who would believe and to show by Jesus' wounds both the seriousness of our sin and the depth of His love.

BHW Therapy is one small way to show Christ that we both recognize and honor this most ultimate sacrifice, and it is also an ideal way to benefit from the therapeutic qualities of essential oils.

Here are the seven basic guidelines for BHW Therapy:

1. With the recipient lying down comfortably, anoint each area in the order presented in this section, starting with the feet and hands and then working your way down the body from the head.

2. The last part of the body to address will be the back and spine. For this area, you will apply the oils with 39 downward motions, representing the 39 stripes Jesus received.

3. For each part of the body, you will use a different oil. See the following table (BHW Therapy Application Chart) for our recommendations.

4. Apply a few drops of a carrier oil and then apply three drops per oil to the area. Note that several of the oils can be applied neat if desired.

5. Rub in the oils seven times using a circular motion (see BHW Therapy Application Chart for specific application suggestions). You can repeat the seven circular motions as many times as desired.

6. During your BHW session, we recommend listening to worship music or the Bible on an app or CD. Third Day has a song entitled "By His Wounds" that is both poignant and fitting.

7. Use light to moderate pressure, depending on the preference of the recipient. Take your time, spending anywhere from one to three minutes on each location for up to 30 minutes total.

BHW THERAPY APPLICATION CHART

Location	Oil	Specific Application
Feet	*Lavender* — Similar to what was used by Mary on Jesus' feet (spikenard). Ideal for greater intuition and clarity.	Apply to both the feet and ankles. Can apply NEAT.
Hands	*Frankincense* — The king of the oils. Can help us release parts of ourselves that hold us back from connecting with our soul, as well as feelings of unworthiness and insecurity.	Apply to both the hands and wrists. Can apply NEAT.
Head	*Myrrh or Rosemary* — A main component in ancient anointing oil for kings. Uplifting to the mind; can relieve stress and relax the body. Rosemary oil also works well because of its neurological and anti-inflammatory benefits.	Apply over the entire head, even dripping the oil onto the top of the head, much like the kings of antiquity were anointed. Can apply NEAT.
Sides	*Thyme* — Similar to hyssop, which was used in the ceremonial cleansing of people and houses in Biblical times.	Apply to one or both sides. Can apply NEAT.

Chest	*Orange* — Uplifts the heart, lends support by uplifting and promoting a positive attitude while calming the spirit.	Apply just above the pectoral muscles. Can apply NEAT.
Neck	*Peppermint* — Can cleanse the spirit and increase attunement with the soul so that intuitive awareness is released.	Dilute with a carrier oil and apply to neck and tops of the shoulders.
Back	*Cedarwood or Cypress* — Great for spinal health. According to some sources, the cross was made of either cedarwood or cypress wood.	Dilute with a carrier oil and apply in a downward motion on the spine 39 times to represent the lashes Jesus received.

You may have noticed that there are seven areas of the body, seven guidelines and a series of seven circular motions used during application. The reason for this is because the number seven is the foundation of God's word. The number was used 735 times in the Bible (54 times in the book of Revelation alone). Seven is the number of completeness and perfection, both physical and spiritual. It derives much of its meaning from being tied directly to God's creation of all things. Therefore, we feel it is a fitting number to bring an even greater sense of spiritual awareness to your practice.

To further enrich and enhance your practice, here are seven verses that can be said at the beginning of the therapy or during application of the oils:

James 5:14-15 (AMP)
Is anyone among you sick? He must call for the elders (spiritual leaders) of the church and they are to pray over him, anointing him with oil in the name of the Lord; and the prayer of faith will restore the one who is sick, and the Lord will raise him up; and if he has committed sins, he will be forgiven.

Isaiah 53:5 (NIV)
But he was pierced for our transgressions, he was crushed for our iniquities; the punishment that brought us peace was on him, and by his wounds we are healed.

Psalms 103:2-5 (NIV)
Praise the Lord, my soul, and forget not all his benefits—who forgives all your sins and heals all your diseases, who redeems your life from the pit and crowns you with love and compassion, who satisfies your desires with good things so that your youth is renewed like the eagle's.

Romans 8:11 (NLT)
The Spirit of God, who raised Jesus from the dead, lives in you. And just as God raised Christ Jesus from the dead, he will give life to your mortal bodies by this same Spirit living within you.

1 Peter 2:24 (NIV)
"He himself bore our sins" in his body on the cross, so that we might die to sins and live for righteousness; "by his wounds you have been healed."

Jeremiah 17:14 (NIV)
Heal me, O LORD, and I shall be healed; save me, and I shall be saved, for You are the one I praise.

Psalm 147:3 (AMP)
He heals the brokenhearted and binds up their wounds [healing their pain and comforting their sorrow].

BHW Therapy can be carried out as a part of your weekly spiritual time with the Lord, as a great way to facilitate healing with your spouse, as a special ceremonial time with your children (young and old) or as a part of a healing regimen.

We recommend performing it at least once weekly. If you are dealing with a serious issue, it is ideal to perform BHW three to seven times a week for 15 to 30 minutes at a time. The oils used can be amended to include other essential oils that may address particular issues you are facing. For example:

» For Hormonal Support: Clary Sage, Ylang Ylang
» For Neurological Support: Helichrysum, Holy Basil
» For Cardiovascular Support: Thyme, Vetiver
» For Immune Support: Ginger, Lemon
» For Chronic Pain: Lemongrass, Turmeric
» For Emotional Trauma: Ylang Ylang, Roman Chamomile

By practicing BHW Therapy, we are putting ourselves in a situation where we fix our eyes on Jesus, the author and perfecter of our faith. We envision people engaging in BHW Therapy with their children and loved ones, and we sincerely hope it can become an incredible healing tool for you and your family. Use it consistently for phenomenal results and an awakened sense of gratitude for Jesus' ultimate sacrifice.

CHAPTER 8

PREGNANCY AND BABY CARE

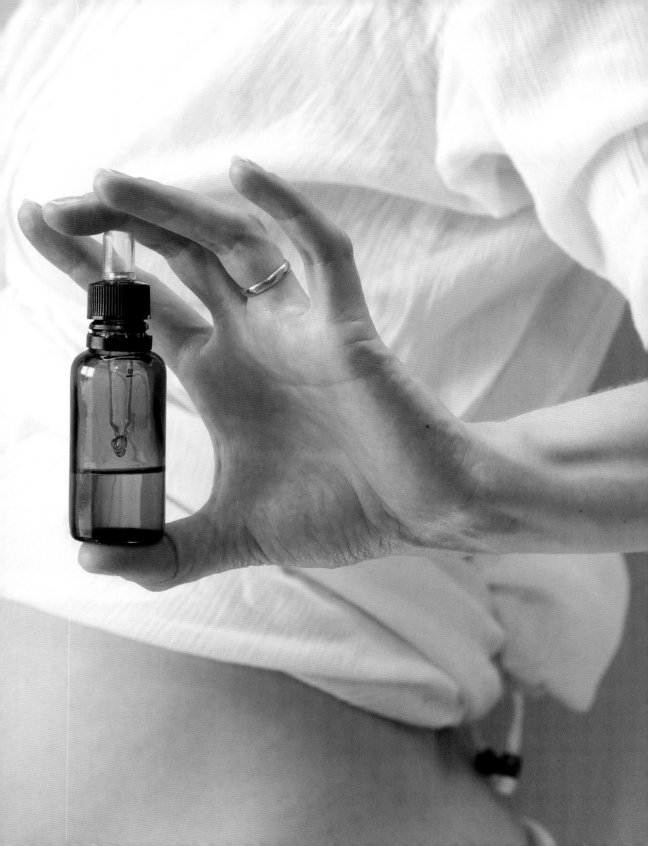

Pregnancy is a joyful time that is also filled with an exhaustive list of unique issues ranging from overall discomfort and fatigue to nausea, constipation and insomnia. When Jordan's wife was pregnant with their first child Joshua, they incorporated essential oils into their daily regimen. They utilized a special blend of Biblical oils including frankincense, myrrh, galbanum and spikenard every morning and evening to provide a calming and soothing effect on both of them.

Ty's wife, Charlene, was incredibly sick during the first trimester of all four of her pregnancies. At the time, they were unaware of how useful essential oils could be during pregnancy, and Charlene certainly wishes she had known about them back then.

This chapter will provide you with a guide to the best essential oils that can help you when you need it most, from the first tinges of morning sickness to some of the more painful complications that arise during breastfeeding, as well as present you with some simple home remedies that are gentle and effective for little ones.

FROM PREGNANCY TO MOTHERHOOD

Essential oils can be tremendous tools for expectant mothers. When used properly, essential oils are safe and gentle, making them useful during the critical time of your baby's growth and development within the womb. Essential oils may help relieve nausea, body aches, fatigue, stress, swelling, infections and elevated blood pressure. They can also assist with some of the uncomfortable changes that occur in a woman's body during labor, postpartum and while breastfeeding.

While some oils are not recommended for use during pregnancy (see a partial list at the end of this chapter, as well as specific safety considerations for each single oil in Part II), other oils may provide you with many benefits. The following is a list of essential oils that are generally considered safe for aromatherapy and topical use while you are expecting:

Beneficial Essential Oils for Pregnancy

+ Frankincense
+ Geranium
+ Ginger
+ Lavender

+ Lemon
+ Orange
+ Peppermint

+ Roman Chamomile
+ Sandalwood
+ Ylang Ylang

Remedies for Pregnancy Discomforts

If you are looking for a remedy for some of pregnancy's most irksome side effects, look no further. This table will provide you with essential oil remedies to help relieve the most common discomforts you may experience during pregnancy.

Pregnancy Issue	Essential Oils Remedy
Anxiety	Add 5 drops of ylang ylang or lavender oil to a warm bath, or diffuse 5 drops of lavender or orange.
Breast Tenderness	Apply 2 to 3 drops of lavender oil to the top of the breasts.
Congestion	Apply 2 to 3 drops of lemon or bergamot oil to the chest or bottoms of the feet.
Constipation	Add 1 drop of ginger oil to a glass of water or tea. Rub 1 to 2 drops of lemon, ginger or frankincense oil onto the stomach.
Cramps	Apply 1 to 2 drops of lavender, peppermint, bergamot or sandalwood oil to the area of concern.
Depression	Diffuse 5 drops of lavender, bergamot or orange oil, or apply 1 to 2 drops of frankincense oil to the bottoms of the feet.

Fatigue	Diffuse 5 drops of lemon or orange oil, or inhale it directly from the bottle.
Headache	Apply 2 to 3 drops of lavender to the back of the neck and temples.
Hemorrhoids	Dilute 2 to 3 drops of geranium oil with equal parts of a carrier oil and apply it to the area of concern, or add 5 drops of geranium oil to a warm-water bath.
High Blood Pressure	Diffuse 5 drops of lavender or ylang ylang oil, or add the drops to a warm-water bath.
Insomnia	Diffuse 5 drops of lavender, Roman chamomile or ylang ylang oil before bed, or apply 1 to 2 drops to the bottoms of the feet.
Irritated or Itchy Skin	Apply 2 to 3 drops of lavender oil, diluted with coconut or jojoba oil, to the area of concern.
Nausea/Morning Sickness	Add 1 to 2 drops of ginger oil to water or tea, or apply 1 to 2 drops of ginger or peppermint oil to the bottoms of the feet.
Stretch Marks	Apply 2 to 3 drops of lavender or sandalwood oil, diluted with coconut or jojoba oil, to the area of concern.
Swelling	Combine 2 drops of lavender oil, 2 drops of ginger oil and 1 teaspoon of a carrier oil and massage it onto the feet and legs.
Urinary Tract Infection	Add 1 to 2 drops of lemon oil to water and drink.

Essential oils not only bring relief from symptoms during pregnancy, but they may also provide you with multiple benefits during labor as well. Here is a list of the essential oils most commonly used during labor.

Beneficial Essential Oils during Labor

+ Basil
+ Bergamot
+ Clary Sage
+ Frankincense

+ Geranium
+ Helichrysum
+ Jasmine

+ Lavender
+ Orange
+ Peppermint

Remedies for Labor and Delivery

The following table offers specific essential oil remedies to help promote a healthy and peaceful labor and delivery.

Labor Discomfort	Essential Oils Remedy
Back Labor	Dilute 3 to 5 drops of peppermint oil and massage onto the back.
Fatigue	Diffuse 5 drops of orange, bergamot, lavender or clary sage oil, or add 5 to 10 drops of orange or bergamot oil to a warm-water bath.
Excessive Bleeding	Apply 3 to 5 drops of helichrysum oil to the area of concern or to the bottoms of the feet.
Overheated	Dilute 2 to 3 drops of peppermint oil and apply to the temples, wrists and bottoms of the feet.
Perineum Prep	Dilute 2 to 3 drops of frankincense or geranium oil and apply it onto the perineum.
Placenta Delivery	Rub 2 to 3 drops of clary sage oil onto the abdomen, or diffuse 5 drops of lavender oil.

Stalled Labor	Massage 3 to 5 drops of clary sage oil onto the lower abdomen.
Stress and Trauma	Diffuse 5 drops of lavender or frankincense oil, or massage 2 to 3 drops onto the wrists, temples and bottoms of the feet.

Once your bundle of joy has arrived, the newness of motherhood can sometimes be overshadowed by the discomfort of sleepless nights and breastfeeding difficulties. Thankfully, essential oils are known to provide nursing mothers with both stress relief and support for common breastfeeding complications. Below is a list of commonly used essential oils while nursing.

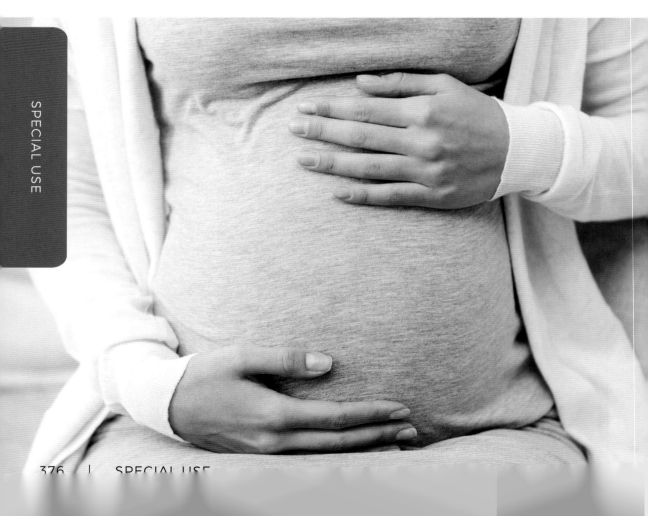

Beneficial Essential Oils for Breastfeeding

+ Basil
+ Clary Sage
+ Fennel
+ Lavender

+ Myrrh
+ Orange
+ Peppermint
+ Roman Chamomile

+ Ylang Ylang
(Note: Avoid excessive peppermint use)

Essential oils can help new moms in many ways. For a lot of women who are new to breastfeeding, common complications such as mastitis and cracked nipples can actually cause them to lose hope that they can successfully breastfeed. Essential oils may help ease some of the pain and discomfort that occurs after your milk comes in, and they could just provide the extra boost you need to keep going past the initial discomforts of nursing your new arrival.

Remedies for Breastfeeding

Here are essential oil remedies to aid in common breastfeeding complications.

Labor Discomfort	Essential Oils Remedy
Cracked Nipples	Dilute 2 to 3 drops of lavender or ylang ylang oil with coconut oil and apply it to the nipples after breastfeeding.
Low Milk Supply	Combine 1 drop each of fennel, basil and clary sage with coconut oil. Rub it into your hands and apply it to the breasts throughout the day. (Fennel can also be used for up to 10 days.)
Mastitis (Breast Inflammation)	Combine lavender, Roman chamomile and coconut oils and gently massage the mixture onto the breast.
Tender Breasts	Combine lavender, Roman chamomile, ylang ylang and coconut oils. Warm up the mixture in your hands and gently massage onto the breasts.

Note: To be safe, we recommend that you gently remove ointments and salves containing essential oils with a damp, soft washcloth (no soap) just prior to breastfeeding.

Now that we've covered how essential oils help moms, we will discuss how oils can benefit their babies as well.

BABIES AND ESSENTIAL OILS

Babies are just tiny humans, which of course means that the same compounds present in essential oils that benefit us adults can benefit them. The difference, however, is in the word "tiny." The average adult weighs 180 pounds, while the average infant weighs in at just 7.5 pounds. For this reason, and because their skin is not mature, essential oil use in babies looks a little different than it does for the rest of us.

For babies under three months of age, we recommend diffusing oils as the safest and effective tool for infant care. When using oils topically, oils should be diluted with a carrier oil and applied to the baby's back, abdomen or feet.

It is a good idea to introduce one essential oil at a time, and then watch how your little one reacts to it. Look for skin irritations and any other signs of a reaction such as rashes, itching and respiratory issues. The following is a list of oils that are generally accepted as safe for use on and around infants, either diffused or applied topically in small doses:

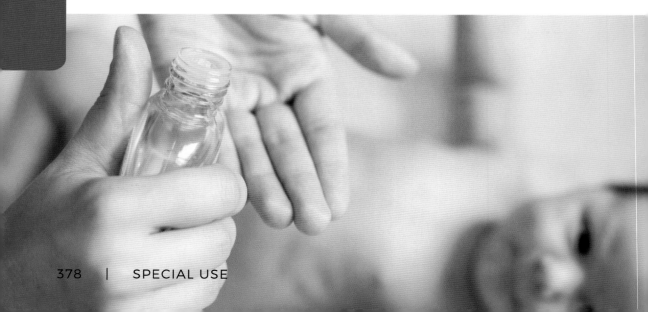

Beneficial Essential Oils for Babies

+ Basil
+ Clove
+ Eucalyptus
+ Fennel

+ Ginger
+ Lavender
+ Lemon

+ Peppermint
+ Roman Chamomile
+ Tea Tree

Remedies for Infant Care

Below are specific essential oil remedies to aid in caring for an infant. Be sure to discuss these and any other natural supplements with your child's pediatrician prior to use.

Infant Discomfort	Essential Oils Remedy
Acid Reflux	Dilute 1 drop of ginger oil and 1 drop of peppermint oil and massage it onto the belly.
Acne	Dilute 1 drop of tea tree oil and apply it to the area of concern.
Allergies	Dilute 1 to 2 drops of lemon, lavender or tea tree oil and apply it to the chest and bottoms of the feet.
Bug Bites	Apply 1 to 2 drops of lavender oil to the area of concern.
Cold/Flu	Dilute 1 to 2 drops of tea tree or eucalyptus oil and apply it to the chest or bottoms of the feet.
Colic	Dilute 1 to 2 drops of fennel or lavender oil and apply it to the chest or bottoms of the feet.

Congestion	Dilute 2 to 3 drops of lemon oil and apply it to the chest, under the nose and to the bottoms of the feet.
Constipation	Dilute 1 to 2 drops of ginger oil and apply it to the stomach.
Cradle Cap	Combine 2 drops of lavender oil and 1 teaspoon of coconut oil and massage it into the scalp before bedtime.
Diaper Rash	Dilute 1 to 2 drops of lavender, tea tree or frankincense oil and apply it to the area of concern.
Dry Skin	Dilute 1 to 2 drops of lavender or lemon oil and apply it to the area of concern.
Earache	Dilute 1 to 2 drops of basil, lavender or Roman chamomile oil and apply it behind the ears.
Fever	Dilute 1 to 2 drops of frankincense or peppermint oil and apply it to the bottoms of the feet.
Headache	Dilute 1 to 2 drops of lavender or peppermint oil and apply it to the temples or bottoms of the feet.
Hiccups	Dilute 1 to 2 drops of fennel or lemon oil and apply it to the chest or bottoms of the feet.
Hives	Dilute 1 to 2 drops of basil, tea tree or Roman chamomile oil and apply it to the area of concern.
Jaundice	Dilute 1 to 2 drops of lemon oil and apply it to the bottoms of the feet.
Rash	Dilute 1 to 2 drops of lavender, lemon or tea tree oil and apply it to the area of concern.

Sleeping Issues	Diffuse 3 to 5 drops of lavender oil beside the infant's crib.
Stomachache	Dilute 1 to 2 drops of ginger oil and apply it to the stomach.
Sunburn	Dilute 1 to 2 drops of lavender or peppermint oil and apply it to the area of concern.
Teething	Using your finger, apply 1 drop of clove or lavender oil to the area of concern.
Vomiting	Dilute 1 to 2 drops of clove or ginger oil and apply it to the bottoms of the feet, or add 1 drop of ginger oil to milk or formula (best if used in a dropper because it will alter the taste and the baby may refuse it).

FINAL THOUGHTS

While essential oils can provide you and your baby with some much needed relief during pregnancy, childbirth and the postpartum period, some general safety guidelines regarding essential oil use should be followed to ensure optimal health and protection for you and your children:

Consult with a healthcare professional. Use caution during the first and second trimesters of pregnancy, as the baby is developing rapidly, and always consult with your healthcare practitioner to ensure essential oil use during pregnancy is right for you. You should also consult with your child's pediatrician for any questions regarding essential oil use with infants.

Use the highest quality oils. When using essential oils during pregnancy and with children, the quality of the oil is of vital importance. Only use organic, pure, therapeutic-grade oils from a brand that has received third party certifications to ensure there are no harmful substances present.

Use sparingly. Use only a drop or two of essential oils on small children, and dilute them with a carrier oil before topical application. It is also important for pregnant women to pay extra attention to how their bodies respond to essential oil use and use only as much as is needed for the desired effect.

Avoid certain oils. Some oils are generally considered safe for use during pregnancy, while others are considered to contain properties that could harm the mother or fetus during pregnancy. This includes, but is not limited to, emmenagogue and abortifacient essential oils, as they have the ability to stimulate contractions and encourage blood flow in the uterus. A few specific oils that are not generally recommended for use during pregnancy include:

» Cinnamon, clove, rosemary and clary sage—all of which can cause contractions
» Hyssop—exhibits abortifacient qualities
» Fennel—encourages estrogen production
» Wintergreen—contains a chemical (methyl salicylate) that may cause allergic reactions and is toxic when ingested

For a more complete list of which oils to avoid during pregnancy, check the specific safety considerations for each single oil in Part II.

Remember: when in doubt, diffuse. The safest way to use oils during pregnancy is to diffuse five to seven drops in order to promote peace and boost energy. If you are interested in using oils internally during pregnancy in small doses, only do so after consulting with your physician.

It's important for expectant and breastfeeding mothers to remember to listen to their own bodies and also consult with a health professional regarding their unique circumstances to best determine whether or not a specific oil is right for them.

Virtually *anything* can become toxic at high levels, which makes proper dosage with any medicine, salve, ointment or remedy—including essential oils—important. When it comes to using essential oils during pregnancy and in caring for your precious little ones, common sense is key!

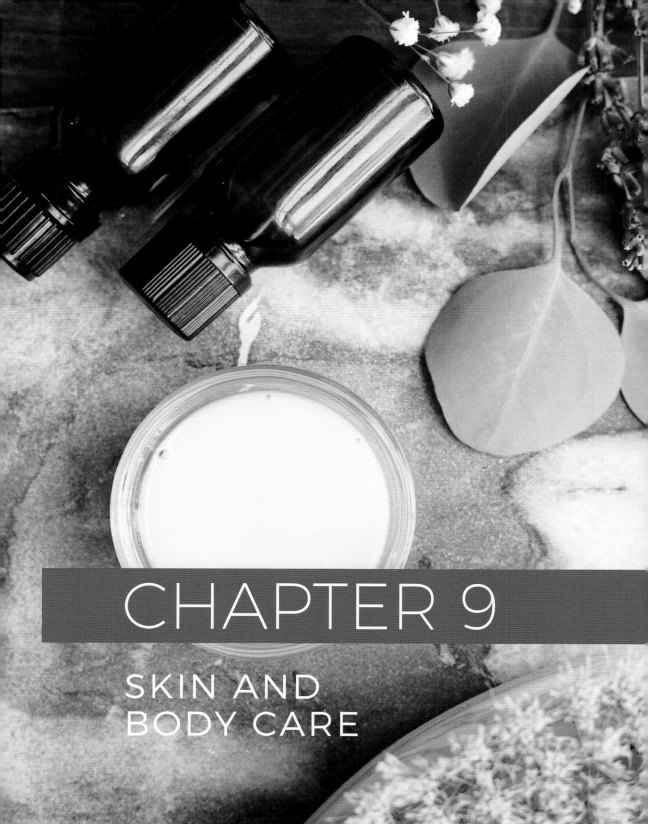

CHAPTER 9

SKIN AND BODY CARE

Essential oils can work wonders on the skin because of their ability to alleviate feelings of stress and anxiety, fight insomnia and sleep deprivation and balance hormone levels. These are some common issues that lead to acne, premature aging and other skin conditions.

Consider using essential oils such as tea tree, lavender, clary sage and juniper berry to address skin conditions first, or use them as a supplement to other skin treatments. They don't come with nasty side effects, and they are safe and gentle enough for topical use.

Each of us uses essential oils as a primary part of our daily personal care, and our wives use oils in their skin and beauty routines with excellent results. We put oils in our shampoos, facial lotions, body butters and washes, and we even apply some of them neat to our faces to help address issues such as premature signs of aging and blemishes.

The following chart lists eight of the most common skincare concerns. Below each one, we have indicated which oils are best known to help alleviate symptoms of the condition and help improve the overall look of your skin.

Some carrier oils are also beneficial for the skin, as they can help to hydrate dry and damaged areas and also slow down the signs of aging. The best carrier oils for skin care include coconut oil, jojoba oil, evening primrose oil, rosehip seed oil, argan oil and pomegranate seed oil. For a complete list of our recommended carrier oils, refer to Part II.

Part V is filled with DIY recipes that can greatly benefit your skin, hair and body. We encourage you to use these easy, beneficial, great smelling recipes to create some natural alternatives to conventional body and personal care products that are too often filled with unpronounceable mystery ingredients.

So let's get mixin'!

The Best Essential Oils for Skin Care

Essential Oil	Acne	Aging	Dry Skin	Oily Skin	Sensitive Skin	Dark Spots	Infections	Elasticity
Bergamot				X				
Cedarwood			X	X				
Clary Sage	X	X	X	X				
Cypress		X		X				
Frankincense		X		X		X	X	X
Geranium	X		X					X
Helichrysum					X			
Jasmine			X		X			
Lavender	X	X		X	X	X	X	X
Lemon						X		
Lemongrass	X					X		
Myrrh		X	X				X	X
Orange	X	X		X				
Patchouli	X	X	X					
Peppermint	X			X				
Roman Chamomile			X	X	X		X	
Rose	X	X			X			
Rosemary				X			X	
Sandalwood		X	X	X				
Tea Tree	X			X			X	
Ylang Ylang		X		X	X			X

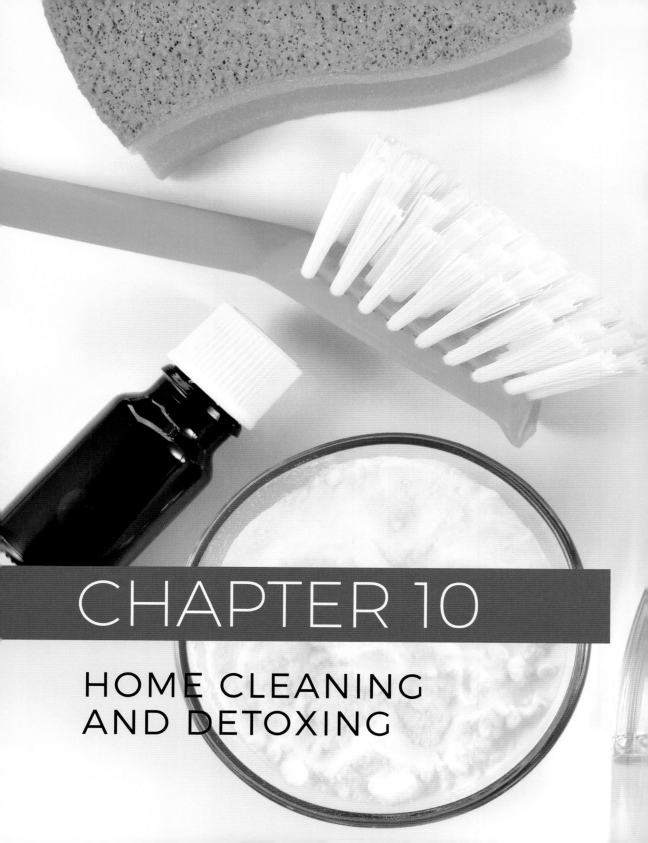

CHAPTER 10

HOME CLEANING AND DETOXING

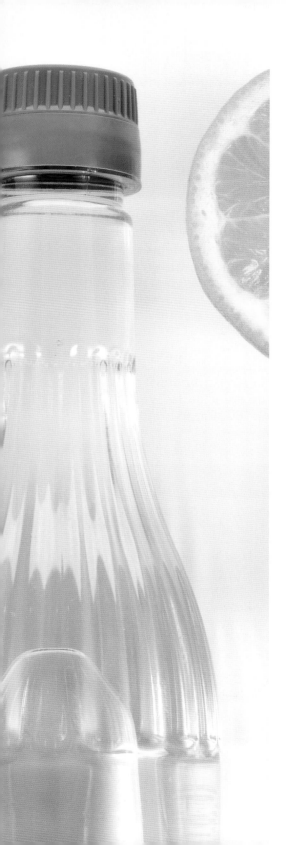

Essential oils offer powerful ways to clean your home and refresh your airspace. We love the difference that essential oils have made in the freshness and cleanliness of our homes.

And because the DIY home care recipes we use have just a few simple ingredients, we feel good about knowing exactly what we and our families are breathing in and touching every single day.

Essential oils are simply some of the best-smelling, naturally anti-bacterial options for homemade cleaning recipes. It is vital to use safe and non-toxic cleaning products in the home that do not contain dangerous ingredients that can build toxicity in the body and be harmful to children and pets.

Add oils to "green" your laundry routine, sanitize the kitchen and fight mold in the bathroom, all while making your house smell clean—no scary fumes needed!

We have found the best essential oils for detoxing and cleaning the home to include:

+ Cinnamon
+ Citrus oils such as lemon and orange
+ Eucalyptus
+ Lemongrass
+ Peppermint
+ Tea tree

It's not just an advertising gimmick that many commercial products contain citrus oils such as lemon or lime—they are natural degreasers and have anti-microbial properties. Oils such as lemongrass are even great for cleaning porous surfaces that trap dirt and grime, such as yoga mats. You can also put a few drops into your shoes to help keep them smelling fresh!

Essential Oil-Based Cleaning Recipes

Using natural products instead of chemically laden commercial ones makes household tasks (dare we say) a pleasure to tackle. Here are some essential oil-based cleaning recipes to help get you started on the path to greener cleaning.

Cleaner	Directions
All-Purpose Spray	Add 5 drops of lemon oil and 5 drops of tea tree oil to a spray bottle filled with warm water.
Bathtub Cleaner	Mix ½ cup of baking soda, ½ cup of vinegar and 5 drops of lemon, lime or bergamot oil. Scrub the bathtub and rinse with water to remove residue.
Carpet Deodorizer	Mix 20 drops of tea tree oil with borax to make a homemade carpet powder. Apply it evenly to the carpet and vacuum.
Dishwasher Detergent	Combine 1 grated bar of castile soap, 2 cups of borax, 2 cups of washing soda, 1 cup of baking soda, 15 drops of lavender oil and 15 drops of peppermint oil.

Cleaner	Directions
Fabric Softener	Combine ½ cup of vinegar, 2 tablespoons of baking soda and 20 drops of lavender oil. Add 2 to 4 tablespoons of the mixture to the rinse cycle.
Floor Cleaner	Combine 2 tablespoons of unscented liquid soap, 10 drops of lemon oil and 5 drops of tea tree oil. This cleaner is safe for most floors.
Home Deodorizer and Freshener	Diffuse 5 to 10 drops of lemon, clove, rosemary or orange oil at home.
Laundry Detergent	Add 10 to 15 drops of lemon oil to each load of laundry.
Mold Eliminator	Diffuse 5 to 10 drops of tea tree oil to kill mold and other pathogens in the air.
Oven Cleaner	Combine 10 drops of lemon oil, ¼ cup of vinegar and 1-½ cups of baking soda. Wipe down the inside and outside of the oven; then wipe it down again with a damp sponge and warm water to remove any residue.
Produce Washer	Add 2 drops of lemon oil to a large bowl of water and scrub the produce with the mixture, and then rinse.
Shower Curtain Cleaner	Add 4 drops of eucalyptus oil and 4 drops of tea tree oil to a spray bottle filled with warm water. Spray the mixture onto the shower curtain to remove mold and buildup.
Smoke Eliminator	Add 3 to 4 drops each of rosemary, tea tree and eucalyptus oils to a spray bottle filled with water and spray around the house or in smoky areas.
Sports Gear Cleaner	Combine 2 drops of tea tree oil, 2 drops of lemon oil, 1 quart of warm water and 4 tablespoons of baking soda. Use the mixture to clean jerseys, cleats and other sports gear.

Cleaner	Directions
Toilet Bowl Cleaner	Mix ½ cup of baking soda, ½ cup of vinegar and 5 drops of lemon, lime or bergamot oil. Scrub the toilet and wipe it down with a damp sponge or paper towel to remove residue.
Trash Can Refresher	Put a cotton ball with 2 drops each of lemon oil and tea tree oil at the bottom of the trashcan to decrease odor and detoxify the air.
Vacuum Cleaner	Add 5 to 10 drops of lemon oil or peppermint oil to a vacuum bag or dust container.
Window Cleaner	Combine 5 tablespoons of vinegar and 15 drops of lemon oil.

Making your own natural cleaning recipes is not time-consuming or expensive. In fact, quite the opposite is true. In less time than it takes to run to the supermarket to buy conventional cleaning supplies, you can fill up a spray bottle with vinegar and water, add a few drops of essential oils, and clean your appliances and all of the glass in your home.

Believe it or not, you can also save a lot of money. The price of commercial cleaners can range from $5 to $8 dollars or more, and let's not forget that a bottle of store-bought laundry detergent can cost as much as $20! A natural alternative, on the other hand, can cost pennies to make. While high-quality essential oils are relatively expensive, they are also highly potent. That means you can use just 5 to 30 drops of an oil (depending on the formula) to make an entire bottle of cleaner than can last for months. Other all-natural ingredients such as vinegar, baking soda, water and castile soap are also inexpensive.

You will be amazed at the amount of "necessary" products you can throw away altogether. According to the book *Toxic Free* by Debra Lynn Dadd, the average kitchen contains 30 or more commercial products! Many of the essential oil-based formulas in this book are multipurpose, so you can ditch all those unnecessary specialty products and simplify your life.

See Part V for more DIY recipes and enjoy a clean, green and less toxic home.

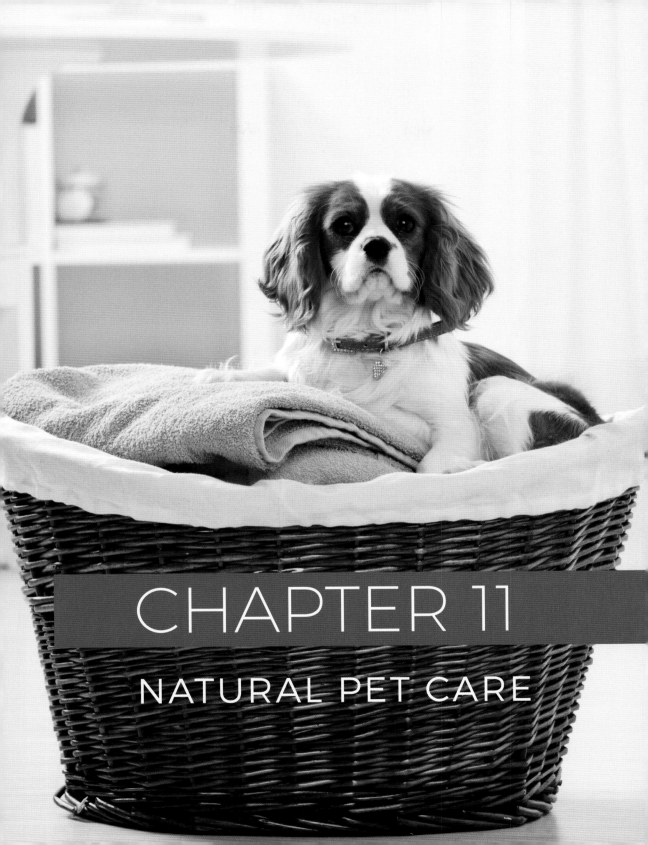

CHAPTER 11

NATURAL PET CARE

America has a love affair with pets—and why wouldn't we? Our furry friends can bring so much joy, fun and happiness into our lives.

Dr. Josh and Chelsea have two dogs named Oakley and Flash. They use essential oils with them on a regular basis. They use a blend of lemongrass, rosemary and geranium to repel fleas and ticks and wash their dogs' hair with a homemade shampoo made with rosemary, Roman chamomile and aloe vera gel. Dr. Josh will also often rub frankincense oil on the hips of their dog Oakley to prevent hip pain.

Jordan and his team at Heal the Planet Farm have used herbs and oils effectively to naturally treat a wide variety of animals, including livestock and guard animals.

The Bollingers own a German shepherd named Grizzly and about a dozen cats that roam their 15 acres. After one of their cats was attacked and severely injured by a neighbor's dog, Charlene actually used a homeopathic remedy (Arnica Montana) to help nurse the feline back to health. The cat, aptly named Miracle, made a full recovery.

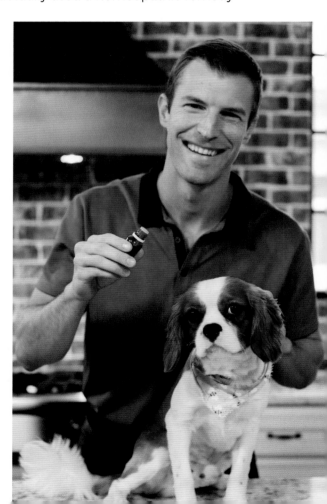

We love our pets—and we also love the fact that we can use the same gentle, natural supplements on them that we use on our human family.

When taken in conjunction with your vet's recommended treatments, essential oils can be used on pets as a natural remedy for a variety of health issues. Essential oils can even be used in combination with medications in order to reduce potential side effects from drugs. It is important for a pet to receive an accurate diagnosis from a veterinarian when health issues are worsening over a short period of time. Together with your veterinarian, you can decide on the best treatment options.

Recommended Essential Oils for Pets

Here is a list of essential oils that are safe for most pets.

Essential Oil	Pet Benefits
Cilantro	Reduces muscle and joint pain, supports circulation and the immune system, detoxifies the body and reduces inflammation.
Frankincense	Supports the liver, brain, bladder and kidney health; reduces sadness; reduces inflammation; detoxifies the body and promotes healthy cell production.
Geranium	Helps to detoxify the body, improves dry skin, supports liver health, stops bleeding and promotes normal hormone production.
Helichrysum	Supports muscle health, stops bleeding, helps circulation and aids in healing wounds.
Lavender	Reduces anxiety, stress, fear and sadness. Helps to heal burns and wounds, supports the immune system, reduces inflammation and promotes skin health.
Lemongrass	Helps to detoxify the body, supports healthy muscles, eliminates parasites and supports the bladder and thyroid health.
Rosemary	Reduces inflammation, relieves pain and discomfort, supports the respiratory system and boosts brain function.

Some essential oils that are NOT recommended for pets include:

X Birch
X Clove

X Oregano
X Tea Tree

X Thyme
X Wintergreen

Once you have determined that an essential oil is safe for topical application, you can apply it to the bottom of the back paws, between toe pads, on the stomach or behind the ears. Avoid putting oils around the face, nose or eyes of your animals. And don't forget that diffusing essential oils at home can also be beneficial to pets. You may also place a few drops in a sprayer with water and gently mist your pet, depending on the condition you are treating. This technique can work well for burns, skin irritations and external infections.

Remedies for Common Pet Health Conditions

Here are some great home remedies for common issues with pets.

Pet Health Issue	Essential Oils Remedy
Arthritis	Dilute 1 to 2 drops of frankincense and apply it to the base of the ears, tail and affected hip/ joint.
Bleeding	Dilute 1 to 2 drops of helichrysum and apply it to the wound.
Burns	Dilute 1 to 2 drops of lavender and apply it to burned area, or add 5 drops of lavender to a spray bottle filled with water and mist it onto the affected area.
Ear Infection	Dilute 1 to 2 drops of geranium or frankincense and apply it to the back and front of the ear.
Fear and Anxiety	Dilute 1 to 2 drops of lavender and apply it to the back of the ears and tail, or diffuse the oil at home.
Fleas	Add 2 to 4 drops of lemongrass to the pet's shampoo.
Fungal Infection	Dilute 1 to 2 drops of geranium or lemongrass and apply it to the affected area twice daily.

Indigestion	Dilute 1 to 2 drops of lavender (or fennel for a dog) and apply it to the stomach and back feet, or diffuse lavender at home.
Infection (external)	Dilute 1 to 2 drops of frankincense or helichrysum and apply it to the infected area twice daily, or add 5 drops of both oils to a spray bottle and mist it onto the area of concern.
Insect Repellent	Add 5 drops of lemongrass to a spray bottle filled with water and mist it onto the animal's coat.
Liver Disorder	Dilute 1 to 2 drops of geranium or helichrysum and apply it over the liver and in-between the back toes.
Malignant Skin Tumors	Apply 1 to 2 drops of frankincense to the tumor twice daily.
Pain	Dilute 1 to 2 drops of frankincense or lavender and apply it to the area of pain.
Vomiting	Dilute 1 to 2 drops of lavender and rub it onto the stomach and in-between the back toes.

TIPS FOR TREATING PETS WITH ESSENTIAL OILS

Essential oils contain a host of biologically active and powerful compounds that when used correctly are an indispensible part of integrative medical care for humans and pets alike. However, they can cause undesirable side effects in animals as well as people, which is why a few precautions must be taken:

Always dilute. Just like when using essential oils on children, the dilution ratio you use depends on the weight of the pet. Smaller pets should only be given diluted essential oils; use 2 tablespoons of coconut oil to 1 to 2 drops of essential oils for pets under 30 pounds. For pets over 30 pounds, a 1:1 ratio is recommended (1 tablespoon of coconut oil for 1 to 2 drops of essential oils).

Perform patch testing. Smaller pets or certain breeds may be more sensitive to essential oils. For this reason, it is important to do a patch test first. Apply 1 to 2 drops, diluted with coconut oil, to the pet's feet and monitor his or her reactions.

Watch for intolerance. Check for irritation or indication of GI upset, itchiness, redness or inflammation. As an added precaution, do not use essential oils on animals that are pregnant, under three months old, ill or epileptic. Some common signs of essential oil intolerance or toxicity in pets include:

- » Change in sleeping or eating patterns/habits
- » Behavior changes, such as fatigue, lack of energy, not wanting to play, confusion or lightheadedness
- » Digestive conditions, such as vomiting, constipation or diarrhea
- » Muscle tremors
- » Increased salivation or drooling

Use only the highest quality oils. Since pets are part of our families, we require the same level of quality in our oils for them as we do for our loved ones. Ensure you are using only 100 percent pure, organic oils that have received third party certifications to ensure there are no harmful substances present within the oils.

Essential oils can help your pets look and feel their best—and they can save you money! Flea and tick shampoo and other pet care items can really be pricey, so save yourself time and money by skipping the big box pet stores and making your own pet care home remedies.

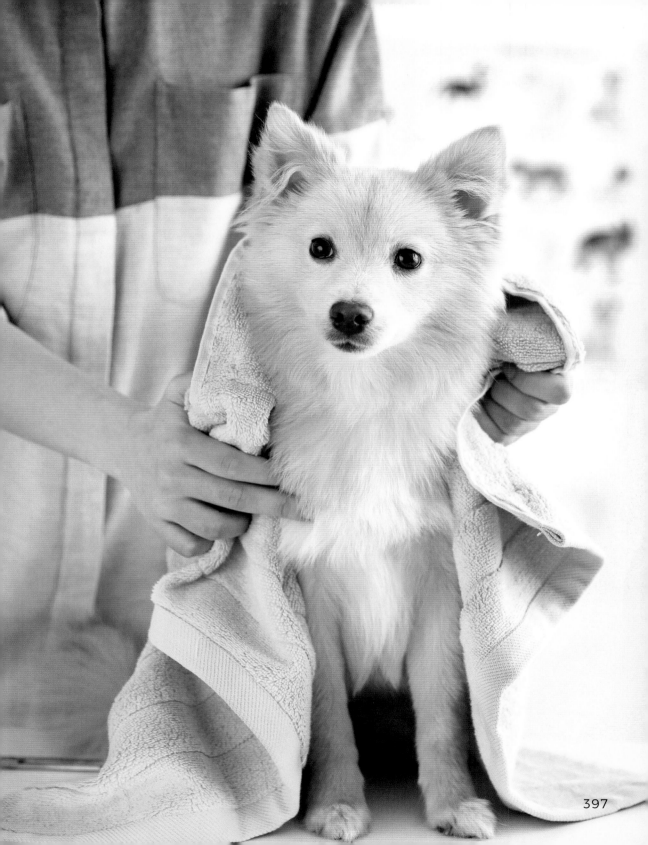

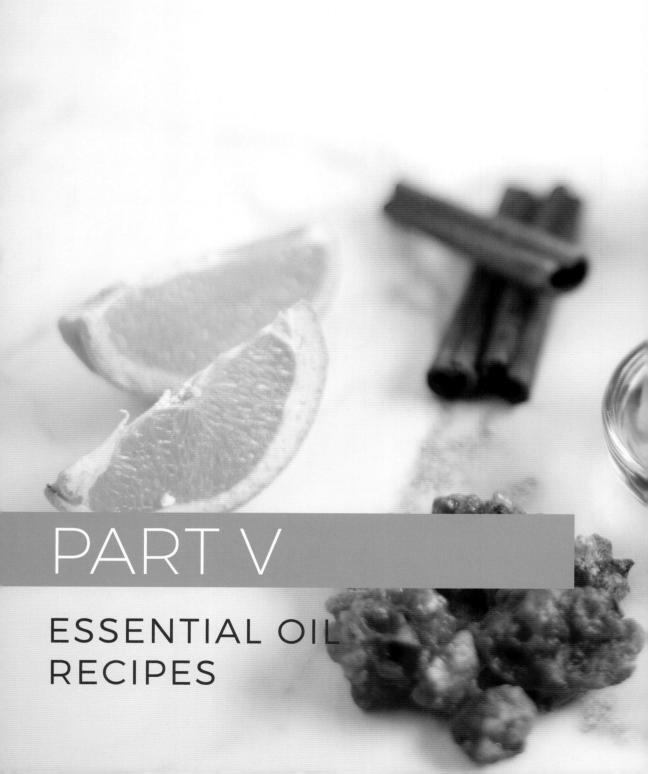

PART V

ESSENTIAL OIL RECIPES

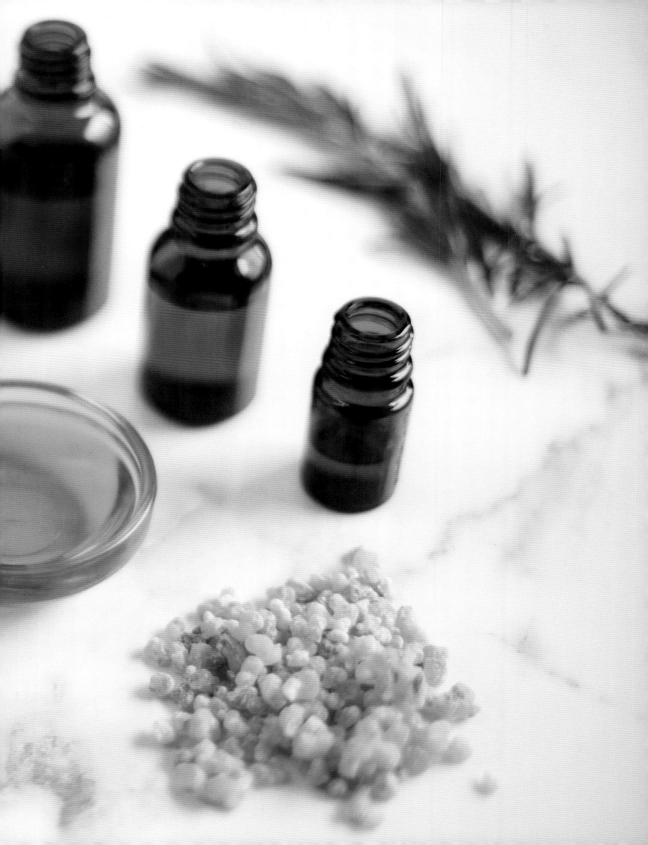

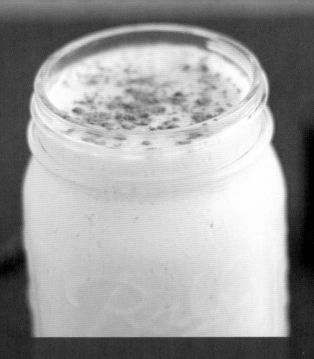

CINNAMON
VANILLA
SMOOTHIE

BREAKFAST

ORANGE
CINNAMON
PANCAKES

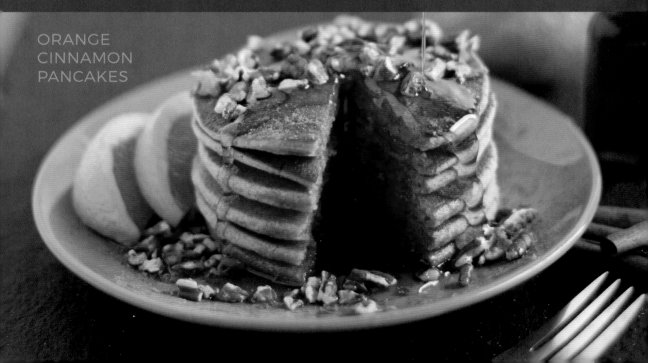

CINNAMON VANILLA SMOOTHIE

TIME: 2 MINUTES   SERVES: 1-2

INGREDIENTS

- 8 ounces coconut milk
- ½ cup ice
- 1-2 scoops vanilla whey protein powder
- 1 drop cinnamon essential oil

DIRECTIONS

1. In a high-speed blender, add all ingredients and purée on high until smooth.

2. Serve immediately.

ORANGE CINNAMON PANCAKES

TIME: 10 MINUTES   SERVES: 6 PANCAKES

INGREDIENTS

- 1 banana
- 1 cup + 2 tablespoons oatmeal
- 2 eggs
- 1 egg white
- 3 tablespoons almond milk
- 1-2 drops orange essential oil
- 1 drop cinnamon essential oil
- Toppings: ghee, cinnamon powder, maple syrup or raw agave (optional)

DIRECTIONS

1. In a high-speed blender, add the banana, oatmeal, eggs, egg white, almond milk and essential oils. Purée on high until smooth.

2. Grease a large frying pan with ghee and place it over medium heat. Cook the pancakes for 3 to 4 minutes, or until small bubbles form. Flip and repeat.

3. Serve the pancakes topped with ghee, cinnamon powder, maple syrup or raw agave.

PINEAPPLE GINGER SMOOTHIE

TIME: 2 MINUTES   SERVES: 2

INGREDIENTS

- 1 cup coconut milk
- 1 cup cubed fresh pineapple
- 1 banana
- ½ cup coconut water
- ½ cup ice
- 2 scoops collagen protein powder
- 1 knob peeled ginger (or 1 drop ginger essential oil)
- 1 drop grapefruit essential oil

DIRECTIONS

1. In a high-speed blender, add all ingredients and purée on high until smooth.

2. Serve immediately.

THIN MINT SMOOTHIE

TIME: 2 MINUTES   SERVES: 1-2

INGREDIENTS

- 1 cup coconut milk
- 1 drop peppermint essential oil
- 2 tablespoons cacao powder
- 1 scoop chocolate Bone Broth Protein powder
- ½ cup ice

DIRECTIONS

1. In a high-speed blender, add all ingredients and purée on high until smooth.

2. Serve immediately.

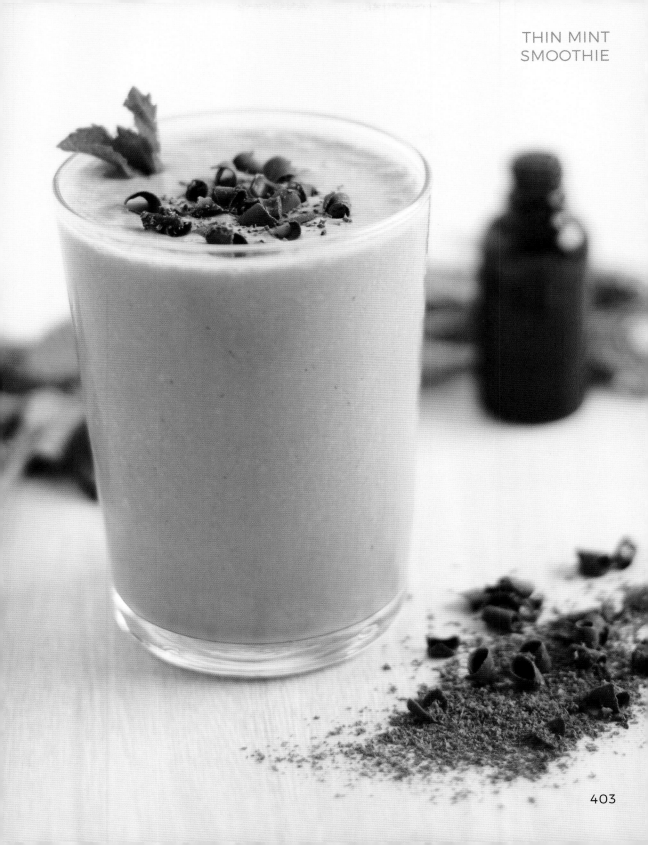

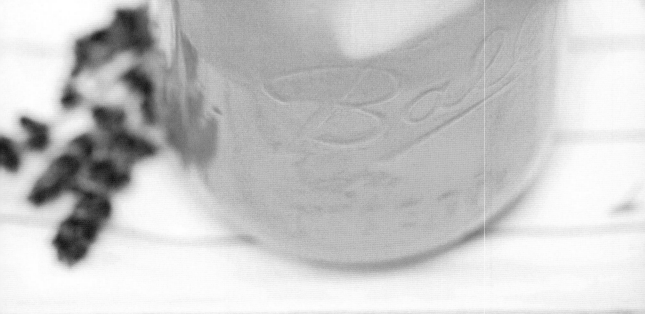

LAVENDER
LEMONADE

DRINKS

LAVENDER LEMONADE

TIME: 10 MINUTES   SERVES: 6-8

INGREDIENTS

- 1 cup water
- 1 cup granulated coconut sugar (or maple or date)
- 1 cup lemon juice
- 4 cups cold water
- 3 drops lavender essential oil
- Ice (optional)

DIRECTIONS

1. In a small pot over high heat, bring the water to a boil.

2. Dissolve the sugar in the boiling water and stir well.

3. Pour the sugar water into a large pitcher.

4. Add in the lemon juice and cold water.

5. Then, add in the lavender essential oil and stir before serving.

6. Add ice to the pitcher, if desired.

TURMERIC TEA

TIME: 5 MINUTES   SERVES: 2

INGREDIENTS

- 1 cup coconut milk
- 1 cup water
- 1 tablespoon ghee
- 1 tablespoon maple syrup
- ⅛ teaspoon turmeric powder (or more, if desired)
- 1 drop ginger essential oil

DIRECTIONS

1. In a small saucepan over medium-low heat, combine the coconut milk and water. Warm for 2 minutes.

2. Add the ghee, syrup and turmeric. Stir and warm for another 2 minutes.

3. Remove from the heat and add the ginger essential oil.

4. Stir and pour into glasses.

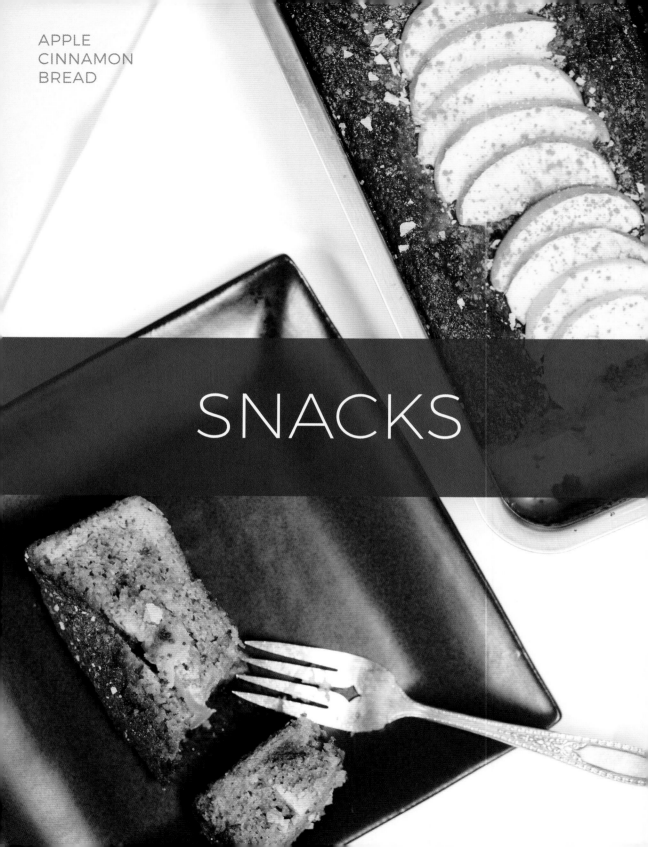

APPLE
CINNAMON
BREAD

SNACKS

APPLE CINNAMON BREAD

TIME: 50 MINUTES   SERVES: 12

INGREDIENTS

- 1 cup cashew butter
- ½ cup unsweetened applesauce
- ½ cup maple syrup
- 2 eggs
- 2 drops cinnamon essential oil
- 1 drop ginger essential oil
- 1 tablespoon apple cider vinegar
- 1 teaspoon baking soda
- ¼ teaspoon nutmeg
- ¼ teaspoon sea salt
- 8-10 thin apple slices (optional)
- Dash of ground cinnamon (optional)

DIRECTIONS

1. Preheat the oven to 350°F.

2. Grease a standard loaf pan with butter or coconut oil and set aside.

3. In a large mixing bowl, add the cashew butter, applesauce, syrup, eggs, essential oils and apple cider vinegar. Stir well.

4. Next, add the baking soda, nutmeg and sea salt. Stir the mixture until well combined.

5. Pour the mixture in the loaf pan.

6. Bake for 35 to 40 minutes.

7. If desired, place the apple slices on top of the loaf 10 to 15 minutes before the loaf is done.

8. Top the finished loaf with ground cinnamon, if desired.

GUACAMOLE

TIME: 5 MINUTES   SERVES: 4

INGREDIENTS

- 3 ripe avocados
- ¾ cup chopped cilantro
- ½ heirloom tomato, guts and membrane removed, chopped
- ½ medium red onion, chopped
- 1 jalapeño, ends and seeds removed, chopped
- Juice of 1 lime
- 1 teaspoon each: garlic powder, cumin, smoked paprika and sea salt
- 1-2 drops cilantro essential oil
- 1 drop lime or lemon essential oil

DIRECTIONS

1. Remove the skin and seeds from the avocados and mash the meat in a bowl.

2. Add in the remaining ingredients and continue to mash/stir.

3. Serve immediately.

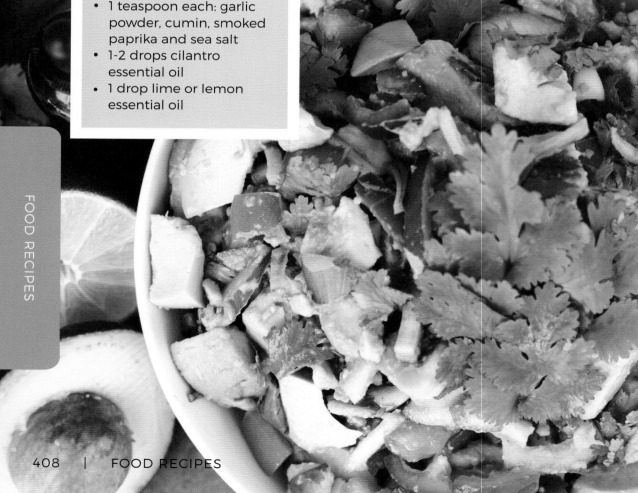

LEMON POPPYSEED MUFFINS

TIME: 45 MINUTES   SERVES: 12 MUFFINS

INGREDIENTS
- ½ cup butter, softened
- ⅔ cup coconut sugar
- 2 eggs, separated
- 1-⅓ cups gluten-free flour
- 1 teaspoon baking powder
- ½ teaspoon baking soda
- ¼ teaspoon sea salt
- 4 tablespoons poppy seeds
- 1 teaspoon lemon zest
- ½ cup goat milk yogurt
- 2 tablespoons lemon juice
- 1 teaspoon vanilla extract
- 3 drops lemon essential oil

DIRECTIONS
1. Preheat the oven to 350°F.

2. In a bowl, cream the butter and sugar.

3. Add the egg yolks, one at time, and mix well after each addition.

4. In a separate bowl, mix the flour, baking powder, baking soda, sea salt, poppy seeds and lemon zest.

5. Combine both mixtures, adding them together slowly and mixing continuously.

6. Next, add the yogurt, lemon juice, vanilla and lemon essential oil.

7. In a separate bowl, beat the egg whites until soft peaks form and fold them into the muffin batter.

8. Fill lined muffin tins and bake for 20 to 25 minutes.

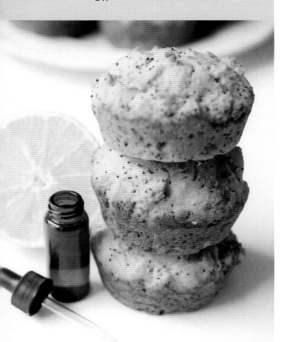

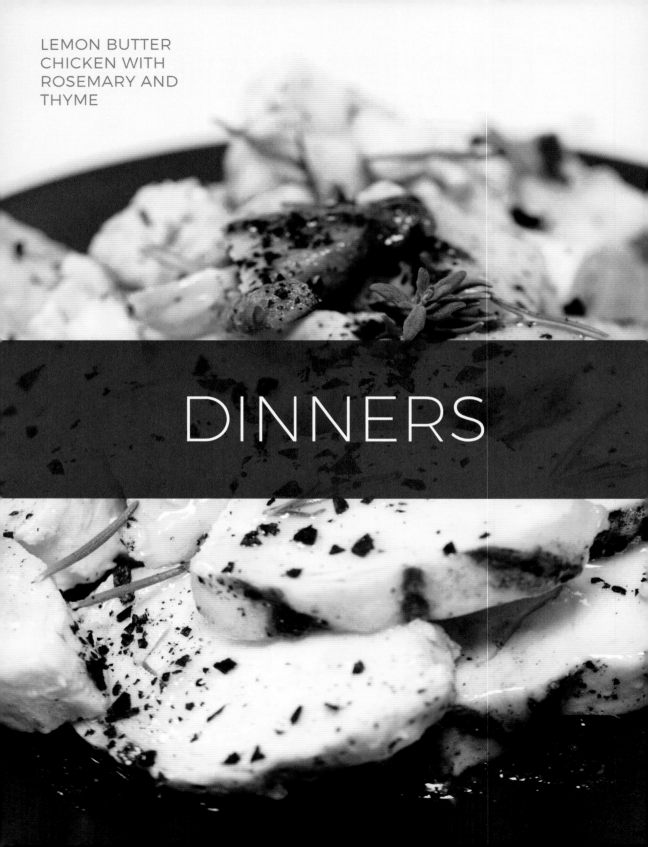

LEMON BUTTER
CHICKEN WITH
ROSEMARY AND
THYME

DINNERS

LEMON BUTTER CHICKEN WITH ROSEMARY AND THYME

TIME: 15 MINUTES   SERVES: 4

INGREDIENTS

- 4 chicken breasts (6 ounces each), cooked and sliced
- ½ cup grass-fed butter
- 4 drops lemon essential oil
- 1 tablespoon fresh rosemary
- 1 tablespoon fresh thyme
- ½ teaspoon sea salt
- Black pepper, to taste
- Lemon wedges (optional)

DIRECTIONS

1. Place the cooked chicken on a pan and set aside.

2. In a small saucepan over medium-low heat, combine the butter and lemon essential oil.

3. Once the butter has melted, add in the rosemary, thyme, sea salt and pepper. Continue cooking until the mixture is fragrant.

4. Pour the mixture over the chicken and stir until completely coated.

5. If desired, garnish the chicken with additional lemon wedges. Serve over a bed of greens or your favorite cooked vegetables.

ORANGE TERIYAKI SALMON

TIME: 15 MINUTES   SERVES: 4

INGREDIENTS

- 4 pieces wild Alaskan salmon (6 ounces each)
- ¼ cup avocado oil
- Juice of 2 orange halves (about ¼ cup)
- ¼ cup coconut aminos
- 1 tablespoon maple syrup
- 1 teaspoon mustard
- 1 teaspoon garlic powder
- 2 drops orange essential oil
- Chopped parsley (optional)
- Sea salt (optional)

DIRECTIONS

1. Place the salmon in a bag or on a pan and set aside.

2. In a small bowl, whisk the avocado oil, orange juice, coconut aminos, maple syrup, mustard, garlic powder and orange essential oil. Pour the mixture over the salmon.

3. Place the salmon in the refrigerator and let it marinate for 1 hour or more.

4. Turn the broiler on high.

5. On a baking sheet lined with foil, place the marinated salmon and broil for 4 to 5 minutes on each side.

6. Top with parsley and sea salt, if desired.

STEAK SALAD WITH ROSEMARY OLIVE OIL

TIME: 20 MINUTES   SERVES: 2-3

INGREDIENTS

Salad

- ½ pound skirt steak
- 2 tablespoons avocado oil
- 2 tablespoons apple cider vinegar
- 1 cup arugula
- 1 zucchini, thinly sliced
- 1 tomato, diced
- ½ avocado, peeled and cubed
- ½ cup chopped curly parsley
- ¼ cup chopped green onion

Dressing

- Juice of ½ lemon
- ¼ cup olive oil
- 2-3 drops rosemary essential oil
- 1 tablespoon apple cider vinegar

DIRECTIONS

1. In a loaf pan, place the steak, avocado oil and apple cider vinegar.

2. Refrigerate for 1 hour, allowing the steak to marinate.

3. In a medium salad bowl, place the arugula, zucchini, tomato, avocado, parsley and onion..

4. In a small bowl, combine the lemon juice, olive oil, rosemary essential oil and apple cider vinegar to create the dressing.

5. Add the dressing to the medium salad bowl, tossing until well combined. Set aside in the refrigerator.

6. Set the oven broiler to high.

7. On a baking sheet lined with foil, place the steak.

8. Broil 4 to 6 minutes on each side, or until the internal temperature reaches 145°F or higher.

TURMERIC BISON BURGERS

TIME: 40 MINUTES   SERVES: 8

INGREDIENTS

- ½ medium red onion, sliced
- 1 clove garlic, peeled
- 1 pound lean bison
- 1 pound lean ground beef
- 1 tablespoon pink Himalayan salt
- ½ teaspoon turmeric
- ½ teaspoon garlic
- ½ teaspoon pepper
- 1 teaspoon dried oregano
- 2 drops fennel essential oil
- ½ teaspoon coconut oil

DIRECTIONS

1. In a food processor, combine the onion and garlic. Pulse until finely chopped.

2. Transfer the mixture to a large mixing bowl along with the bison, ground beef, spices and fennel essential oil, using your hands to combine all ingredients. Form 8 patties.

3. Chill the patties in the refrigerator for 15 to 20 minutes, or until firm.

4. In a large nonstick skillet over medium-high heat, melt the coconut oil. Fry the burgers for 7 to 8 minutes per side, or until firm to the touch and nicely browned.

5. Serve hot with your favorite toppings on a gluten-free bun, bed of lettuce or lettuce wrap.

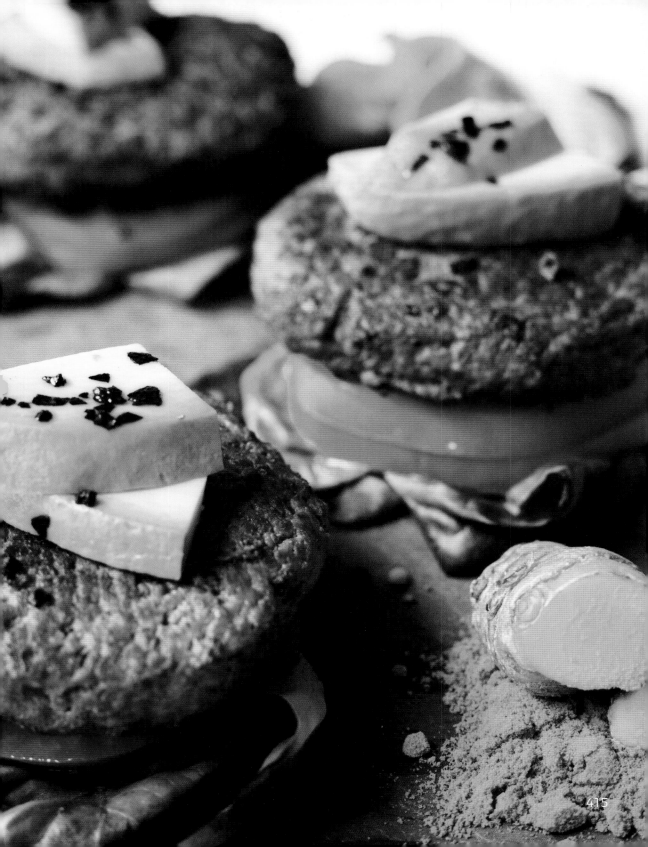

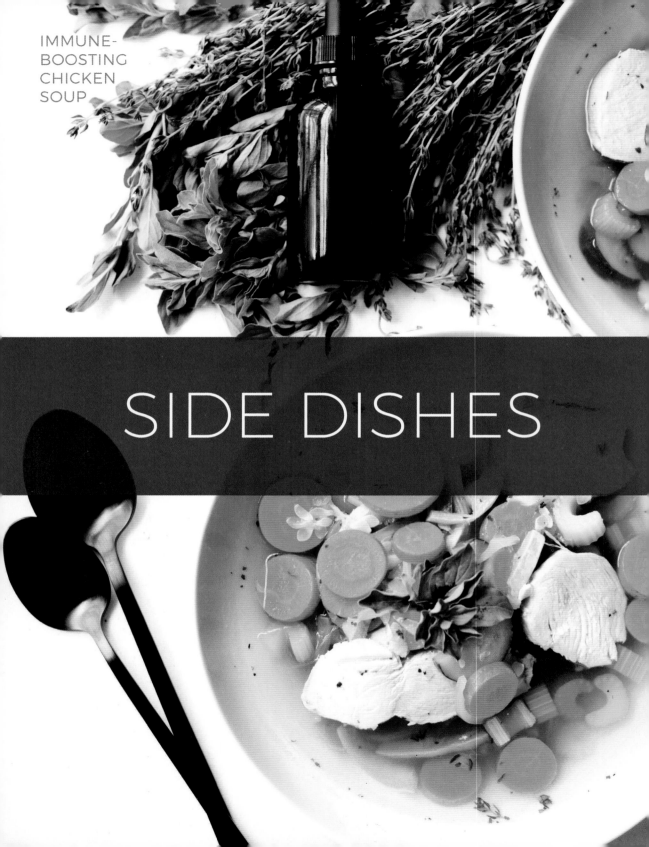

IMMUNE-
BOOSTING
CHICKEN
SOUP

SIDE DISHES

IMMUNE-BOOSTING CHICKEN SOUP

TIME: 2 HOURS   SERVES: 3-4

INGREDIENTS

- 6 cups bone broth
- 1 cup water
- 3 stalks celery, trimmed and coarsely chopped
- 4 carrots, trimmed and coarsely chopped
- 1 tablespoon ghee
- 1 zucchini, chopped
- 1 yellow squash, chopped
- ½ red onion, finely chopped
- 1 teaspoon sea salt
- 1 teaspoon black pepper
- 2 teaspoons oregano
- 3-4 drops thyme essential oil
- 3 cups cooked and shredded chicken

DIRECTIONS

1. In a large stockpot, place all ingredients, except the chicken and thyme essential oil, and allow them to marinate overnight.

2. Add the shredded chicken to the stockpot and cook over medium heat for 1 hour, or until the vegetables are fork tender.

3. Add more sea salt and pepper to taste.

4. Allow the soup to rest for 10 minutes, and then add the thyme essential oil. Serve and enjoy!

LIME CILANTRO CAULIFLOWER RICE

TIME: 15 MINUTES   SERVES: 6-8

INGREDIENTS

- 2 tablespoons ghee
- 6 cups grated cauliflower
- 3 garlic cloves, minced
- 2-3 drops lime essential oil
- Juice of ½ lime
- ½ cup chopped cilantro
- 2 very ripe avocados, pitted, peeled and diced
- ½ teaspoon smoked paprika
- ½ teaspoon cumin
- Sea salt and pepper, to taste

DIRECTIONS

1. In a large pan over medium-high heat, melt the ghee.

2. Add the cauliflower and garlic, stirring occasionally.

3. Cook for 5 to 10 minutes, and then remove from the heat.

4. In a large mixing bowl, place the cauliflower mixture.

5. Pour in the lime essential oil and lime juice, mixing well.

6. Stir in the chopped cilantro, avocados, smoked paprika and cumin.

7. Add the sea salt and pepper. Serve immediately.

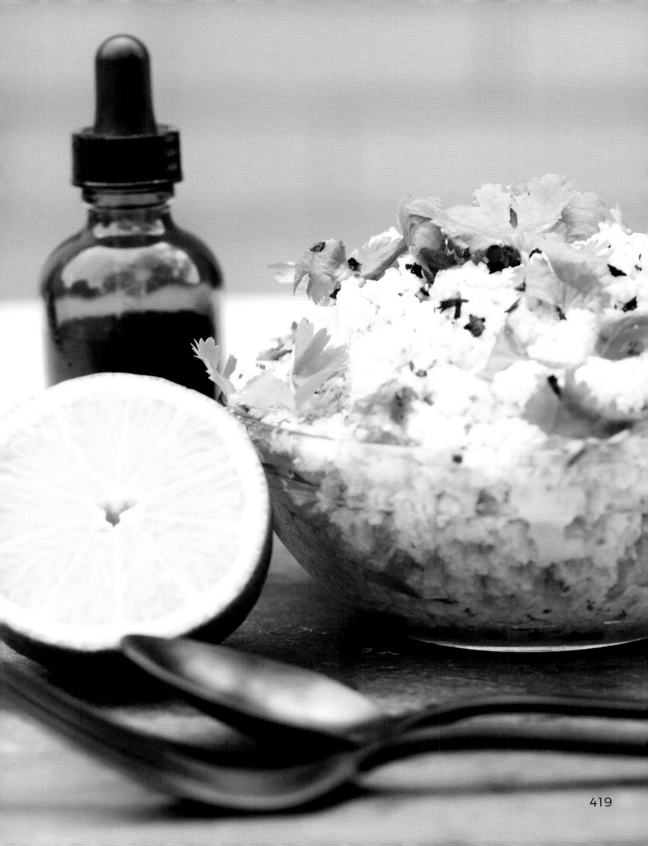

PUMPKIN GINGER SOUP

TIME: 1 HOUR 5 MINUTES   SERVES: 6-8

INGREDIENTS

- 1 tablespoon coconut oil
- 2 sugar pumpkins
- 1 butternut squash
- Salt and pepper, to taste
- 3 carrots, chopped
- ½ white onion, sliced
- 1 clove garlic, peeled and chopped
- 1 green apple, peeled, cored and sliced
- 1 tablespoon grass-fed butter
- ½ tablespoon ground ginger
- ½ tablespoon ground cinnamon
- ½ tablespoon nutmeg
- 5 cups vegetable broth
- 5 drops ginger essential oil

DIRECTIONS

1. Preheat the oven to 425°F.

2. Grease two baking sheets with the coconut oil.

3. Slice the pumpkins and butternut squash lengthwise (through the stem) and remove the seeds.

4. Season the pumpkin and squash with the salt and pepper.

5. Place the pumpkin and squash halves facedown on the baking sheets.

6. Arrange the carrots, onion and garlic around and in between the squash halves on the baking sheets. Bake for 40 minutes.

7. Remove the baking sheets from the oven and allow the squash to cool slightly before handling.

8. Carefully scoop the flesh from the pumpkin and squash halves and add it to a high-powered blender.

9. Add the carrots, onion, garlic, apple, butter, ginger, cinnamon and nutmeg to the blender. Blend well and set aside.

10. In a medium saucepan over medium-high heat, bring the vegetable broth to a boil.

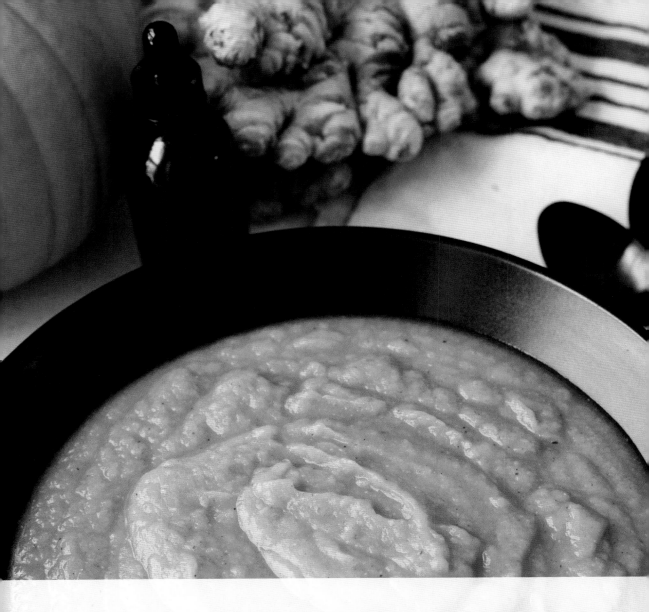

11. Reduce the heat to medium and stir in the blended pumpkin and squash mixture until well incorporated.

12. Cook the bisque for 5 minutes, then reduce the heat and simmer for 10 minutes.

13. Remove from the heat. Add the ginger essential oil and stir until well combined. Add more salt and pepper to taste. Serve warm.

ROSEMARY ORANGE GLAZED CARROTS

TIME: 50 MINUTES   SERVES: 4-6

INGREDIENTS

- 12-14 carrots, peeled
- 3 tablespoons coconut oil
- ¼ cup chopped fresh rosemary
- 2-4 drops orange essential oil
- 1 teaspoon sea salt
- 1 teaspoon black pepper

DIRECTIONS

1. Preheat the oven to 350°F.

2. On a 9x13 baking sheet lined with parchment paper, place the carrots and set aside.

3. In a 12-inch skillet over medium-high heat, melt the coconut oil. Add the rosemary and pan-fry for about 5 minutes, or until the rosemary is crisp.

4. Allow the rosemary to cool and add the orange essential oil, stirring until well combined.

5. Gently pour the oil mixture over the carrots, making sure it is evenly distributed, and bake for 45 minutes, or until the carrots are fork tender.

6. Allow the carrots to cool for 5 to 10 minutes before serving.

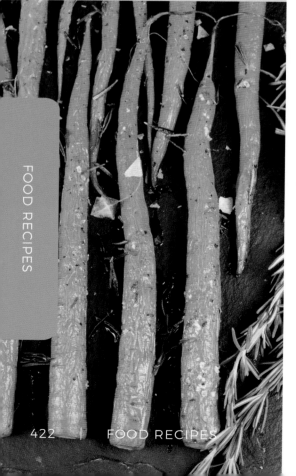

ROSEMARY SUN-DRIED TOMATOES WITH FETA

TIME: 5 MINUTES   SERVES: 2-3

INGREDIENTS
- 1 jar (5 ounces) sun-dried tomatoes, drained
- 4 ounces goat feta
- 1 cup spinach
- 2 tablespoons olive oil
- 1 tablespoon maple syrup
- 1 drop rosemary essential oil
- 1 teaspoon crushed red pepper flakes
- Sea salt, to taste

DIRECTIONS
1. In a medium-sized mixing bowl, place the drained sun-dried tomatoes.

2. Crumble the goat feta over the tomatoes.

3. Add in the spinach and toss it with the tomatoes and feta.

4. In a small bowl, whisk the olive oil, syrup and rosemary essential oil.

5. Drizzle the olive oil mixture over the tomato mixture and toss again.

6. Sprinkle with the red pepper flakes and sea salt.

7. Serve and enjoy!

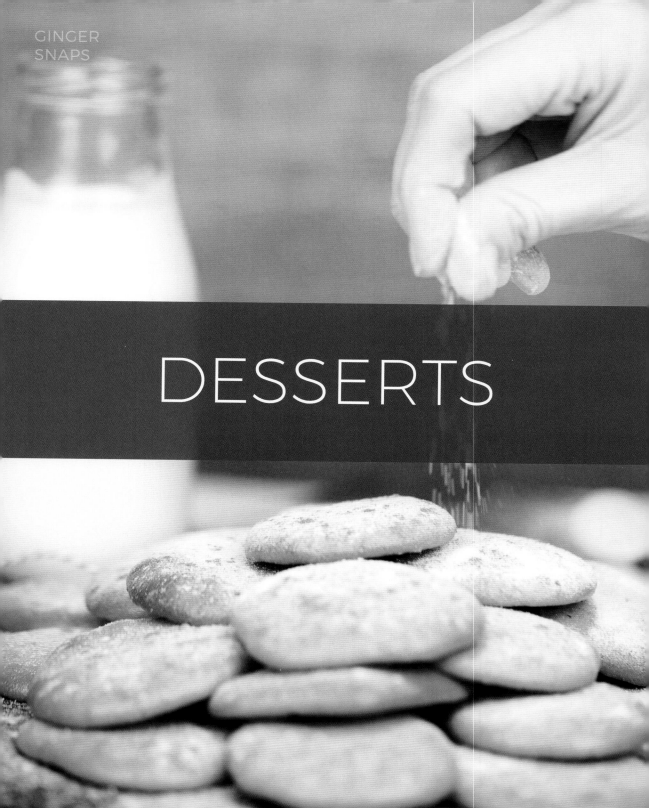

GINGER
SNAPS

DESSERTS

GINGER SNAPS

TIME: 20 MINUTES   SERVES: 40 COOKIES

INGREDIENTS

- 1 cup cashew butter
- ¾ cup maple sugar
- 3 tablespoons molasses
- 2 eggs
- 2 teaspoons fresh grated ginger
- 1 drop ginger essential oil (or 1 teaspoon ground ginger)
- 1 drop cinnamon essential oil
- Juice from ½ lemon
- ½ cup cassava flour
- ½ teaspoon cinnamon powder
- ½ teaspoon sea salt
- Powdered coconut sugar, for topping (optional)

DIRECTIONS

1. Preheat to 350°F.

2. Prepare two baking sheets with parchment paper and set aside.

3. In a large mixing bowl, combine the butter, sugar, molasses, eggs, ginger, ginger essential oil, cinnamon essential oil and lemon juice.

4. In a separate bowl, combine the flour, cinnamon and sea salt.

5. Slowly add the dry mixture to the wet mixture, and stir until well combined.

6. On the baking sheets, spoon out 1 to 2 teaspoons for each cookie.

7. Bake 8 minutes, or until cookies are golden brown.

8. Let cool before serving. Top with the powdered sugar, if desired.

KEY LIME CHEESECAKE

TIME: 2 HOURS 20 MINUTES   SERVES: 10-12

INGREDIENTS

For the crust:

- 3 cups walnuts
- 2-½ cups Medjool dates, pitted
- Dash of Himalayan salt
- 1 teaspoon vanilla (optional)

For the filling:

- 1-½ cups cashews, soaked overnight
- 2 cups fresh coconut meat (or meat of 2 young coconuts)
- 1 can full-fat coconut milk
- ¼ cup coconut nectar
- ⅓ cup melted coconut oil
- 1 tablespoon vanilla extract
- 1 teaspoon Himalayan salt
- Zest and juice of 2 limes
- 5 drops lime essential oil

DIRECTIONS

1. In a food processor, place the ingredients for the crust and blend on high until a dough is formed.

2. In a medium springform pan lined with parchment paper, spread the dough evenly. Place in the freezer while making the filling.

3. In a food processor, place the ingredients for the filling and blend on high until well combined.

4. Remove the pan from the freezer and fill with the filling mixture.

5. Place the pan in the freezer for 2 hours.

6. Defrost the cake in the refrigerator for 20 minutes before serving. Enjoy!

LEMON BARS

TIME: 50 MINUTES   SERVES: 12

INGREDIENTS

For the crust:
- 1 cup coconut oil, room temperature
- ½ cup coconut sugar
- 1 egg
- 2 cups cassava flour
- ½ teaspoon sea salt

For the filling:
- 1 egg
- 5 egg yolks
- 1 cup coconut sugar
- 2 teaspoons lemon zest
- 1 cup lemon juice
- 3 drops lemon essential oil
- 1 teaspoon vanilla extract
- ¾ cup cassava flour

For the topping:
- Powdered sugar (optional)

DIRECTIONS

1. Preheat the oven to 350°F.

2. Line an 8x8 baking dish with parchment paper and set aside.

3. In a large mixing bowl, place the coconut oil, sugar and egg.

4. Whisk or beat until creamy and slowly add in the flour and sea salt until well combined.

5. Pour the crust mixture into the baking dish, pressing down and against the edges.

6. Bake the crust for 12 to 15 minutes, or until slightly golden brown.

7. Meanwhile, in a large mixing bowl, beat the egg, egg yolks and sugar together.

8. Add the lemon zest, lemon juice, lemon essential oil, vanilla and flour. Mix until smooth and creamy.

9. Remove the crust from the oven and pour the filling over the crust.

10. Place the dish back in the oven for another 20 minutes, or until a toothpick inserted comes out clean.

11. Cut into bars and serve. If desired, top the bars with powdered sugar.

ORANGE ZEST CHOCOLATE CAKE

TIME: 45 MINUTES   SERVES: 8-12

INGREDIENTS

For the cake:
- 2 cups gluten-free flour
- 2 cups coconut sugar
- ¾ cup cacao powder
- 2 teaspoons baking powder
- 1-½ teaspoons baking soda
- Zest and juice of ½ orange, separated
- 1 teaspoon sea salt
- 1 cup coconut milk
- ½ cup melted coconut oil
- 2 eggs
- 1 tablespoon vanilla extract
- 3-5 drops orange essential oil

For the frosting:
- 1 cup butter, softened
- ⅓ cup coconut milk
- ⅔ cup cacao powder
- 1 cup honey
- 1 teaspoon vanilla extract
- ½ teaspoon sea salt

DIRECTIONS

1. Preheat the oven to 350°F.

2. Grease and flour two 9-inch cake pans.

3. In a large bowl, mix the flour, sugar, cacao powder, baking powder, baking soda, orange zest and sea salt.

4. Next, add the orange juice, coconut milk, coconut oil, eggs, vanilla and orange essential oil. Mix until combined.

5. Distribute the batter evenly between the pans and bake for 30 to 35 minutes, or until cooked through.

6. Remove the pans from the oven and allow the cakes to cool completely before removing from cake pans.

7. While the cakes are cooling, prepare the frosting. In a medium bowl, combine all frosting ingredients and mix with a whisk or handheld blender until a smooth consistency is achieved.

8. Spread the frosting evenly over one cake and then stack the other cake on top. Cover the cake with the frosting again and serve.

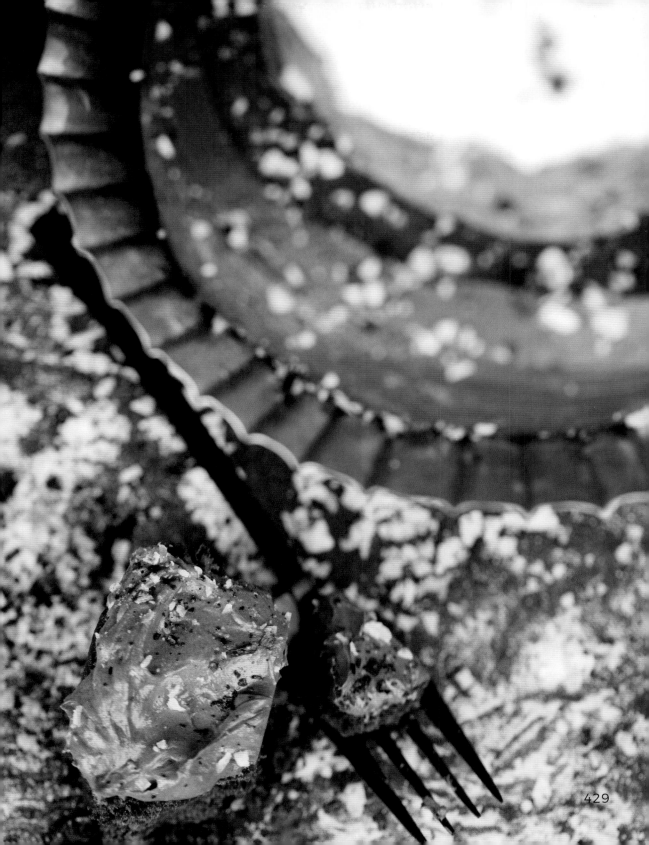

PEPPERMINT PATTIES

TIME: 30 MINUTES   SERVES: 12

INGREDIENTS

- 2 cups coconut oil (at room temperature)
- ½ cup honey
- 5-10 drops peppermint essential oil
- 3 dark chocolate bars (3 ounces each), minimum 72% cacao

DIRECTIONS

1. In a bowl, mix the oil, honey and peppermint essential oil.

2. Form patties out of the mixture and place them on a plate covered with parchment paper. Place in the freezer to harden.

3. Meanwhile, in a saucepan over medium-low heat, melt the chocolate bars. Remove the pan from the heat and allow it to cool for 5 to 10 minutes.

4. Next, dip the hardened patties in the chocolate until covered and place them back on the plate. Place the plate back in the freezer until the chocolate has hardened.

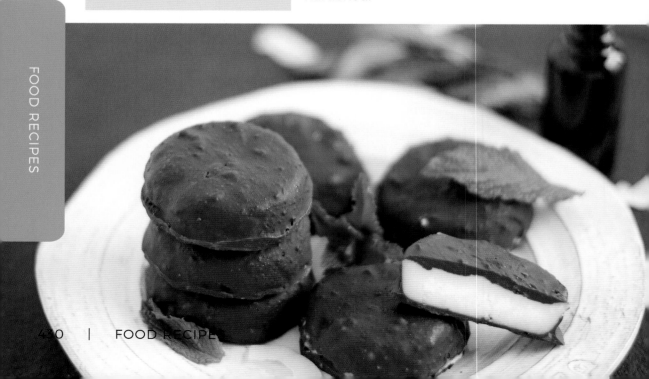

VANILLA LAVENDER MINI CHEESECAKES

TIME: 2 HOURS 20 MINUTES   **SERVES: 24 MINI CHEESECAKES**

INGREDIENTS

For the crust:
- 3 cups walnuts
- 2-½ cups Medjool dates, pitted
- 1 teaspoon vanilla
- Dash of Himalayan salt

For the filling:
- 1-½ cups cashews, soaked overnight
- 2 cups of fresh coconut meat (or meat of 2 young coconuts)
- ½ can full-fat coconut milk
- ½ cup maple syrup
- ⅓ cup melted coconut oil
- 1 tablespoon vanilla extract
- 1 tablespoons dried lavender
- 2-3 drops lavender essential oil
- 1 teaspoon Himalayan salt
- Juice of 1 lemon
- Zest of ½ lemon

For the topping:
- 4 dried figs, sliced
- 8 cherries, sliced
- 6 macadamia nuts, crushed

DIRECTIONS

1. In a food processor, place the ingredients for the crust and blend until a dough is formed.

2. In two muffin pans filled with liners, spread the dough evenly. Place in the freezer while making the filling.

3. In a food processor, place the ingredients for the filling and blend on high until well combined.

4. Remove the pans from the freezer and fill about three-quarters full with the filling mixture.

5. Add the toppings and place the pans back in the freezer for an additional 2 hours.

6. Defrost the mini cheesecakes in the refrigerator for 20 minutes before serving. Enjoy!

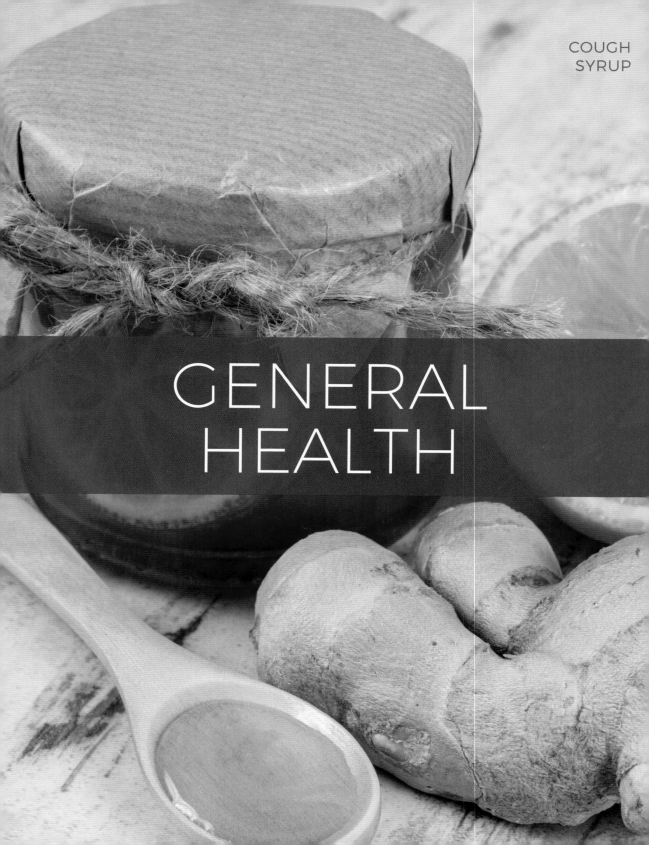

GENERAL HEALTH

COUGH SYRUP

TIME: 2 MINUTES   SERVES: 1 USE

INGREDIENTS
- 1 drop lemon essential oil
- 1 drop ginger essential oil
- 1 drop peppermint essential oil
- 1 drop lavender essential oil
- 1 spoonful honey

DIRECTIONS
1. In a small glass jar, combine all ingredients.

2. Mix well, and then consume.

VAPOR RUB

TIME: 30 MINUTES   SERVES: 30-60 USES

INGREDIENTS
- ¼ cup olive oil
- ½ cup coconut oil
- ¼ cup grated beeswax
- 20 drops peppermint essential oil
- 20 drops eucalyptus essential oil

DIRECTIONS
1. In a medium glass jar, combine the olive oil, coconut oil and beeswax.

2. Fill a saucepan with 2 inches of water and place it over medium-low heat.

3. Place the jar in the saucepan and allow the oils to melt. Stir to combine well.

4. Once combined, allow the mixture to cool slightly and add in the essential oils.

5. Pour the mixture into metal tins or storage containers and allow it to set.

ANOINTING OIL BLEND

TIME: 2 MINUTES   SERVES: 30-60 USES

INGREDIENTS

- ¼ cup + 2 tablespoons olive oil
- 12 drops cinnamon essential oil
- 12 drops frankincense essential oil
- 12 drops myrrh essential oil
- 12 drops rosemary essential oil
- 12 drops orange essential oil

DIRECTIONS

1. In a 4-ounce glass dropper bottle, add all ingredients.

2. Shake gently to mix the oils together.

3. Place 12 drops, or 1 dropper full, on your head and massage into your scalp. Then place 12 drops, or 1 dropper full, on your neck. Do this once daily.

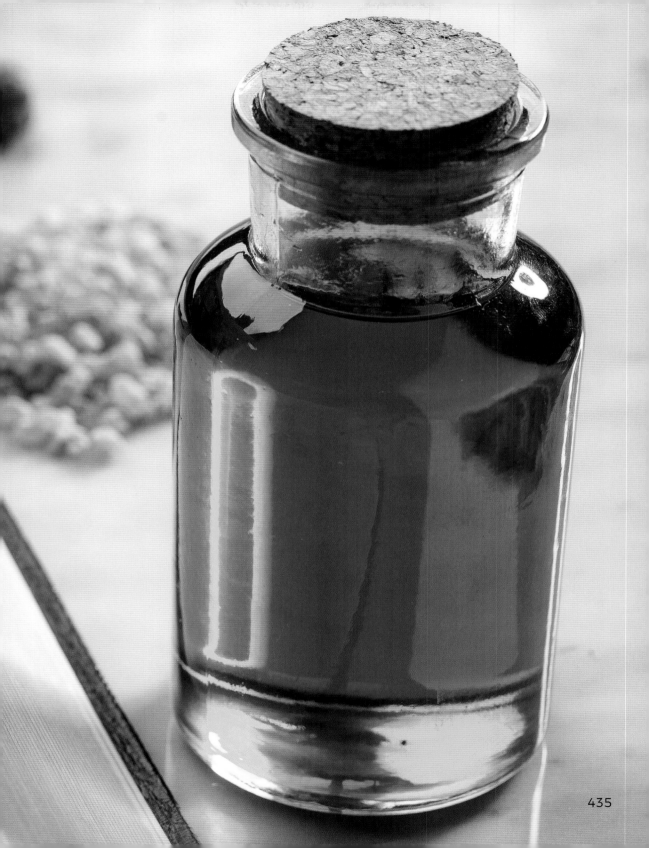

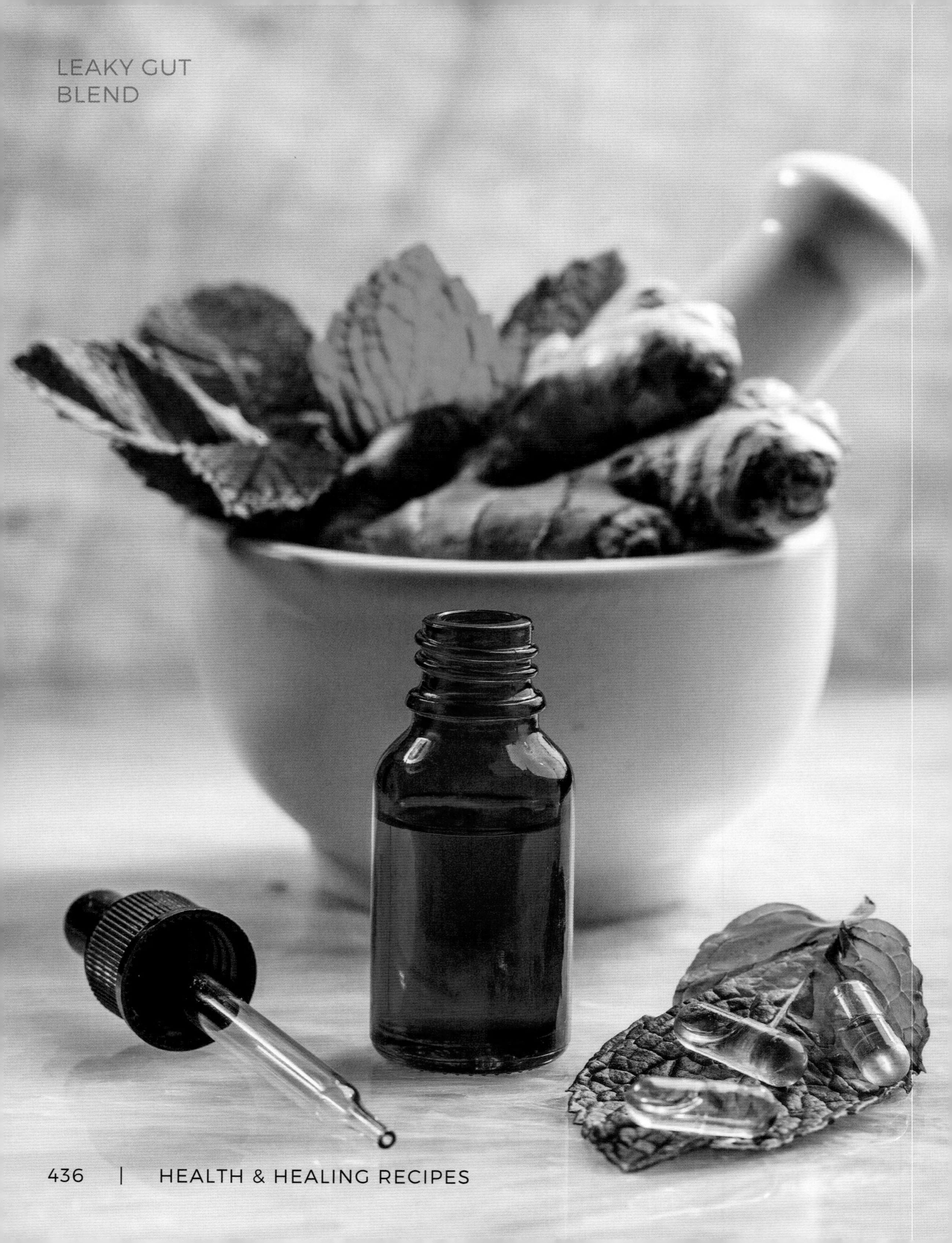

LEAKY GUT BLEND

TIME: 2 MINUTES   SERVES: 1 USE

INGREDIENTS

- 2 drops peppermint essential oil
- 2 drops ginger essential oil
- 2 drops Roman chamomile essential oil
- 2 drops lemon essential oil

DIRECTIONS

1. In an empty vegetable capsule, add all ingredients.

2. Consume with an 8-ounce glass of water 15-20 minutes before you eat.

HAND SANITIZER

TIME: 2 MINUTES   SERVES: 30 USES

INGREDIENTS

- 3 tablespoons aloe vera gel
- 1 tablespoon filtered water
- 5 drops tea tree essential oil
- 1 teaspoon vitamin E

DIRECTIONS

1. In a small bowl, add all ingredients and mix.

2. Transfer the mixture into a BPA-free plastic squeeze bottle and use as needed.

MUSCLE RUB

TIME: 30 MINUTES   SERVES: 30 USES

INGREDIENTS
- ½ cup coconut oil or arnica oil
- ¼ cup grated beeswax
- 2 teaspoons cayenne powder
- 15 drops ginger essential oil
- 15 drops peppermint essential oil
- 15 drops helichrysum essential oil

DIRECTIONS
1. In a small saucepan, add 2 inches of water. Place over medium-low heat.

2. In a glass jar, add the coconut oil and beeswax. Place the jar in the saucepan and stir, allowing the mixture to melt. Add the cayenne and ginger.

3. Once combined, allow the mixture to cool slightly. Mix in the essential oils.

4. Pour the mixture into metal tins or glass storage containers. Allow it to set.

STUDY BLEND

TIME: 2 MINUTES   SERVES: 30-60 USES

INGREDIENTS
- 2 drops vetiver essential oil
- 2 drops rosemary essential oil
- 2 drops cedarwood essential oil
- 2 drops peppermint essential oil (for energy) OR 2 drops Roman chamomile essential oil (to calm)
- Fractionated coconut oil, as needed

DIRECTIONS
1. In a small roll-on glass bottle, combine the essential oils.

2. Top off the mixture with the fractionated coconut oil.

3. Roll the mixture onto the back of your neck before studying or working.

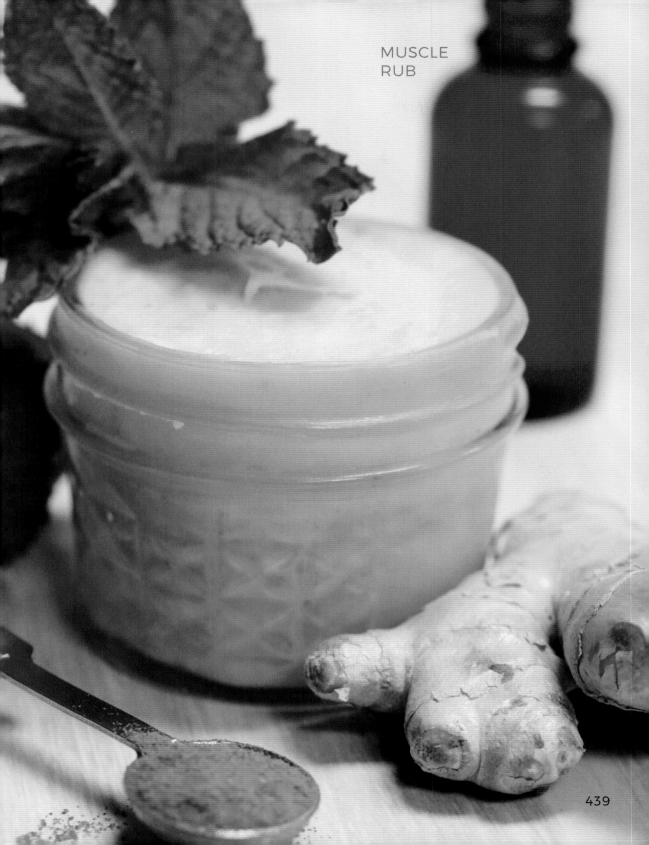

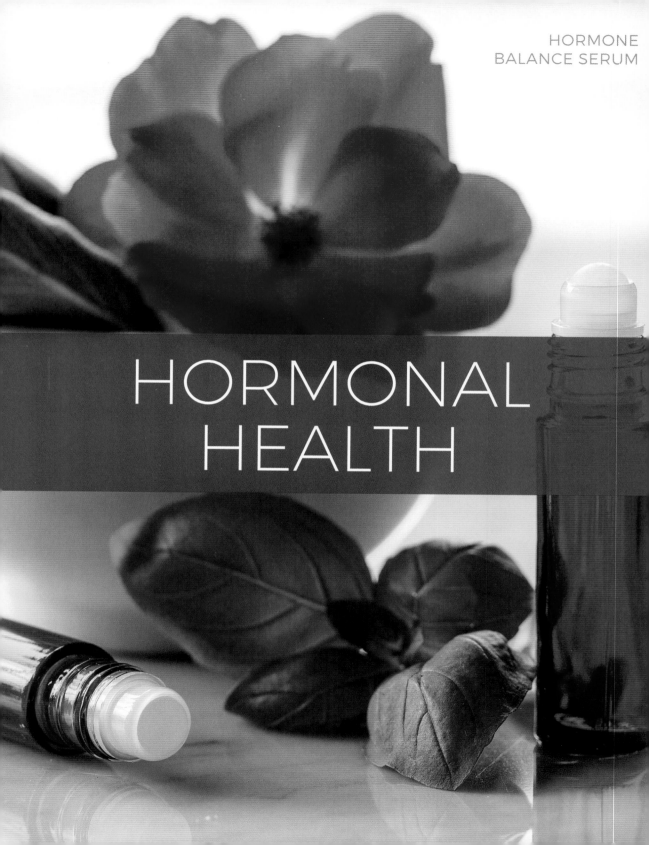

HORMONAL
HEALTH

HORMONE BALANCE SERUM

TIME: 2 MINUTES   SERVES: 30-60 USES

INGREDIENTS

- 2 tablespoons evening primrose oil
- 30 drops clary sage essential oil
- 30 drops thyme essential oil
- 30 drops ylang ylang essential oil

DIRECTIONS

1. In a small glass bottle, mix all ingredients.

2. Pour into a glass vial with a dropper.

3. Rub 5 drops onto your neck twice daily.

ADRENAL REJUVENATING BLEND

TIME: 2 MINUTES   SERVES: 30-60 USES

INGREDIENTS

- 15 drops jojoba oil
- 15 drops holy basil essential oil
- 2 drops rosemary essential oil
- 2 drops peppermint essential oil

DIRECTIONS

1. In a roll-on glass bottle, combine all ingredients.

2. Roll the mixture onto your back (right above your kidneys) up to three times daily.

SLEEP SERUM

TIME: 2 MINUTES   SERVES: 30-60 USES

INGREDIENTS
- 2 drops Roman chamomile essential oil
- 2 drops lavender essential oil
- 2 drops ylang ylang essential oil
- Fractionated coconut oil, as needed

DIRECTIONS
1. In a small roll-on glass bottle, combine the essential oils.

2. Top off the mixture with the fractionated coconut oil.

3. Roll the mixture onto your neck at night right before going to sleep.

THYROID RESTORE BLEND

TIME: 2 MINUTES   SERVES: 30-60 USES

INGREDIENTS
- 15 drops holy basil essential oil
- 2 drops frankincense essential oil
- 2 drops myrrh essential oil
- 2 drops lavender essential oil

DIRECTIONS
1. In a roll-on glass bottle, combine the essential oils.

2. Roll the mixture onto your neck and the area over your thyroid up to three times daily.

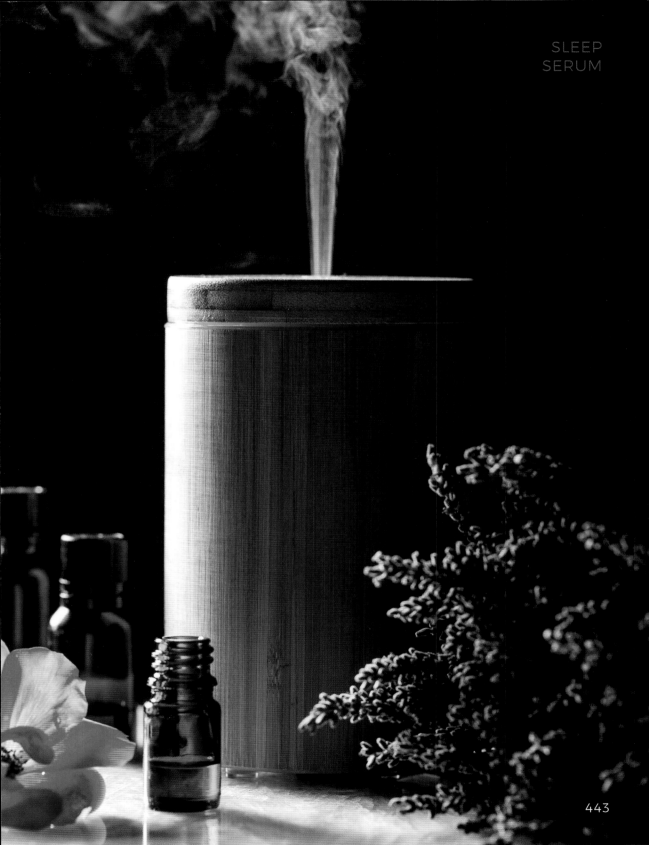

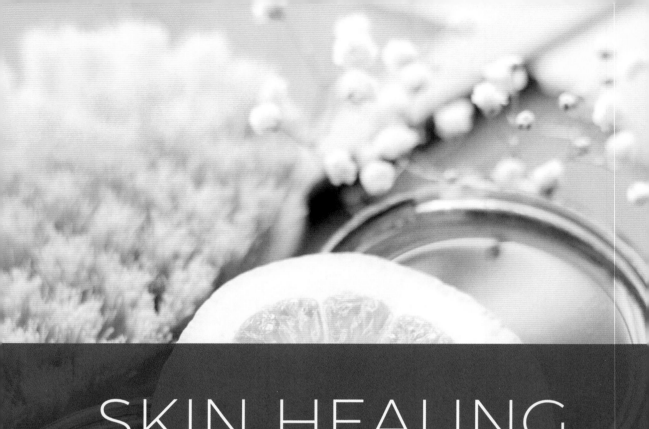

SKIN HEALING

ACNE SCAR REMOVAL
FACE MASK

ACNE SCAR REMOVAL FACE MASK

TIME: 10 MINUTES   SERVES: 10 USES

INGREDIENTS

- 3 tablespoons lemon juice
- 3 tablespoons honey
- 2 tablespoons almond oil or olive oil
- ¼ teaspoon vitamin E oil
- 8-10 drops myrrh essential oil
- 8-10 drops frankincense essential oil
- 6-8 drops helichrysum essential oil

DIRECTIONS

1. In a small glass jar, combine all ingredients and mix well.

2. Apply the mixture onto your face daily, and leave it on for 10 to 15 minutes.

3. Afterward, wash your face thoroughly.

4. Use this mask once daily for 8 to 10 days. If you notice any discomfort, discontinue use or apply it every other day.

ANTI-AGING SERUM

TIME: 2 MINUTES   SERVES: 15 USES

INGREDIENTS

- ½ tablespoon jojoba oil
- ½ tablespoon evening primrose oil
- ½ tablespoon pomegranate oil
- 20 drops lavender essential oil or frankincense essential oil
- 15 drops vitamin E oil
- 10 drops carrot seed essential oil

DIRECTIONS

1. In a small bowl, mix all ingredients.

2. Transfer the serum into a dark glass bottle. Use it every morning and night on your face, neck and chest.

BURN SALVE

TIME: 2 MINUTES   SERVES: 30 USES

INGREDIENTS

- ¼ cup honey
- 2 tablespoons extra virgin olive oil
- 20 drops lavender essential oil

DIRECTIONS

1. In a small bowl, combine all ingredients and mix well.

2. Spread the salve lavishly over the injury.

3. Cover the injury site with a dressing or adhesive bandage.

CELLULITE CREAM

TIME: 2 MINUTES   SERVES: 30 USES

INGREDIENTS

- 30 drops grapefruit essential oil
- 1 cup coconut oil

DIRECTIONS

1. In a glass container, mix the grapefruit essential oil and coconut oil.

2. Rub a small amount onto any areas of cellulite for 5 minutes daily.

ECZEMA CREAM

TIME: 40 MINUTES   SERVES: 25 USES

INGREDIENTS

- ½ cup raw shea butter
- ½ cup coconut oil (alternatives: ¼ cup olive oil or almond oil)
- 1 tablespoon local honey
- 20 drops lavender essential oil
- 20 drops geranium essential oil
- 20 drops myrrh essential oil or tea tree essential oil

DIRECTIONS

1. In a double boiler, melt the shea butter and coconut oil until they are well combined.

2. Add the honey and continue to stir.

3. Once it is well blended, add the essential oils. Continue to stir.

4. Slightly cool the ingredients so that the mixture will begin to thicken, but keep it soft. You can put the solution in the refrigerator for up to 5 minutes to speed up this process.

5. Using a mixer (either a hand-held or stand mixer), mix it for several minutes until the mixture has a frothy appearance, eventually developing the consistency of lotion. You can achieve this by continuing to mix about every 10 minutes.

6. Transfer the cream to a glass mason jar or similar container.

7. Store at room temperature or in the refrigerator. It will stay a bit softer at room temperature, which may make it easier to apply.

STRETCH MARK CREAM

TIME: 20 MINUTES   SERVES: 30-40 USES

INGREDIENTS

- ¼ cup + 2 tablespoons unrefined coconut oil
- 1-½ tablespoons unrefined cocoa butter
- 1-½ tablespoons unrefined shea butter
- 3 tablespoons sweet almond oil
- 6 tablespoons water
- 2 teaspoons vitamin E oil
- 20 drops lavender essential oil
- 20 drops cypress essential oil
- 10 drops grapefruit essential oil
- 10 drops helichrysum essential oil

DIRECTIONS

1. In a small saucepan over low heat, melt the coconut oil, cocoa butter, shea butter and almond oil.

2. Once the oils are completely melted, mix in the water until the oils and water are combined and smooth.

3. Remove the pan from the heat and continue to mix the oil and water until the mixture cools to room temperature and develops a creamy consistency.

4. Once the mixture reaches room temperature, stir in the vitamin E oil and the lavender, cypress, grapefruit and helichrysum essential oils.

5. Apply over the areas of concern.

6. Store the cream in a dark glass container. If you use a clear glass container, store it in a dark place.

SUNBURN SPRAY

TIME: 10 MINUTES   SERVES: 30 USES

INGREDIENTS

- ½ cup liquid aloe vera juice
- ⅛ cup fractionated coconut oil
- 10 drops lavender essential oil
- 10 drops peppermint essential oil

DIRECTIONS

1. In a small saucepan, add 2 inches of water. Place over medium heat.

2. In a glass jar, add the aloe vera juice and coconut oil. Place the jar in the saucepan and stir, allowing the mixture to liquefy and combine.

3. Once combined, remove from saucepan and add in the essential oils, mixing well.

4. Pour the mixture into a glass spray bottle and store in a cool place.

VARICOSE VEIN BLEND

TIME: 2 MINUTES   SERVES: 30-60 USES

INGREDIENTS

- 2 drops frankincense essential oil
- 2 drops cypress essential oil
- 2 drops grapefruit essential oil
- 2 drops lemon essential oil
- Fractionated coconut oil, as needed

DIRECTIONS

1. In a roll-on glass bottle, combine the essential oils.

2. Top off the mixture with the fractionated coconut oil.

3. Roll the mixture onto the affected areas as needed.

LAUNDRY
SOAP

HOME

LAUNDRY SOAP

TIME: 5 MINUTES   SERVES: 12-15 USES

INGREDIENTS

- 1 bar Castile soap, grated
- 2 cups borax
- 2 cups washing soda
- 1 cup baking soda
- 15 drops lavender essential oil
- 15 drops peppermint essential oil

DIRECTIONS

1. In an airtight container, combine all ingredients and store.

2. Use ¼ cup per large load of laundry (adjust accordingly for smaller loads).

BUG SPRAY

TIME: 2 MINUTES   SERVES: 30-60 USES

INGREDIENTS

- ½ cup witch hazel
- ½ cup apple cider vinegar
- 40 drops essential oils (eucalyptus, lemongrass, citronella, tea tree or rosemary)

DIRECTIONS

1. In an 8-ounce glass spray bottle, mix all ingredients.

2. Spray the mixture over all portions of your body, except in your eyes and mouth.

HOUSEHOLD CLEANER

TIME: 2 MINUTES   SERVES: 30-60 USES

INGREDIENTS
- 8 ounces water
- 4 ounces distilled white vinegar
- 15 drops melaleuca essential oil
- 15 drops lemon essential oil

DIRECTIONS
1. In a glass spray bottle, mix all ingredients.

2. Swirl or shake the bottle before each spray.

HOLIDAY HOME CLEANER

TIME: 2 MINUTES   SERVES: 30-60 USES

INGREDIENTS
- 1-1/2 cup distilled white vinegar
- 5 drops cinnamon essential oil
- 5 drops fir essential oil
- 5 drops orange essential oil

DIRECTIONS
1. In a glass spray bottle, add all ingredients.

2. Shake the bottle gently to mix well before using.

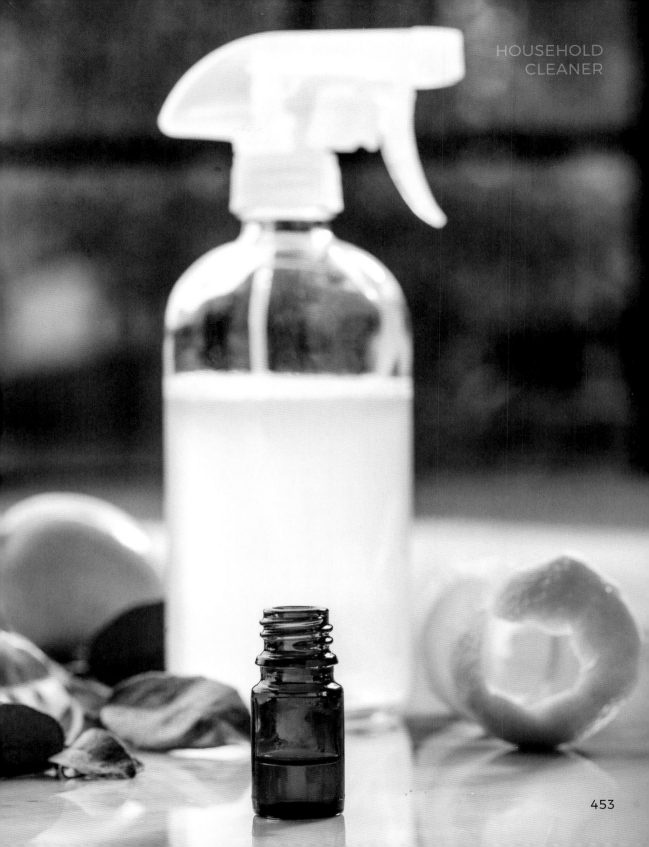

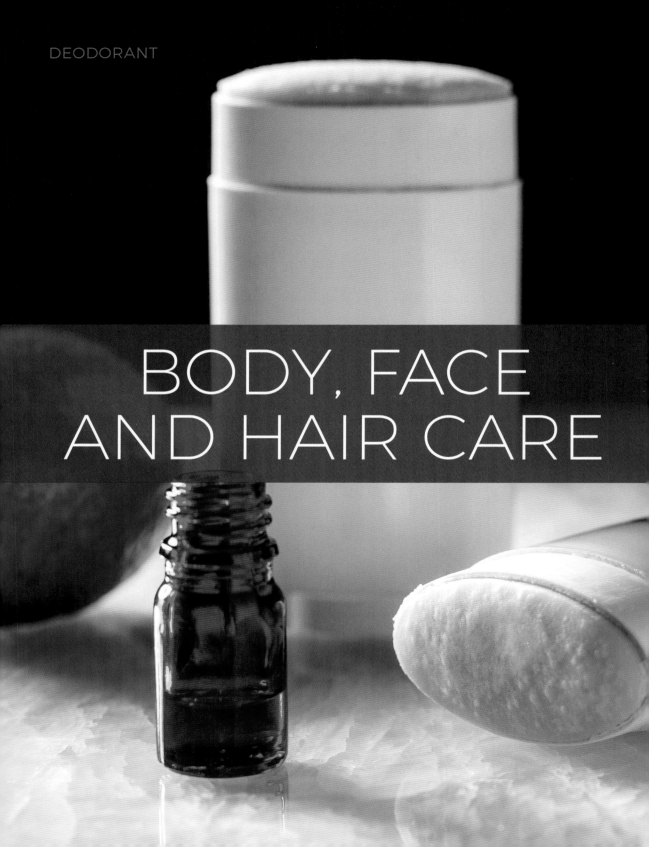

BODY, FACE AND HAIR CARE

DEODORANT

TIME: 5 MINUTES   SERVES: 30-90 USES

INGREDIENTS
- ¼ cup baking soda
- ¼ cup coconut oil
- ¼ cup grated beeswax
- ¼ cup shea butter
- 3 tablespoons arrowroot powder
- 40 drops essential oils of your choice*

  *Note: Recommended female oils scents—ylang ylang, jasmine, lavender and lemon; recommended male oils scents—sandalwood, bergamot, black pepper and cypress.

DIRECTIONS
1. Over a double broiler, melt the coconut or arnica oil and beeswax together. Stir gently until completely melted.

2. Add in the remaining ingredients and stir again.

3. Once mixed, quickly poor the mixture into an empty deodorant container.

4. Keep the container upright and allow the mixture to cool and harden before use.

BATH SALTS

TIME: 2 MINUTES   SERVES: 4 USES

INGREDIENTS
- 3 cups Epsom salt
- 1 cup baking soda
- 40 drops lavender essential oil

DIRECTIONS
1. In a large glass jar with a lid, combine the Epsom salt and baking soda and store.

2. At bath time, add 1 cup of dry ingredients mixture and the lavender into your bath water. (Note: For optimal use, make your bath water as hot as possible without burning yourself.)

3. Soak for 20-40 minutes.

EYE CREAM

TIME: 15 MINUTES   SERVES: 30 USES

INGREDIENTS

- 10 drops frankincense essential oil
- 2 tablespoons pure aloe vera gel
- 2 tablespoons unrefined shea butter
- 2 tablespoons unrefined coconut oil
- ½ teaspoon vitamin E oil

DIRECTIONS

1. In a small bowl, mix all ingredients.

2. If needed (for colder months when the coconut oil is solid), gently heat the shea butter and coconut oil in a small pan, and then add the remaining ingredients so that it blends easily.

3. Once well blended, transfer the cream into a glass jar with a lid.

4. Use it every morning and night around your eyes.

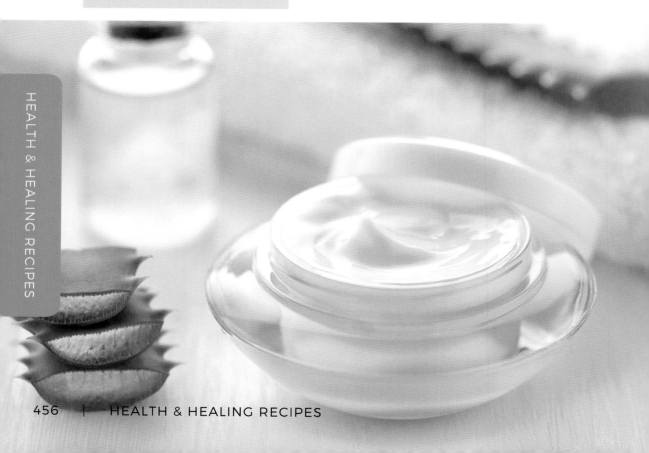

FACE MASK

TIME: 10 MINUTES   SERVES: 1-2 USES

INGREDIENTS

- 1 tablespoon organic, raw, local honey
- ½ teaspoon turmeric powder
- ½ teaspoon organic apple cider vinegar
- ½ teaspoon milk or yogurt
- 1 drop lemon essential oil or fresh lemon juice (for additional skin brightening; optional)

DIRECTIONS

1. To begin, wash your face and hands to remove impurities and any make-up.

2. In a small bowl or jar, mix the honey, turmeric powder, apple cider vinegar, milk or yogurt and optional lemon oil. Aim for a consistency that will stick to your face.

3. Apply the mask carefully, avoiding your eyes.

4. Allow the mask to sit on your face for 15-20 minutes, and then rinse with warm water.

5. If any mixture is left in the bowl, cover and store it in the fridge for your next application.

LIP BALM

TIME: 15 MINUTES   SERVES: 2-3 LIP BALM TINS

INGREDIENTS

- 3 tablespoons beeswax
- 4 tablespoons coconut oil
- 2 drops vitamin E
- 7 drops lavender essential oil
- 7 drops lemon essential oil

DIRECTIONS

1. In a small pot over medium-low heat, melt the beeswax, coconut oil and vitamin E. Stir frequently, using a chopstick or similar long, narrow stick.

2. Remove the pot from the heat and add in the essential oils. Whisk well with the chopstick, distributing the oils throughout the mixture.

3. Pour the mixture quickly into lip balm tins or small glass jars. Let the balm cool on a counter until it hardens.

HAND SOAP

TIME: 2 MINUTES   SERVES: 30-60 USES

INGREDIENTS

- ¼ cup Castile soap
- ¾ cup water
- 10 drops peppermint essential oil
- 10 drops grapefruit essential oil

DIRECTIONS

1. In a small bowl, mix the soap and water together. Add in the essential oils and mix again.

2. Pour the soap into glass bottle or BPA-free plastic dispenser.

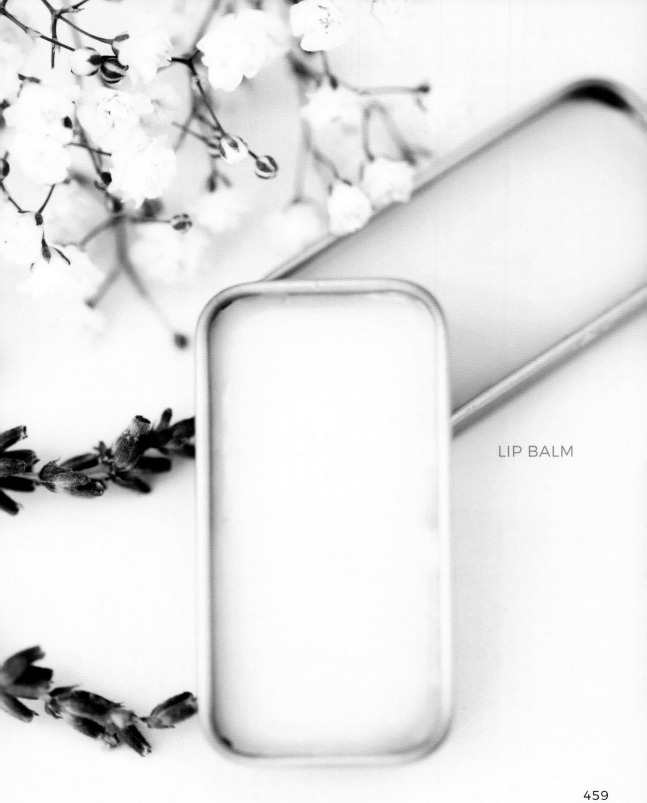

LIP BALM

FRANKINCENSE AND MYRRH BODY LOTION

TIME: 90 MINUTES   SERVES: 30 USES

INGREDIENTS
- ¼ cup olive oil
- ¼ cup coconut oil
- ¼ cup beeswax
- ¼ cup shea butter
- 2 tablespoons vitamin E
- 20 drops frankincense essential oil
- 20 drops myrrh essential oil
- 20 drops lavender essential oil

DIRECTIONS

1. In a small glass bowl, combine the olive oil, coconut oil, beeswax and shea butter.

2. Place the bowl in a saucepan with 2 inches of water and over medium heat. Stir to combine well.

3. Place the bowl in the refrigerator for 1 hour, or until solid.

4. With a regular mixer or hand mixer, beat the mixture until it is whipped and fluffy. Mix in the vitamin E and essential oils.

5. Put the lotion in a BPA-free plastic lotion bottle or glass container. Store it in a cool place.

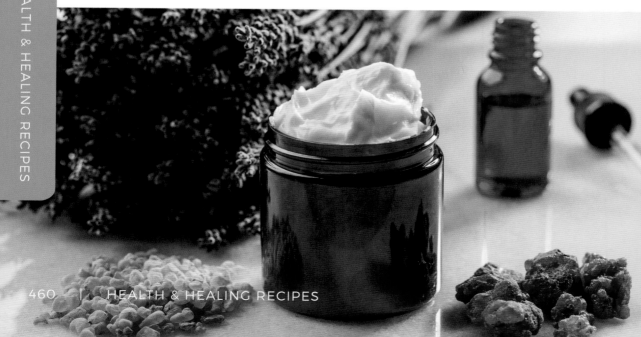

MAGNESIUM BODY BUTTER

TIME: 45 MINUTES   SERVES: 30 USES

INGREDIENTS

- ¾ cup cocoa butter
- ¼ cup magnesium oil
- ¼ cup avocado oil
- 30 drops lavender essential oil

DIRECTIONS

1. Put the cocoa butter in a medium glass jar.

2. Place the jar in a saucepan with 2 inches of water and over low heat.

3. Once melted, pour the cocoa butter into a bowl. Let it cool in the fridge for 30 minutes.

4. Next, using a standard mixer, whip the cocoa butter. Then mix in the magnesium oil, avocado oil and lavender essential oil.

5. Transfer the mixture into a glass jar or BPA-free plastic container. Store in the fridge.

WOMEN'S PERFUME

TIME: 2 MINUTES   SERVES: 30-60 USES

INGREDIENTS

- 20 drops ylang ylang essential oil
- 20 drops jasmine essential oil
- 20 drops vanilla essential oil
- Fractionated coconut oil, as needed

DIRECTIONS

1. In a roll-on glass bottle, combine the essential oils.

2. Top off the mixture with the fractionated coconut oil.

3. Roll the mixture onto your wrists or neck as needed.

MOISTURIZER

TIME: 10 MINUTES   SERVES: 12-15 LIP BALM TINS

INGREDIENTS

- 15-20 drops lavender essential oil
- ¼ cup + 2 tablespoons unrefined coconut oil
- 2 tablespoons shea butter
- 2 tablespoons jojoba oil
- 2 tablespoons pure aloe
- ½ teaspoon vitamin E oil

DIRECTIONS

1. In a small bowl, combine all ingredients.

2. Using a hand mixer, blend the mixture until it is whipped to a light and fluffy consistency.

3. Place the moisturizer in a glass jar with a lid, and apply it once or twice daily to the skin. If possible, apply it to damp skin to help seal in the moisture.

MEN'S COLOGNE

TIME: 2 MINUTES   SERVES: 30-60 USES

INGREDIENTS

- 10 drops sandalwood essential oil
- 10 drops bergamot essential oil
- 10 drops cypress oil
- 1 cup 70 percent alcohol or vodka

DIRECTIONS

1. In a glass cologne spray bottle, combine all ingredients.

2. Spray the mixture onto your wrists or neck as needed.

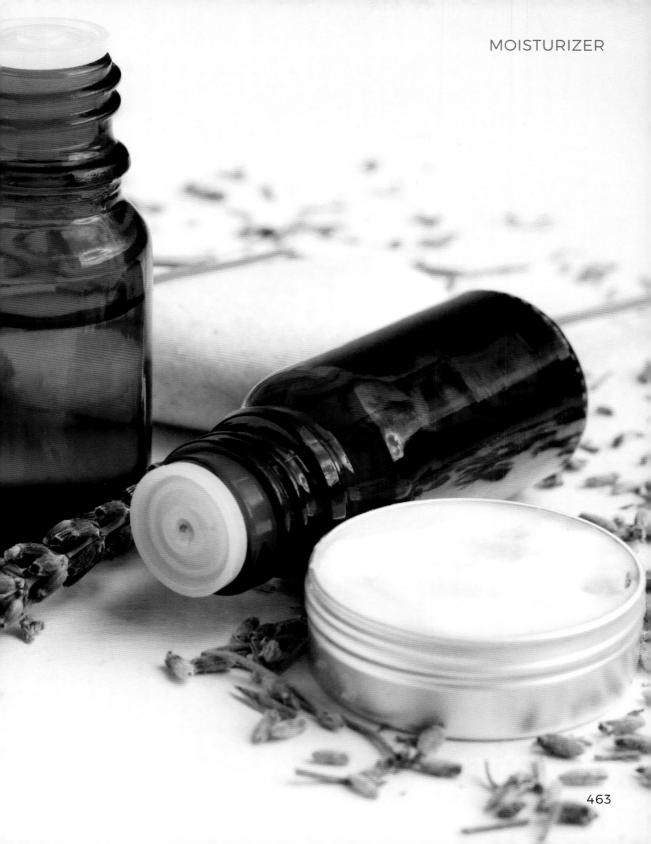

SUNSCREEN

TIME: 20 MINUTES   SERVES: 10 USES

INGREDIENTS

- ¾ cup coconut oil
- 2 tablespoons shea butter
- 1 tablespoon pomegranate oil
- 20 drops lavender essential oil
- 10 drops myrrh essential oil
- 2 tablespoons zinc oxide

DIRECTIONS

1. In a small saucepan, add 2 inches of water. Place over medium-low heat.

2. In a glass jar, add the coconut oil, shea butter, pomegranate oil and essential oils. Place the jar in the saucepan and stir, allowing the mixture to melt and combine.

3. Once combined, add in the zinc oxide and stir well.

4. Remove from the saucepan and store in a cool place.

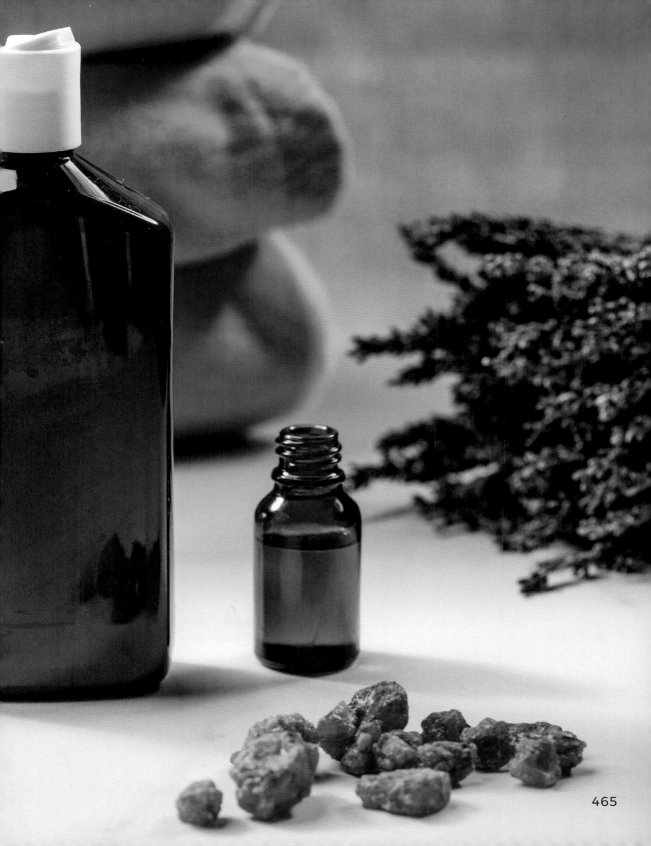

465

DRY SHAMPOO

TIME: 2 MINUTES   SERVES: 3-5 USES

INGREDIENTS

- 2 tablespoons cornstarch or arrowroot powder (for lighter hair colors)
  OR 2 tablespoons cocoa or cinnamon powder (for darker hair colors)
- 2 drops lavender essential oil
- 1 drop peppermint essential oil

DIRECTIONS

1. In a small bowl or a container with a lid, blend all ingredients together.

2. Sprinkle the mixture onto your scalp and hair roots, then work it in with your fingertips. You may also use a clean makeup brush to apply it to your roots. Apply evenly.

3. Allow the product to sit for at least 2 minutes before styling.

4. When styling, make sure to comb or blow-dry your hair to help the dry shampoo blend in.

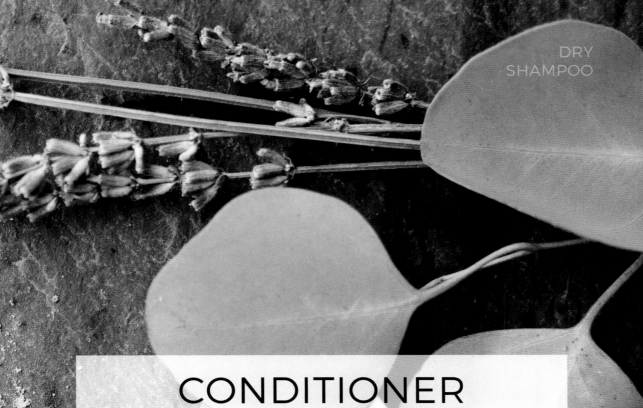

CONDITIONER

TIME: 2 MINUTES   SERVES: 20-30 USES

INGREDIENTS
- 1 cup water
- 2 tablespoons apple cider vinegar
- 10 drops essential oils (see Customize Your Conditioner)

DIRECTIONS
1. In an 8-ounce glass or BPA-free plastic spray bottle, mix all ingredients together.

2. Shake the bottle before using, and then spray the conditioner into your hair.

3. Leave the conditioner in your hair for 5 minutes, and then rinse.

Customize Your Conditioner:
Rosemary or sage essential oils for all types of hair; lemon, bergamot or tea tree essential oils for oily hair; lavender, sandalwood or geranium essential oils for dry hair or dandruff.

BODY WASH

TIME: 2 MINUTES   SERVES: 30 USES

INGREDIENTS

- 1 cup water
- ¼ cup honey
- ⅔ cup liquid Castile soap
- 30 drops lavender, grapefruit, peppermint or geranium essential oil
- 1 teaspoon vitamin E
- 2 teaspoons jojoba oil

DIRECTIONS

1. In a small bowl, combine all ingredients and mix until smooth.

2. Store in an 8-ounce glass or BPA-free plastic bottle.

OILY HAIR SHAMPOO

TIME: 15 MINUTES   SERVES: 10-12 USES

INGREDIENTS

- 1 tablespoon green clay
- 6 teaspoons strongly brewed organic green tea, cooled
- 2 tablespoons liquid Castile soap
- 1 tablespoon raw honey
- 2 tablespoons raw apple cider vinegar
- ½ cup pure water
- 10-12 drops tea tree essential oil

DIRECTIONS

1. In a small bowl, combine the green clay and green tea and mix well. Add the Castile soap and mix again.

2. Next, add the honey and apple cider vinegar, and continue mixing until well blended.

3. Mix in the pure water and essential oil until the mixture is smooth.

4. Place in a BPA-free plastic bottle or glass container. Store in the fridge up to three weeks.

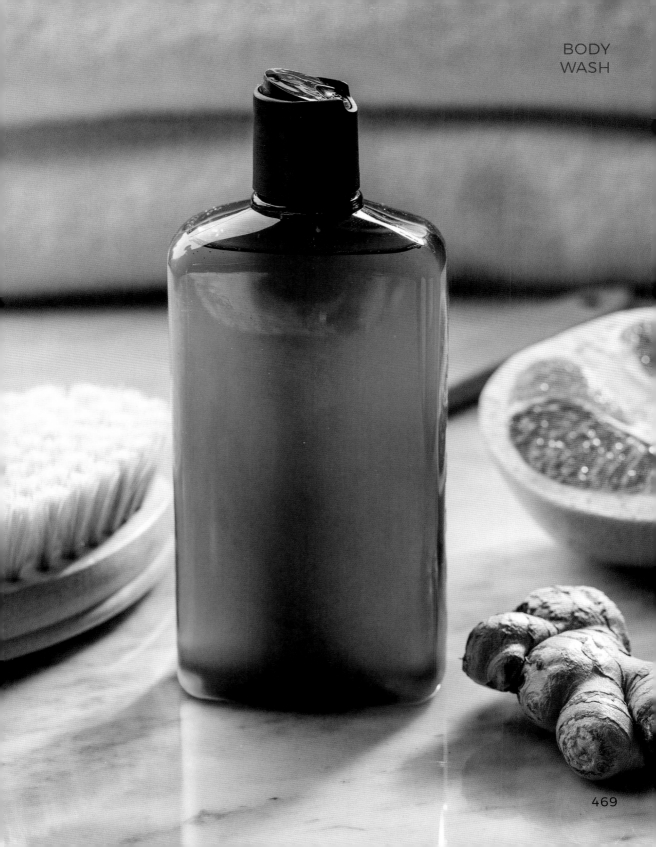

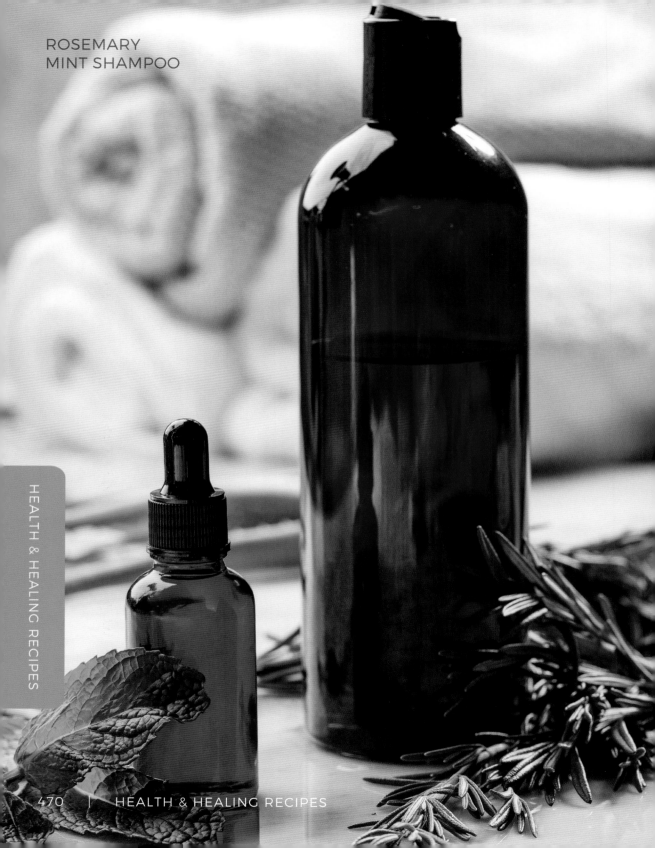

ROSEMARY MINT SHAMPOO

ROSEMARY MINT SHAMPOO

TIME: 2 MINUTES   SERVES: 10-15 USES

INGREDIENTS
- ¾ cup aloe vera gel
- 3 tablespoons olive oil
- ½ cup baking soda
- 25 drops rosemary essential oil
- 12 drops peppermint essential oil

DIRECTIONS
1. In a small bowl, mix all ingredients together.

2. Store in an 8-ounce glass or BPA-free plastic bottle.

BAKING SODA SHAMPOO

TIME: 5 MINUTES   SERVES: 14-16 USES

INGREDIENTS
- ¼ cup baking soda
- ¾ cup purified water
- 10 drops lavender essential oil

DIRECTIONS
1. Place the baking soda in a clean shampoo bottle.

2. Add the purified water and shake well.

3. Add the lavender and shake again, making sure all ingredients are well blended.

4. Gently massage a dollop or two into your hair and scalp.

5. Rinse well.

HAIR THICKENER

TIME: 5 MINUTES   **SERVES: 8-10 USES**

INGREDIENTS

- 3 tablespoons jojoba oil
- 3 tablespoons grapeseed oil
- 30 drops pure cedarwood essential oil
- 30 drops pure rosemary essential oil
- 30 drops pure sage essential oil

DIRECTIONS

1. In a glass jar, combine the jojoba and grapeseed oils. Add the essential oils.

2. Place a lid securely on the jar and shake vigorously to blend the mixture.

3. Apply the mixture generously onto your hair and massage into your scalp and hair, wet or dry. The mixture can be applied daily or at least three times a week.

4. Leave it in your hair for at least 20 minutes (longer, if possible); or apply it before bed and leave it in overnight. You may want to use a towel or shower cap to prevent staining any bed linens.

5. Afterward, shampoo, rinse and style as usual.

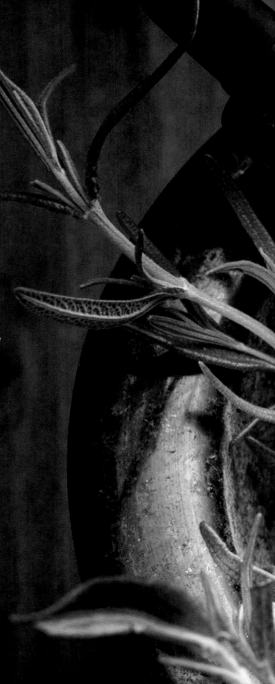

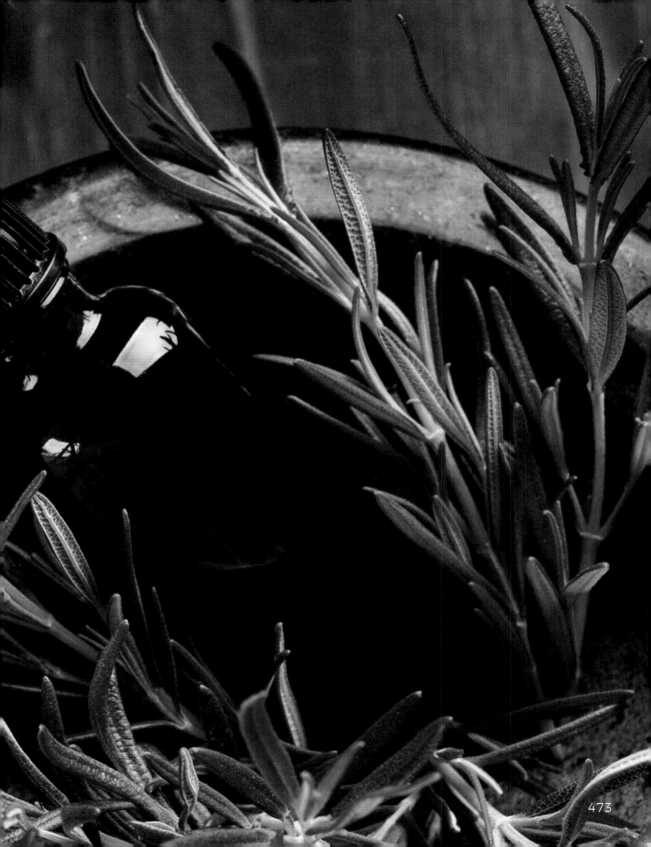

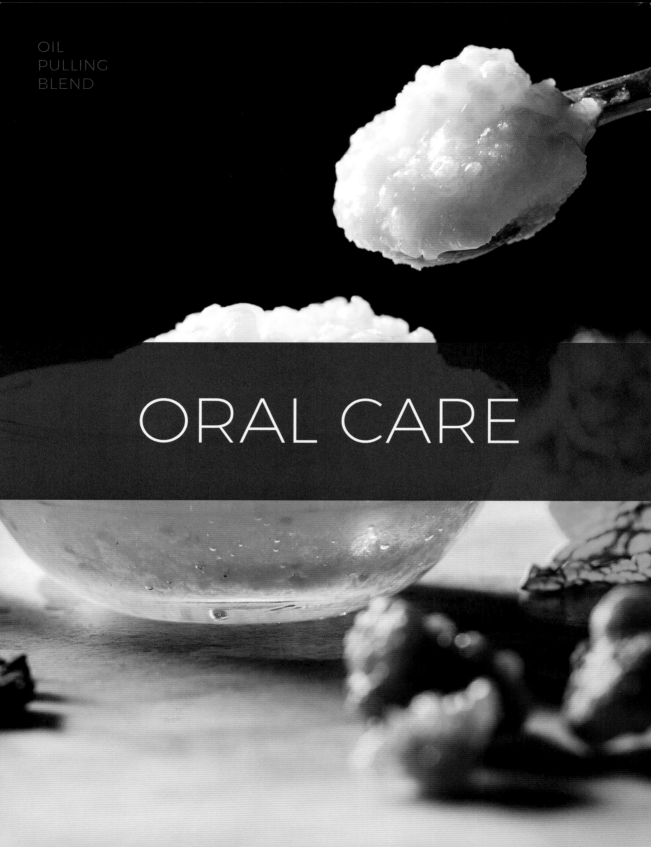

OIL
PULLING
BLEND

ORAL CARE

OIL PULLING BLEND

TIME: 2 MINUTES   SERVES: 1 USES

INGREDIENTS

- 1 tablespoon coconut oil
- 3 drops myrrh essential oil
- 3 drops peppermint essential oil
- 2 drops clove essential oil

DIRECTIONS

1. In a small jar, add all ingredients and mix well.

2. Spoon out the mixture and put it into your mouth, swishing for 5 to 20 minutes.

3. Spit it out into a trashcan. Do not swallow.

MOUTHWASH

TIME: 1 MINUTES   SERVES: 30 USES

INGREDIENTS

- 2 cups spring water
- 5 drops peppermint essential oil
- 5 drops tea tree essential oil

DIRECTIONS

1. In a BPA-free plastic dispenser bottle, add all ingredients. Shake to mix.

2. Take a small sip, swish mixture around in your mouth, gargle for 30 seconds and spit out. Do not swallow.

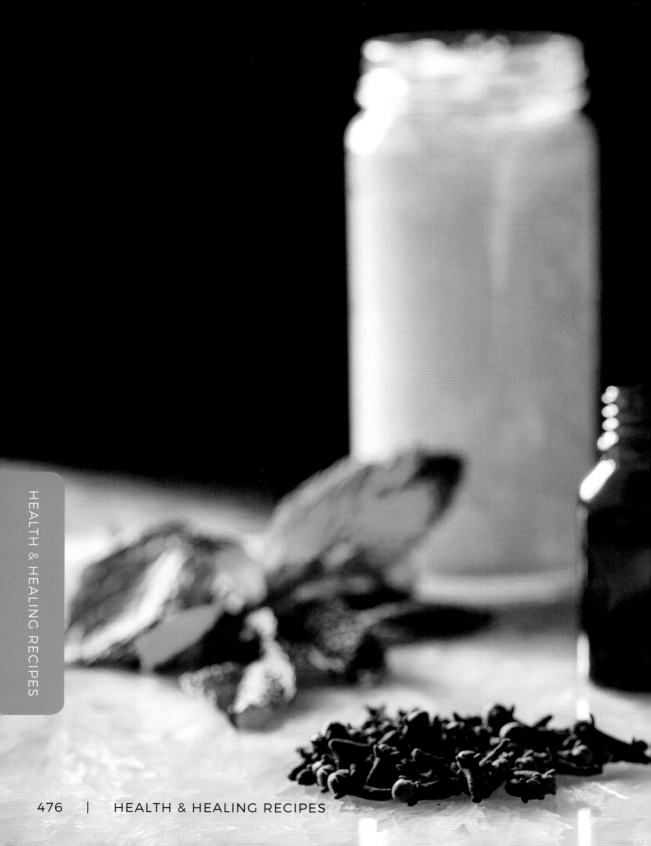

TOOHPASTE

INGREDIENTS

- ¼ cup coconut oil
- 1 tablespoon baking soda
- 2 tablespoons bentonite clay
- 10 drops peppermint essential oil
- 10 drops clove essential oil
- 1 tablespoon xylitol or ½ teaspoon stevia (optional)

DIRECTIONS

1. In a small bowl, mix all ingredients together.

2. Put into a rubber tube or sealed glass container.

3. Brush your teeth for 2 minutes, two to three times daily.

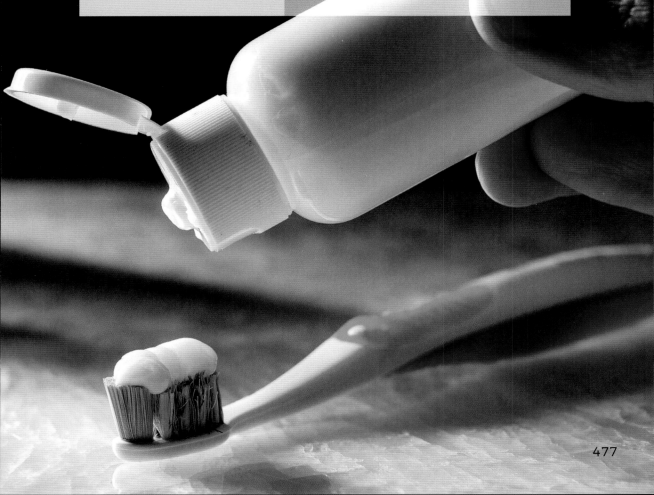

REFERENCES

PART I

CHAPTER 1

[1] Light, Donald W. (June, 2014). New Prescription Drugs: A Major Health Risk With Few Offsetting Advantages. *Harvard University Edmond J. Safra Center for Ethics.* Retrieved from http://ethics.harvard.edu/blog/new-prescription-drugs-major-health-risk-few-offsetting-advantages

[2] Sayorwan, W., Siripornpanich, V., Piriyapunyaporn, T., Hongratanaworakit, T., Kotchabhakdi, N., & Ruangrungsi, N. (April, 2012). The effects of lavender oil inhalation on emotional states, autonomic nervous system, and brain electrical activity. *Journal of the Medical Association of Thailand.* Retrieved from http://www.ncbi.nlm.nih.gov/pubmed/22612017

[3] Amsterdam, J.D., Shults, J., Soeller, I., Mao, J.J., Rockwell, K., & Newberg, A.B. (2012). Chamomile (Matricaria recutita) may provide antidepressant activity in anxious, depressed humans: an exploratory study. *Alternative Therapies in Health and Medicine.* Retrieved from http://www.ncbi.nlm.nih.gov/pubmed/22894890

[4] Takahashi, M., Yoshino, A., Yamanaka, A., Asanuma, C., Satou, T., Hayashi, S., … Koike, K. (November, 2012). Effects of inhaled lavender essential oil on stress-loaded animals: changes in anxiety-related behavior and expression levels of selected mRNAs and proteins. *Natural Product Communications.* Retrieved from http://www.ncbi.nlm.nih.gov/pubmed/23285826

[5] Stewart, David. *Healing Oils of the Bible.* Marble Hill, MO: Center for Aromatherapy Research & Education, 2002. Print.

CHAPTER 2

[6] Jeena, K., Liju, V.B., & Kuttan, R. (2013). Antioxidant, anti-inflammatory and antinociceptive activities of essential oil from ginger. *Indian Journal of Physiology and Pharmacology.* Retrieved from http://www.ncbi.nlm.nih.gov/pubmed/24020099

[7] Liju, V.B., & Jenna, K. (2015). Gatroprotective Activity of Essential Oils from Turmeric and Ginger. *Journal of Basic and Clinical Physiology and Pharmacology.* Retrieved from http://www.ncbi.nlm.nih.gov/pubmed/24756059

[8] Chamovitz, David. *What A Plant Knows: A Field Guide to the Senses.* New York: Scientific American, 2012. Print.

CHAPTER 3

[9] Dinstel, R. R., Cascio, J., & Koukel, S. (2013). The antioxidant level of Alaska's wild berries: high, higher and highest. *International Journal of Circumpolar Health, 72,* 10.3402/ijch.v72i0.21188. Retrieved from http://doi.org/10.3402/ijch.v72i0.21188

CHAPTER 4

[10] Null, G., Dean, C., Feldman, M., & Rasio, D. (2005). *Journal of Orthomolecular Medicine, Vol. 20.* Retrieved from http://orthomolecular.org/library/jom/2005/pdf/2005-v20n01-p021.pdf

[11] Chen, Y., Zhou, C., Ge, Z., Liu, Y., Liu, Y., Fend, W., & Wei, T. (2013). Composition and potential anticancer activities of essential oils obtained from myrrh and frankincense. *Oncology Letters.* Retrieved from http://doi.org/10.3892/ol.2013.1520

[12] Kirste, S., Treier, M., Wehrle, S.J., Becker, G., Abdel-Tawab, M., Gerbeth, K., … Momm, F. (2011). Boswellia serrata acts on cerebral edema in patients irradiated for brain tumors: a prospective, randomized, placebo-controlled, double-blind pilot trial. *Cancer.* Retrieved from http://www.ncbi.nlm.nih.gov/pubmed/21287538

[13] Suhail, M., Wu, W., Cao, A., Mondalek, F., Fung, K., Shih, P., … Lin, H. (2011). Boswellia sacra essential oil induces tumor cell-specific apoptosis and suppresses tumor aggressiveness in cultured human breast cancer cells. *The official journal of the International Society for Complementary Medicine Research.* Retrieved from http://bmccomplementalternmed.biomedcentral.com/articles/10.1186/1472-6882-11-129

[14] Takahashi, M., Sung, B., Shen, Y., Hur, K., Link, A., Boland, C.R., … Goel, A. (2012). Boswellic acid exerts antitumor effects in colorectal cancer cells by modulating expression of the let-7 and miR-200 microRNA family. *Carcinogenisis.* Retrieved from http://www.ncbi.nlm.nih.gov/pubmed/22983985

[15] Park, B., Prasad, S., Yadav, V., Sung, B., & Aggarawal, B. (2011). Boswellic Acid Suppresses Growth and Metastasis of Human Pancreatic Tumors in an Orthotopic Nude Mouse Model through Modulation of Multiple Targets. *PLOS One.* Retrieved from http://www.ncbi.nlm.nih.gov/pmc/articles/PMC3204996/

[16] Modzelewska, A., Sur, S., Kumar, S.K., & Khan, S.R. (September, 2005). Sesquiterpenes: natural products that decrease cancer growth. *Current Medicinal Chemistry. Anti-Cancer Agents.* Retrieved from http://www.ncbi.nlm.nih.gov/pubmed/16178774

[17] Cirić, A., Karioti, A., Koukoulitsa, C., Soković, M., & Skaltsa, H. (December, 2012). Sesquiterpene lactones from Centaurea zuccariniana and their antimicrobial activity. *Chemistry & Biodiversity, Volume 9*. Retrieved from http://onlinelibrary.wiley.com/doi/10.1002/cbdv.201100405/abstract

CHAPTER 5

[18] Koulivand, P.H., Khaleghi Ghadiri, M., & Gorji, A. (March, 2013). Lavender and the nervous system. *Evidence Based Complementary and Alternative Med*. Retrieved from http://www.ncbi.nlm.nih.gov/pmc/articles/PMC3612440/

PART II

[1] Fyfe, L., Armstrong, F., Stewart, J. (1997, January). Inhibition of Listeria monocytogenes and Salmonella enteriditis by combinations of plant oils and derivatives of benzoic acid: the development of synergistic antimicrobial combinations. *Int J Antimicrob Agents*. Retrieved from http://www.ncbi.nlm.nih.gov/pubmed/9552716

[2] Joshi, R.K. (2014, January). Chemical composition and antimicrobial activity of the essential oil of Ocimum basilicum L. (sweet basil) from Western Ghats of North West Karnataka, India. *Anc Sci Life*. Retrieved from http://www.ncbi.nlm.nih.gov/pmc/articles/PMC4264302/

[3] Kristinsson, K.G., Magnusdottir, A.B., Petersen, H., Hermansson, A. (2005, January 12). Effective Treatment of Experimental Acute Otitis Media by Application of Volatile Fluids into the Ear Canal. *Infectious Diseases Society of America*. Retrieved from http://jid.oxfordjournals.org/content/191/11/1876.full

[4] Hongratanaworakit, T. (2011, August). Aroma-therapeutic effects of massage blended essential oils on humans. *Nat Prod Commun*. Retrieved from http://www.ncbi.nlm.nih.gov/pubmed/21922934

[5] Bagetta, G., Morrone, L.A., Rombolà, L., Amantea, D., Russo, R., Berliocchi, L., Sakurada, S., Sakurada, T., Rotiroti, D., Corasaniti, M.T. (2010, September). Neuropharmacology of the essential oil of bergamot. *Fitoterapia*. Retrieved from http://www.ncbi.nlm.nih.gov/pubmed/20093169

[6] Russo, R., Cassiano, M.G.V., Ciociaro, A., Adornetto, A., Varano, G.P., Chiappini, C., Berliocchi, L., Tassorelli, C., Bagetta, G., Tiziana Corasaniti, M. (2014, November 24). Role of D-Limonene in Autophagy Induced by Bergamot Essential Oil in SH-SY5Y Neuroblastoma Cells. *PLoS One*. Retrieved from http://www.ncbi.nlm.nih.gov/pmc/articles/PMC4242674/

[7] (2011). Health Benefits of Bergamot Essential Oil. *Organic Facts*. Retrieved from https://www.organicfacts.net/health-benefits/essential-oils/health-benefits-of-bergamot-essential-oil.html

[8] Maruzzella, J., Sicurella, N. (2006, September). Antibacterial Activity of Essential Oil Vapors. *Journal of Pharmaceutical Sciences. Volume 49, Issue 11, Pages 692-694*. Retrieved from http://onlinelibrary.wiley.com/doi/10.1002/jps.3030491103/abstract

[9] Radentz, L.M. (1995, March 28). Birch Used To Shrink Melanoma In Mice. *New York Times*. Retrieved from http://www.nytimes.com/1995/03/28/science/birch-used-to-shrink-melanoma-in-mice.html, http://www.google.ch/patents/US20140170249

[10] Dehelean, C.A., Şoica, C., Ledeţi, I., Aluaş, M., Zupko, I., Găluşcan, A., Cinta-Pinzaru, S., Munteanu, M. (2012, November 19). Study of the betulin enriched birch bark extracts effects on human carcinoma cells and ear inflammation. *Chem Cent J*. Retrieved from http://www.ncbi.nlm.nih.gov/pmc/articles/PMC3527166/

[11] Rose, J.E., Behm, F.M. (1994, February). Inhalation of vapor from black pepper extract reduces smoking withdrawal symptoms. *Drug Alcohol Depend*. Retrieved from http://www.ncbi.nlm.nih.gov/pubmed/8033760

[12] Ou, M.C., Lee, Y.F., Li, C.C., Wu, S.K. (2014, October). The effectiveness of essential oils for patients with neck pain: a randomized controlled study. *J Altern Complement Med*. Retrieved from http://www.ncbi.nlm.nih.gov/pubmed/25192562

[13] McNamara, F.N., Randall, A., Gunthorpe, M.J. (2005, March). Effects of piperine, the pungent component of black pepper, at the human vanilloid receptor (TRPV1). *Br J Pharmacol*. Retrieved from http://www.ncbi.nlm.nih.gov/pmc/articles/PMC1576058/

[14] al-Zuhair, H., el-Sayeh. B., Ameen. H.A., al-Shoora, H. (1996, July). Pharmacological studies of cardamom oil in animals. *Pharmacol Res*. Retrieved from http://www.ncbi.nlm.nih.gov/pubmed/8981560

[15] Sharma, R. (2012, March). Cardamom comfort. Dent Res J (Isfahan). Retrieved from http://www.ncbi.nlm.nih.gov/pmc/articles/PMC3353705/

[16] Lee, J.J., Lee, J.H., Cho, W.K., Han, J.H., Ma, J.Y. (2016, July 28). Herbal composition of Cinnamomum cassia, Pinus densiflora, Curcuma longa and Glycyrrhiza glabra prevents atherosclerosis by upregulating p27 (Kip1) expression. *BMC Complement Altern Med*.

Retrieved from http://www.ncbi.nlm.nih.gov/pubmed/27465365

[17] Ooi, L.S., Li, Y., Kam, S.L., Wang, H., Wong, E.Y., Ooi, V.E. (2006). Antimicrobial activities of cinnamon oil and cinnamaldehyde from the Chinese medicinal herb Cinnamomum cassia Blume. *Am J Chin Med*. Retrieved from http://www.ncbi.nlm.nih.gov/pubmed/16710900

[18] Yao, Y., Huang, H.Y., Yang, Y.X., Guo, J.Y. (2015, March 13). Cinnamic aldehyde treatment alleviates chronic unexpected stress-induced depressive-like behaviors via targeting cyclooxygenase-2 in mid-aged rats. *J Ethnopharmacol*. Retrieved from http://www.ncbi.nlm.nih.gov/pubmed/25556926

[19] Chaudhari, L.K., Jawale, B.A., Sharma, S., Sharma, H., Kumar, C.D., Kulkarni, P.A. (2012, January 1). Antimicrobial activity of commercially available essential oils against Streptococcus mutans. *J Contemp Dent Pract*. Retrieved from http://www.ncbi.nlm.nih.gov/pubmed/22430697

[20] Friedmann, T.S. (2009). Attention Deficit and Hyperactivity Disorder (ADHD). *Int J Clin Aromather*. Retrieved from http://files.meetup.com/1481956/ADHD%20Research%20by%20Dr.%20Terry%20Friedmann.pdf

[21] Sreelatha, S., Inbavalli, R. (2012, July). Antioxidant, antihyperglycemic, and antihyperlipidemic effects of Coriandrum sativum leaf and stem in alloxan-induced diabetic rats. *J Food Sci*. Retrieved from http://www.ncbi.nlm.nih.gov/pubmed/22671941

[22] Omura, Y., Beckman, S.L. (1995, August). Role of mercury (Hg) in resistant infections & effective treatment of Chlamydia trachomatis and Herpes family viral infections (and potential treatment for cancer) by removing localized Hg deposits with Chinese parsley and delivering effective antibiotics using various drug uptake enhancement methods. *Acupunct Electrother Res*. Retrieved from http://www.ncbi.nlm.nih.gov/pubmed/8686573

[23] Chung, J.W., Kim, J.J., Kim, S.J. (2011, October). Antioxidative effects of cinnamomi cortex: A potential role of iNOS and COX-II. *Pharmacogn Mag*. Retrieved from http://www.ncbi.nlm.nih.gov/pmc/articles/PMC3261065/

[24] Al-Mariri, A., Saour, G., Hamou, R. (2012, June). In Vitro Antibacterial Effects of Five Volatile Oil Extracts Against Intramacrophage Brucella Abortus 544. *Iran J Med Sci*. Retrieved from http://www.ncbi.nlm.nih.gov/pmc/articles/PMC3470071/

[25] Choi, H.S., Song, H.S., Ukeda, H., Sawamura, M. (2000, September). Radical-scavenging activities of citrus essential oils and their components: detection using 1,1-diphenyl-2-picrylhydrazyl. *J Agric Food Chem*. Retrieved from http://www.ncbi.nlm.nih.gov/pubmed/10995330

[26] Kumaran, A.M., D'Souza, P., Agarwal, A., Bokkolla, R.M., Balasubramaniam, M. (2003). Geraniol, the putative anthelmintic principle of Cymbopogon martinii. *Phytother. Res.*, 17: 957. doi: 10.1002/ptr.1267.

[27] Burns, E., Blamey, C., Ersser, S.J., Lloyd, A.J., Barnetson, L. (2000, February). The use of aromatherapy in intrapartum midwifery practice an observational study. *Complement Ther Nurs Midwifery*. Retrieved from http://www.ncbi.nlm.nih.gov/pubmed/11033651

[28] Sienkiewicz, M., Głowacka, A., Poznańska-Kurowska, K., Kaszuba, A., Urbaniak, A., Kowalczyk, E. (2015, February 3). The effect of clary sage oil on staphylococci responsible for wound infections. *Postepy Dermatol Alergol*. Retrieved from http://www.ncbi.nlm.nih.gov/pmc/articles/PMC4360007/

[29] Fu, Y., Zu, Y., Chen, L., Shi, X., Wang, Z., Sun, S., Efferth, T. (2007, October). Antimicrobial activity of clove and rosemary essential oils alone and in combination. *Phytother Res*. Retrieved from http://www.ncbi.nlm.nih.gov/pubmed/17562569

[30] Marya, C.M., Satija, G., J.A., Nagpal, R., Kapoor, R., Ahmad, A. (2012). In vitro inhibitory effect of clove essential oil and its two active principles on tooth decalcification by apple juice. *Int J Dent*. Retrieved from http://www.ncbi.nlm.nih.gov/pubmed/22997520

[31] Freires Ide, A., Murata, R.M., Furletti, V.F., Sartoratto, A., Alencar, S.M., Figueira, G.M., de Oliveira Rodrigues, J.A., Duarte, M.C., Rosalen, P.L.. (2014, June). Coriandrum sativum L. (Coriander) essential oil: antifungal activity and mode of action on Candida spp., and molecular targets affected in human whole-genome expression. *PLoS One*. Retrieved from http://www.ncbi.nlm.nih.gov/pmc/articles/PMC4047076/

[32] Silva, F., Ferreira, S., Queiroz, J.A., Domingues, F.C. (2012, February). Coriander (Coriandrum sativum L.) essential oil: its antibacterial activity and mode of action evaluated by flow cytometry. *J Med Microbiol*. Retrieved from http://www.ncbi.nlm.nih.gov/pubmed/21862758

[33] Iacobellis, N.S., Lo Cantore, P., Capasso, F., Senatore, F. (2005, January). Antibacterial activity of Cuminum cyminum L. and Carum carvi L. essential oils. *J Agric Food Chem*. Retrieved from http://www.ncbi.nlm.nih.gov/pubmed/15631509

[34] Lee, H.S. (2005, April 6). Cuminaldehyde: Aldose Reductase and alpha-Glucosidase Inhibitor Derived from Cuminum cyminum L. Seeds. *J Agric*

Food Chem. Retrieved from http://www.ncbi.nlm.nih.gov/pubmed/15796577

[35] Alma, M.H., Nitz, S., Kollmannsberger, H., Digrak, M., Efe, F.T., Yilmaz, N. (2004, June). Chemical composition and antimicrobial activity of the essential oils from the gum of Turkish pistachio (Pistacia vera L.). *J Agric Food Chem.* Retrieved from http://www.ncbi.nlm.nih.gov/pubmed/15186116

[36] Ibrahim, N.A., El-Seedi, H.R., Mohammed, M.M. (2007, August). Phytochemical investigation and hepatoprotective activity of Cupressus sempervirens L. leaves growing in Egypt. **Nat Prod Res.** Retrieved from http://www.ncbi.nlm.nih.gov/pubmed/17680494

[37] Jun, Y.S., Kang, P., Min, S.S., Lee, J.M., Kim, H.K., Seol, G.H. (2013). Effect of eucalyptus oil inhalation on pain and inflammatory responses after total knee replacement: a randomized clinical trial. *Evid Based Complement Alternat Med.* Retrieved from http://www.ncbi.nlm.nih.gov/pubmed/23853660

[38] Sudhoff, H., Klenke, C., Greiner, J.F.W., Müller, J., Brotzmann, V., Ebmeyer, J., Kaltschmidt, B., Kaltschmidt, C. (2015). 1,8-Cineol Reduces Mucus-Production in a Novel Human Ex Vivo Model of Late Rhinosinusitis. *PLoS One.* Retrieved from http://www.ncbi.nlm.nih.gov/pmc/articles/PMC4514714/

[39] Alexandrovich, I., Rakovitskaya, O., Kolmo, E., Sidorova, T., Shushunov, S. (2003, July). The effect of fennel (Foeniculum Vulgare) seed oil emulsion in infantile colic: a randomized, placebo-controlled study. *Altern Ther Health Med.* Retrieved from http://www.ncbi.nlm.nih.gov/pubmed/12868253

[40] Mohamad, R.H., El-Bastawesy, A.M., Abdel-Monem, M.G., Noor, A.M., Al-Mehdar, H.A., Sharawy, S.M., El-Merzabani, M.M. (2011, September). Antioxidant and anticarcinogenic effects of methanolic extract and volatile oil of fennel seeds (Foeniculum vulgare). *J Med Food.* Retrieved from http://www.ncbi.nlm.nih.gov/pubmed/21812646

[41] Mahmoudi, Z., Soleimani, M., Saidi, A., Khamisipour, G., Azizsoltani, A. (2013). Effects of Foeniculum vulgare ethanol extract on osteogenesis in human mecenchymal stem cells. *Avicenna J Phytomed.* Retrieved from http://www.ncbi.nlm.nih.gov/pmc/articles/PMC4075705/

[42] Legault, J., Dahl, W., Debiton, E., Pichette, A., Madelmont, J.C. (2003, May). Antitumor activity of balsam fir oil: production of reactive oxygen species induced by alpha-humulene as possible mechanism of action. *Planta Med.* Retrieved from http://www.ncbi.nlm.nih.gov/pubmed/12802719

[43] Pichette, A., Larouche, P.L., Lebrun, M., Legault, J. (2006, May). Composition and antibacterial activity of Abies balsamea essential oil. *Phytother Res.* Retrieved from http://www.ncbi.nlm.nih.gov/pubmed/16619365

[44] Suhail, M.M., Wu, W., Cao, A., Mondalek, F.G., Fung, K.M., Shih, P.T., Fang, Y.T., Woolley, C., Young, G., Lin, H.K. (2011, December). Boswellia sacra essential oil induces tumor cell-specific apoptosis and suppresses tumor aggressiveness in cultured human breast cancer cells. *BMC Complement Altern Med.* Retrieved from http://www.ncbi.nlm.nih.gov/pubmed/22171782

[45] Khosravi Samani, M., Mahmoodian, H., Moghadamnia, A., Poorsattar Bejeh Mir, A., Chitsazan, M. (2011). The effect of Frankincense in the treatment of moderate plaque-induced gingivitis: a double blinded randomized clinical trial. *Daru.* Retrieved from http://www.ncbi.nlm.nih.gov/pubmed/22615671

[46] Maruyama, N., Takizawa, T., Ishibashi, H., Hisajima, T., Inouye, S., Yamaguchi, H., Abe, S. (2008, August). Protective activity of geranium oil and its component, geraniol, in combination with vaginal washing against vaginal candidiasis in mice. *Biol Pharm Bull.* Retrieved from http://www.ncbi.nlm.nih.gov/pubmed/18670079

[47] Reh, D.D., Hur, K., Merlo, C.A. (2013, April). Efficacy of a topical sesame/rose geranium oil compound in patients with hereditary hemorrhagic telangiectasia associated epistaxis. *Laryngoscope.* Retrieved from http://www.ncbi.nlm.nih.gov/pubmed/23401038

[48] Stea, S., Beraudi, A., De Pasquale, D. (2014). Essential oils for complementary treatment of surgical patients: state of the art. *Evid Based Complement Alternat Med.* Retrieved from http://www.ncbi.nlm.nih.gov/pmc/articles/PMC3953654/

[49] Jeena, K., Liju, V.B., Kuttan, R. (2013, January). Antioxidant, anti-inflammatory and antinociceptive activities of essential oil from ginger. *Indian J Physiol Pharmacol.* Retrieved from http://www.ncbi.nlm.nih.gov/pubmed/24020099

[50] Haze, S., Sakai, K., Gozu, Y. (2002, November). Effects of fragrance inhalation on sympathetic activity in normal adults. *Jpn J Pharmacol.* Retrieved from http://www.ncbi.nlm.nih.gov/pubmed/12499579

[51] Niijima, A., Nagai, K. (2003, November). Effect of olfactory stimulation with flavor of grapefruit oil and lemon oil on the activity of sympathetic branch in the white adipose tissue of the epididymis. *Exp Biol Med.* Retrieved from http://www.ncbi.nlm.nih.gov/pubmed/14610259

[52] Antunes Viegas, D., Palmeira-de-Oliveira, A., Salgueiro, L., Martinez-de-Oliveira, J., Palmeira-de-Oliveira, R. (2013). Helichrysum italicum: from traditional use to scientific data. *J Ethnopharmacol.* Retrieved from http://www.ncbi.nlm.nih.gov/pubmed/?term=Antunes%20Viegas%20D%5BAuthor%5D&cauthor=true&cauthor_uid=24239849

[53] Rigano, D., Formisano, C., Senatore, F., Piacente, S., Pagano, E., Capasso, R., Borrelli, F., Izzo, A.A. (2013, December). Intestinal antispasmodic effects of Helichrysum italicum (Roth) Don ssp. italicum and chemical identification of the active ingredients. *J Ethnopharmacol.* Retrieved from http://www.ncbi.nlm.nih.gov/pubmed/24140587

[54] Agrawal, P., Rai, V., Singh, R.B. (1996, September). Randomized placebo-controlled, single blind trial of holy basil leaves in patients with noninsulin-dependent diabetes mellitus. *Int J Clin Pharmacol Ther.* Retrieved from http://www.ncbi.nlm.nih.gov/pubmed/8880292/

[55] Yamani, H.A., Pang, E.C., Mantri, N., Deighton, M.A. (2016, May 17). Antimicrobial Activity of Tulsi (Ocimum tenuiflorum) Essential Oil and Their Major Constituents against Three Species of Bacteria. *Front Microbiol.* Retrieved from http://www.ncbi.nlm.nih.gov/pubmed/27242708

[56] Lu, M., Battinelli, L., Daniele, C., Melchioni, C., Salvatore, G., Mazzanti, G. (2002, March). Muscle relaxing activity of Hyssopus officinalis essential oil on isolated intestinal preparations. *Planta Med.* Retrieved from http://www.ncbi.nlm.nih.gov/pubmed/11914956

[57] Koch, C., Reichling, J., Schneele, J., Schnitzler, P. (2008, January). Inhibitory effect of essential oils against herpes simplex virus type 2. *Phytomedicine.* Retrieved from http://www.ncbi.nlm.nih.gov/pubmed/17976968

[58] Hongratanaworakit, T. (2010, January). Stimulating effect of aromatherapy massage with jasmine oil. *Nat Prod Commun.* Retrieved from http://www.ncbi.nlm.nih.gov/pubmed/?term=Hongratanaworakit%20T%5BAuthor%5D&cauthor=true&cauthor_uid=20184043

[59] Hur, M.H., Yang, Y.S., Lee, M.S. (2008, September). Aromatherapy massage affects menopausal symptoms in korean climacteric women: a pilot-controlled clinical trial. *Evid Based Complement Alternat Med.* Retrieved from http://www.ncbi.nlm.nih.gov/pmc/articles/PMC2529395/

[60] Filipowicz, N., Kamiński, M., Kurlenda, J., Asztemborska, M., Ochocka, J.R. (2003, March). Antibacterial and antifungal activity of juniper berry oil and its selected components. *Phytother Res.* Retrieved from http://www.ncbi.nlm.nih.gov/pubmed/12672151

[61] Yang, W.Z., Benchaar, C., Ametaj, B.N., Chaves, A.V., He, M.L., McAllister, T.A. (2007, December). Effects of garlic and juniper berry essential oils on ruminal fermentation and on the site and extent of digestion in lactating cows. *J Dairy Sci.* Retrieved from http://www.ncbi.nlm.nih.gov/pubmed/18024759

[62] Sebai, H., Selmi, S., Rtibi, K., Souli, A., Gharbi, N., Sakly, M. (2013, December 28). Lavender (Lavandula stoechas L.) essential oils attenuate hyperglycemia and protect against oxidative stress in alloxan-induced diabetic rats. *Lipids Health Dis.* Retrieved from http://www.ncbi.nlm.nih.gov/pmc/articles/PMC3880178/

[63] Hossein Koulivand, P., Khaleghi Ghadiri, M., Gorji, A. (2013). Lavender and the Nervous System. *Evid Based Complement Alternat Med.* Retrieved from http://www.ncbi.nlm.nih.gov/pmc/articles/PMC3612440/

[64] Uehleke, B., Schaper, S., Dienel, A., Schlaefke, S., Stange, R. (2012, June 15). Phase II trial on the effects of Silexan in patients with neurasthenia, post-traumatic stress disorder or somatization disorder. *Unbound MEDLINE.* Retrieved from http://www.unboundmedicine.com/medline/citation/22475718/Phase_II_trial_on_the_effects_of_Silexan_in_patients_with_neurasthenia_post_traumatic_stress_disorder_or_somatization_disorder_

[65] Yavari Kia, P., Safajou, F., Shahnazi, M., Nazemiyeh, H. (2014, March). The effect of lemon inhalation aromatherapy on nausea and vomiting of pregnancy: a double-blinded, randomized, controlled clinical trial. *Iran Red Crescent Med J.* Retrieved from http://www.ncbi.nlm.nih.gov/pubmed/24829772

[66] Komiya, M., Takeuchi, T., Harada, E. (2006, September). Lemon oil vapor causes an anti-stress effect via modulating the 5-HT and DA activities in mice. *Behav Brain Res.* Retrieved from http://www.ncbi.nlm.nih.gov/pubmed/16780969

[67] Adukwu, E.C., Allen, S.C., Phillips, C.A. (2012, November). The anti-biofilm activity of lemongrass (Cymbopogon flexuosus) and grapefruit (Citrus paradisi) essential oils against five strains of Staphylococcus aureus. *J Appl Microbiol.* Retrieved from http://www.ncbi.nlm.nih.gov/pubmed/22862808

[68] Silva Cde, B., Guterres, S.S., Weisheimer, V., Schapoval, E.E. (2008, February). Antifungal activity

of the lemongrass oil and citral against Candida spp. *Braz J Infect Dis*. Retrieved from http://www.ncbi.nlm.nih.gov/pubmed/18553017

[69] Asnaashari, S., Delazar, A., Habibi, B., Vasfi, R., Nahar, L., Hamedeyazdan, S. and Sarker, S. D. (2010), Essential Oil from Citrus aurantifolia prevents ketotifen-induced weight-gain in mice. *Phytother*. Res., 24: 1893–1897. doi: 10.1002/ptr.3227

[70] Prabuseenivasan, S., Jayakumar, M., & Ignacimuthu, S. (2006). In vitro antibacterial activity of some plant essential oils. *BMC Complementary and Alternative Medicine, 6, 39.* http://doi.org/10.1186/1472-6882-6-39

[71] Chen, C.C., Yan, S.H., Yen, M.Y., Wu, P.F., Liao, W.T., Huang, T.S., Wen, Z.H., David Wang, H.M. (2016, February). Investigations of kanuka and manuka essential oils for in vitro treatment of disease and cellular inflammation caused by infectious microorganisms. *J Microbiol Immunol Infect*. Retrieved from http://www.ncbi.nlm.nih.gov/pubmed/24582465

[72] Takarada, K., Kimizuka, R., Takahashi, N., Honma, K., Okuda, K., Kato, T. (2004, February). A comparison of the antibacterial efficacies of essential oils against oral pathogens. *Oral Microbiol Immunol*. Retrieved from http://www.ncbi.nlm.nih.gov/pubmed/14678476

[73] Takarada, K., Kimizuka, R., Takahashi, N., Honma, K., Okuda, K., Kato, T. (2004, February). A comparison of the antibacterial efficacies of essential oils against oral pathogens. *Oral Microbiol Immunol*. Retrieved from http://www.ncbi.nlm.nih.gov/pubmed/14678476

[74] Kim, M.J., Nam, E.S., Paik, S.I. (2005, February). The effects of aromatherapy on pain, depression, and life satisfaction of arthritis patients. *Taehan Kanho Hakhoe Chi*. Retrieved from http://www.ncbi.nlm.nih.gov/pubmed/15778570

[75] Ou, M.C., Lee, Y.F., Li, C.C., Wu, S.K. (2014, October). The effectiveness of essential oils for patients with neck pain: a randomized controlled study. *J Altern Complement Med*. Retrieved from http://www.ncbi.nlm.nih.gov/pubmed/25192562

[76] Enshaieh, S., Jooya, A., Siadat, A.H., Iraji, F. (2007, January). The efficacy of 5% topical tea tree oil gel in mild to moderate acne vulgaris: a randomized, double-blind placebo-controlled study. *Indian J Dermatol Venereol Leprol*. Retrieved from http://www.ncbi.nlm.nih.gov/pubmed/17314442

[77] Ramage, G., Milligan, S., Lappin, D.F., Sherry, L., Sweeney, M., Williams, C., Bagg, J., Culshaw, S. (2012, June 18). Antifungal, Cytotoxic, and Immunomodulatory Properties of Tea Tree Oil and Its Derivative Components: Potential Role in Management of Oral Candidosis in Cancer Patients. *Front Microbiol*. Retrieved from http://www.ncbi.nlm.nih.gov/pmc/articles/PMC3376416/

[78] de Sousa, A.C., Alviano, D.S., Blank, A.F., Alves, P.B., Alviano, C.S., Gattass, C.R. (2004, May). Melissa officinalis L. essential oil: antitumoral and antioxidant activities. *J Pharm Pharmacol*. Retrieved from http://www.ncbi.nlm.nih.gov/pubmed/15142347

[79] Jun, H.J., Lee, J.H., Jia, Y., Hoang, M.H., Byun, H., Kim, K.H., Lee, S.J. (2012, March). Melissa officinalis essential oil reduces plasma triglycerides in human apolipoprotein E2 transgenic mice by inhibiting sterol regulatory element-binding protein-1c-dependent fatty acid synthesis. *J Nutr*. Retrieved from http://jn.nutrition.org/content/142/3/432.long

[80] Chen, Y., Zhou, C., Ge, Z., Liu, Y., Liu, Y., Fend, W., Wei, T. 2013. Composition and potential anticancer activities of essential oils obtained from myrrh and frankincense. *Oncology Letters, 6(4), 1140–1146.* Retrieved from http://doi.org/10.3892/ol.2013.1520

[81] Haffor, A.S. (2010, March). Effect of myrrh (Commiphora molmol) on leukocyte levels before and during healing from gastric ulcer or skin injury. *J Immunotoxicol*. Retrieved from http://www.ncbi.nlm.nih.gov/pubmed/19995243

[82] Qiu, P., Dong, P., Guan, H., Li, S., Ho, C.-T., Pan, M.-H., McClements, D. J. and Xiao, H. (2010). Inhibitory effects of 5-hydroxy polymethoxyflavones on colon cancer cells. *Mol. Nutr. Food Res., 54: S244–S252.* doi: 10.1002/mnfr.200900605

[83] Igarashi, M., Ikei, H., Song, C., Miyazaki, Y. (2014, December). Effects of olfactory stimulation with rose and orange oil on prefrontal cortex activity. *Complement Ther Med*. Retrieved from http://www.ncbi.nlm.nih.gov/pubmed/25453523

[84] Sienkiewicz, M., Wasiela, M., Głowacka, A. (2012). The antibacterial activity of oregano essential oil (Origanum heracleoticum L.) against clinical strains of Escherichia coli and Pseudomonas aeruginosa. *Med Dosw Mikrobiol*. Retrieved from http://www.ncbi.nlm.nih.gov/pubmed/23484421

[85] Gilling, D.H., Kitajima, M., Torrey, J.R., Bright. K.R. (2014, May). Antiviral efficacy and mechanisms of action of oregano essential oil and its primary component carvacrol against murine norovirus. *J Appl Microbiol*. Retrieved from http://www.ncbi.nlm.nih.gov/pubmed/24779581

[86] Yang, X., Zhang, X., Yang, S.-P., & Liu, W.-Q. (2013). Evaluation of the Antibacterial Activity of Patchouli Oil. *Iranian Journal of Pharmaceutical Research : IJPR, 12(3), 307–316.*

[87] Jeong, J.B., Shin, Y.K., Lee, S.H. (2013, May). Anti-inflammatory activity of patchouli alcohol in RAW264.7 and HT-29 cells. *Food Chem Toxicol.* Retrieved from http://www.ncbi.nlm.nih.gov/pubmed/23348408

[88] Cappello, G., Spezzaferro, M., Grossi, L., Manzoli, L., Marzio, L. (2007, June). Peppermint oil (Mintoil) in the treatment of irritable bowel syndrome: a prospective double blind placebo-controlled randomized trial. *Dig Liver Dis.* Retrieved from http://www.ncbi.nlm.nih.gov/pubmed/17420159

[89] Göbel, H., Schmidt, G., Soyka, D. (1994, June). Effect of peppermint and eucalyptus oil preparations on neurophysiological and experimental algesimetric headache parameters. *Cephalalgia.* Retrieved from http://www.ncbi.nlm.nih.gov/pubmed/7954745

[90] Mossa,M., Howartha, R., Wilkinsona, L., Wesnesa, K. (2006, July 21). Expectancy and the aroma of Roman chamomile influence mood and cognition in healthy volunteers. *International Journal of Aromatherapy.* Retrieved from http://www.sciencedirect.com/science/article/pii/S0962456206000245

[91] Cho, M.Y., Min, E.S., Hur, M.H., Lee, M.S. (2013). Effects of Aromatherapy on the Anxiety, Vital Signs, and Sleep Quality of Percutaneous Coronary Intervention Patients in Intensive Care Units. *Evidence-Based Complementary and Alternative Medicine : eCAM, 2013, 381381.* Retrieved from http://doi.org/10.1155/2013/381381

[92] Hongratanaworakit, T. (2009, February). Relaxing effect of rose oil on humans. *Nat Prod Commun.* Retrieved from http://www.ncbi.nlm.nih.gov/pubmed/19370942

[93] Nazıroğlu, M., Kozlu, S., Yorgancıgil, E., Uğuz, A.C., Karakuş, K. (2013, January). Rose oil (from Rosa × damascena Mill.) vapor attenuates depression-induced oxidative toxicity in rat brain. *J Nat Med.* Retrieved from http://www.ncbi.nlm.nih.gov/pubmed/22484603

[94] Moss, M., Oliver, L. (2012). Plasma 1,8-cineole correlates with cognitive performance following exposure to rosemary essential oil aroma. *Therapeutic Advances in Psychopharmacology, 2(3), 103–113.* http://doi.org/10.1177/2045125312436573

[95] Luqman, S., Dwivedi, G.R., Darokar, M.P., Kalra. A., Khanuja, S.P. (2007, September). Potential of rosemary oil to be used in drug-resistant infections. *Altern Ther Health Med.* Retrieved from http://www.ncbi.nlm.nih.gov/pubmed/17900043

[96] Dwivedi, C., Zhang, Y. (1999, October). Sandalwood oil prevent skin tumour development in CD1 mice. *Eur J Cancer Prev.* Retrieved from http://www.ncbi.nlm.nih.gov/pubmed/10548401

[97] Santha, S., Dwivedi, C. (2015, June). Anticancer Effects of Sandalwood (Santalum album). *Anticancer Res.* Retrieved from http://www.ncbi.nlm.nih.gov/pubmed/26026073

[98] Takemoto, H., Ito, M., Shiraki, T., Yagura, T., Honda, G. (2008, January). Sedative effects of vapor inhalation of agarwood oil and spikenard extract and identification of their active components. *J Nat Med.* Retrieved from http://www.ncbi.nlm.nih.gov/pubmed/18404340

[99] Gottumukkala, V.R., Annamalai, T., Mukhopadhyay, T. (2011). Phytochemical investigation and hair growth studies on the rhizomes of Nardostachys jatamansi DC. *Pharmacognosy Magazine, 7(26), 146–150.* Retrieved from http://doi.org/10.4103/0973-1296.80674

[100] Sienkiewicz M, Łysakowska M, Ciećwierz J, Denys P, Kowalczyk E. (2011, November). Antibacterial activity of thyme and lavender essential oils. *Med Chem.* Retrieved from http://www.ncbi.nlm.nih.gov/pubmed/22313307

[101] Bukovská, A., Cikos, S., Juhás, S., Il'ková, G., Rehák, P., Koppel, J. (2007). Effects of a combination of thyme and oregano essential oils on TNBS-induced colitis in mice. *Mediators Inflamm.* Retrieved from http://www.ncbi.nlm.nih.gov/pmc/articles/PMC2233768/

[102] Higdon, J., Drake, V.J., Delage, B., Howells, L. (2005-2016). Curcumin. *Linus Pauling Institute.* Retrieved from http://lpi.oregonstate.edu/mic/dietary-factors/phytochemicals/curcumin#authors-reviewers

[103] Orellana-Paucar, A.M., Afrikanova, T., Thomas, J., Aibuldinov, Y.K., Dehaen, W., de Witte, P.A., Esguerra, C.V. (2013, December 13). Insights from zebrafish and mouse models on the activity and safety of ar-turmerone as a potential drug candidate for the treatment of epilepsy. *PLoS One.* Retrieved from http://www.ncbi.nlm.nih.gov/pubmed/24349101

[104] Friedmann, T.S. (2009). Attention Deficit and Hyperactivity Disorder (ADHD). *Int J Clin Aromather.* Retrieved from http://files.meetup.com/1481956/ADHD%20Research%20by%20Dr.%20Terry%20Friedmann.pdf

[105] Sinha, S., Jothiramajayam, M., Ghosh, M., Jana, A., Chatterji, U., Mukherjee, A. (2015, July). Vetiver oil (Java) attenuates cisplatin-induced oxidative stress, nephrotoxicity and myelosuppression in Swiss albino mice. *Food Chem Toxicol.* Retrieved from http://www.ncbi.nlm.nih.gov/pubmed/25910835

[106] Vergnes, S., Ladouce, N., Fournier, S., Ferhout, H., Attia, F., & Dumas, B. (2014). Foliar treatments with Gaultheria procumbens essential oil induce defense responses and resistance against a fungal pathogen in Arabidopsis. *Frontiers in Plant Science, 5, 477.* http://doi.org/10.3389/fpls.2014.00477

[107] Barbar, A., Raouf, M., Plakogiannis, F.M. (1990). In vitro release studies of methyl salicylate from the ointment bases and the commercial dermatological products. *Pharm Acta Helv.* Retrieved from http://www.ncbi.nlm.nih.gov/pubmed/2371308

[108] Hongratanaworakit, T., Buchbauer, G. (2006, September). Relaxing effect of ylang ylang oil on humans after transdermal absorption. *Phytother Res.* Retrieved from http://www.ncbi.nlm.nih.gov/pubmed/16807875

[109] Jung, D.J., Cha, J.Y., Kim, S.E., Ko, I.G., Jee, Y.S. (2013). Effects of Ylang-Ylang aroma on blood pressure and heart rate in healthy men. *Journal of Exercise Rehabilitation, 9(2), 250–255.* Retrieved from http://doi.org/10.12965/jer.130007

PART III

[1] Braden, R., Reichow, S., Halm, MA. (2009, December 24). The use of the essential oil lavandin to reduce preoperative anxiety in surgical patients. *Journal of PeriAnesthesia Nursing.* Retrieved from http://www.ncbi.nlm.nih.gov/pubmed/19962101

[2] Tournaire, M., Theau-Yonneau, A. (2007, December 4). Complementary and Alternative Approaches to Pain Relief During Labor. *Evid Based Complement Alternat Med.* Retrieved from http://www.ncbi.nlm.nih.gov/pmc/articles/PMC2176140/

[3] Willette, RC., Barrow, L., Doster, R, Wilkins, J., Wilkins, JS., Heggers, JP. Purified d-limonene: an effective agent for the relief of occasional symptoms of heartburn. Retrieved from a proprietary study, WRC Laboratories, Inc. Galveston, TX.

[4] Liju, V.B., Jenna, K. (2015, January 26). Gatroprotective Activity of Essential Oils from Turmeric and Ginger. *Pubmed, 24756059.* Retrieved from http://www.ncbi.nlm.nih.gov/pubmed/24756059

[5] Gavini, E., Sanna, V., Sharma, R., Juliano, C., Usai, M., Marchetti, M., Karlsen, J., Giunchedi, P. (2005). Solid lipid microparticles (SLM) containing juniper oil as anti-acne topical carriers: preliminary studies. *Pharm Dev Technol.* Retrieved from http://www.ncbi.nlm.nih.gov/pubmed/16370177

[6] Mori, HM., Kawanami, H., Kawahata, H., Aoki, M. (2016, May 26). Wound healing potential of lavender oil by acceleration of granulation and wound contraction through induction of TGF-ßin a rat model. *BMC Complement Altern Med.* Retrieved from http://www.ncbi.nlm.nih.gov/pubmed/27229681

[7] Enshaieh, S., Jooya, A., Siadat, AH., Iraji, F. (2007, February). The efficacy of 5% topical tea tree oil gel in mild to moderate acne vulgaris: a randomized, double-blind placebo-controlled study. *Indian J Dermatol Venereol Leprol.* Retrieved from http://www.ncbi.nlm.nih.gov/pubmed/17314442

[8] (2015) About ADHD. *CHADD.* According to the National Resource Center on ADHD. Retrieved from http://www.chadd.org/About-CHADD/National-Resource-Center.aspx

[9] Friedmann, T. Attention Deficit and Hyperactivity Disorder (ADHD). Retrieved from http://files.meetup.com/1481956/ADHD%20Research%20by%20Dr.%20Terry%20Friedmann.pdf

[10] Richardson, A., Montgomery, P. (2005, May). The Oxford-Durham Study: A Randomized, Controlled Trial of Dietary Supplementation With Fatty Acids in Children With Developmental Coordination Disorder. *Pediatrics, Volume 115, Issue 5.* Retrieved from http://pediatrics.aappublications.org/content/115/5/1360

[11] Pedram, P., Wadden, D., Amini, P., Gulliver, W., Randell, E., Cahill, F., Vasdev, S., Goodridge, A., Carter, J., Zhai, G., Ji, Y., Sun, G. (2014, September 4). Food Addiction: Its Prevalence and Significant Association with Obesity in the General Population. *PLoS ONE 8(9): e74832.* Retrieved from http://journals.plos.org/plosone/article/asset?id=10.1371/journal.pone.0074832.PDF

[12] Sayorwan, W., Siripornpanich, V., Piriyapunyaporn, T., Hongratanaworakit, T., Kotchabhakdi, N., Ruangrungsi, N. (2012, April) The effects of lavender oil inhalation on emotional states, autonomic nervous system, and brain electrical activity. *J Med Assoc Thai.* Retrieved from http://www.ncbi.nlm.nih.gov/pubmed/22612017

[13] Komiya, M., Takeuchi, T., Harada, E. (2006, September). Lemon oil vapor causes an anti-stress effect via modulating the 5-HT and DA activities in mice. *Behav Brain Res. Pubmed, 16780969.* Retrieved from http://www.ncbi.nlm.nih.gov/pubmed/16780969

[14] Blum, K., Ross, J., Reuben, C., Gastelu, D., Miller, DK. (2001, February). Nutritional Gene Therapy: Natural Healing in Recovery. *Counselor Magazine.* Retrieved from http://www.counselormagazine.com/

[15] Gholap, S., Kar, A. (2004). Hypoglycaemic effects of some plant extracts are possibly mediated through inhibition in corticosteroid concentration. *Pharmazie; 59(11):876-878*. Retrieved from http://www.ingentaconnect.com/contentone/govi/pharmaz/2004/00000059/00000011/art00014?crawler=true

[16] Hongratanaworakit, T. (2009, February 4). Relaxing effect of rose oil on humans. *Nat Prod Commun*. Retrieved by http://www.ncbi.nlm.nih.gov/pubmed/19370942

[17] Matsumoto, T., Nakamura, S., Nakashima, S., Fujimoto, K., Yoshikawa, M., Ohta, T., Ogawa, K., Matsuda, H. (2014, April 25) Lignan dicarboxylates and terpenoids from the flower buds of Cananga odorata and their inhibitory effects on melanogenesis. *J Nat Prod*. Retrieved from http://www.ncbi.nlm.nih.gov/pubmed/24601675

[18] Mikhaeil, B., Maatooq, G., Badria, F., Amer, M. (2002, November 4). Chemistry and Immunomodulatory Activity of Frankincense Oil. Department of Pharmacognosy, Faculty of Pharmacy, Mansoura University. Retrieved from http://www.znaturforsch.com/ac/v58c/s58c0230.pdf

[19] Glaser, G. (2002, December 17). Doctors Rethinking Treatments for Sick Sinuses. Wayne State University. Retrieved from http://www.nytimes.com/2002/12/17/health/doctors-rethinking-treatments-for-sick-sinuses.html?pagewanted=all

[20] Cingi, C., Conk-Dalay, M., Cakli, H., Bal, C. (2008, October). The effects of spirulina on allergic rhinitis. *Eur Arch Otorhinolaryngol*. Retrieved from http://www.ncbi.nlm.nih.gov/pubmed/18343939

[21] Moss, M., Cook, J., Wesnes, K., Duckett, P. (2003, January). Aromas of rosemary and lavender essential oils differentially affect cognition and mood in healthy adults. *Int J Neurosci*. Retrieved from http://www.ncbi.nlm.nih.gov/pubmed/12690999

[22] Jimbo D, Kimura Y, Taniguchi M, Inoue M, Urakami K. (2009, December). Effect of aromatherapy on patients with Alzheimer's disease. Psychogeriatrics. *Pubmed, 20377818*. Retrieved from http://www.ncbi.nlm.nih.gov/pubmed/20377818

[23] Kasper, S. (2013, November). An orally administered lavandula oil preparation (Silexan) for anxiety disorder and related conditions: an evidence based review. *Int J Psychiatry Clin Pract*. Retrieved from http://www.ncbi.nlm.nih.gov/pubmed/?term=International+Journal+of+Psychiatry+in+Clinical+Practice+lavender+anxiety

[24] Cooley, K., Szczurko, O., Perri, D., Mills, E.,

Bernhardt, B., Zhou, Q., Seely, D. (2009, August 31). Naturopathic Care for Anxiety: A Randomized Controlled Trial ISRCTN78958974. *PLoS One*. Retrieved from http://www.ncbi.nlm.nih.gov/pmc/articles/PMC2729375/

[25] Thomson, M., Al-Qattan, KK., Al-Sawan, SM., Alnaqeeb, MA., Khan, I., Ali, M. (2002 December). The use of ginger (Zingiber officinale Rosc.) as a potential anti-inflammatory and antithrombotic agent. *Prostaglandins Leukot Essent Fatty Acids*. Retreived by http://www.ncbi.nlm.nih.gov/pubmed/12468270

[26] Jeena K, Liju VB, Kuttan R. (2013, March). Antioxidant, anti-inflammatory and antinociceptive activities of essential oil from ginger. *Indian J Physiol Pharmacol. Pubmed, 24020099*. Retrieved from http://www.ncbi.nlm.nih.gov/pubmed/24020099

[27] Reed, GW., Leung, K., Rossetti, RG., Vanbuskirk, S., Sharp, JT., Zurier, RB. (2014, March 19). Treatment of rheumatoid arthritis with marine and botanical oils: an 18-month, randomized, and double-blind trial. *Evid Based Complement Alternat Med*. Retrieved by http://www.ncbi.nlm.nih.gov/pubmed/24803948

[28] Lee, HS., Park, DE., Song, WJ., Park, HW., Kang, HR., Cho, SH., Sohn, SW. (2016). Effect of 1,8-Cineole in Dermatophagoides pteronyssinus-Stimulated Bronchial Epithelial Cells and Mouse Model of Asthma. Biol Pharm Bull. Retrieved from http://www.ncbi.nlm.nih.gov/pubmed/27251496

[29] Gupta, K., Kumar, S., Gupta, RK., Sharma, A., Verma, AK., Stalin, K., Chaudhari, BP., Das, M., Singh, SP., Dwivedi, PD. (2016 April). Reversion of Asthmatic Complications and Mast Cell Signalling Pathways in BALB/c Mice Model Using Quercetin Nanocrystals. *J Biomed Nanotechnol*. Retrieved from http://www.ncbi.nlm.nih.gov/pubmed/27301198

[30] Li, WR., Li, HL., Shi, QS., Sun, TL., Xie, XB., Song, B., Huang, XM. (2016, July 7). The dynamics and mechanism of the antimicrobial activity of tea tree oil against bacteria and fungi. *Appl Microbiol Biotechnol*. Retrieved by http://www.ncbi.nlm.nih.gov/pubmed/27388769

[31] Moore-Neibel, K., Gerber, C., Patel, J., Friedman, M., Jaroni, D., Ravishankar, S. (2013 May). Antimicrobial activity of oregano oil against antibiotic-resistant Salmonella enterica on organic leafy greens at varying exposure times and storage temperatures. *Food Microbiol. Pubmed, 23498188*. Retrieved from http://www.ncbi.nlm.nih.gov/pubmed/23498188

[32] O'Connor, A. (2011, January 7). Remedies: Garlic

for Athlete's Foot. *NY Times*. Retrieved from http://well.blogs.nytimes.com/2011/01/06/remedies-garlic-for-athletes-foot/?_r=2

[33] Kokkiripati, PK., Bhakshu, LM., Marri, S., Padmasree, K., Row, AT., Raghavendra, AS., Tetali, SD. (2011, September 1). Gum resin of Boswellia serrata inhibited human monocytic (THP-1) cell activation and platelet aggregation. *J Ethnopharmacol*. Retrieved from http://www.ncbi.nlm.nih.gov/pubmed/?term=Frankincense+heart+blood

[34] Moss, M., Cook, J., Wesnes, K., Duckett, P. (2003, January). Aromas of rosemary and lavender essential oils differentially affect cognition and mood in healthy adults. *Int J Neurosci*. Retrieved from http://www.ncbi.nlm.nih.gov/pubmed/12690999

[35] Parletta, N., Niyonsenga, T., Duff, J. (2016, May 27). Omega-3 and Omega-6 Polyunsaturated Fatty Acid Levels and Correlations with Symptoms in Children with Attention Deficit Hyperactivity Disorder, Autistic Spectrum Disorder and Typically Developing Controls. *PLoS One*. Retrieved from http://www.ncbi.nlm.nih.gov/pubmed/27232999

[36] Karthivashan, G., Kura, AU., Arulselvan, P., Md Isa, N., Fakurazi, S. (2016, July 7). The modulatory effect of Moringa oleifera leaf extract on endogenous antioxidant systems and inflammatory markers in an acetaminophen-induced nephrotoxic mice model. *PeerJ*. Retrieved from http://www.ncbi.nlm.nih.gov/pubmed/27441110

[37] Barbar, A., Raouf, M., Plakogiannis, FM. (1990). In vitro release studies of methyl salicylate from the ointment bases and the commercial dermatological products. *Pharm Acta Helv*. Retrieved from http://www.ncbi.nlm.nih.gov/pubmed/2371308

[38] Lacy, B., Gabbard, S., Crowell, M. (2011, November). Pathophysiology, Evaluation, and Treatment of Bloating: Hope, Hype, or Hot Air? *Gastroenterol Hepatol (NY)*. Retrieved from http://www.ncbi.nlm.nih.gov/pmc/articles/PMC3264926/

[39] Yang, WZ., Benchaar, C., Ametaj, BN., Chaves, AV., He, ML., McAllister, TA. (2007, December). Effects of garlic and juniper berry essential oils on ruminal fermentation and on the site and extent of digestion in lactating cows. *J Dairy Sci*. Retrieved from http://www.ncbi.nlm.nih.gov/pubmed/18024759

[40] Glynn, S. (2013, January 18). Two Percent Of People Have Armpits That Never Smell. Medical News Today. Retrieved from http://www.medicalnewstoday.com/articles/255147.php

[41] Carson, C.F., Hammer, K.A., Riley, T.V. (2006, January). Melaleuca alternifolia (Tea Tree) Oil: a Review of Antimicrobial and Other Medicinal Properties. *Clin Microbiol Rev*. Retrieved from http://www.ncbi.nlm.nih.gov/pmc/articles/PMC1360273/

[42] Ben-Arye, E., Dudai, N., Eini, A., Torem, M., Schiff, E., Rakover, Y. (2010, November 1). Treatment of Upper Respiratory Tract Infections in Primary Care: A Randomized Study Using Aromatic Herbs. *Evid Based Complement Alternat Med*. Retrieved from http://www.ncbi.nlm.nih.gov/pmc/articles/PMC2967840/

[43] Worth, H., Schacher, C., Dethlefsen, U. (2009, July 22). Concomitant therapy with Cineole (Eucalyptole) reduces exacerbations in COPD: A placebo-controlled double-blind trial. *Respir Res*. Retrieved from http://www.ncbi.nlm.nih.gov/pmc/articles/PMC2720945/

[44] Selim, S., Adam, M., Hassan, S., Albalawi, A. (2014, June 2). Chemical composition, antimicrobial and antibiofilm activity of the essential oil and methanol extract of the Mediterranean cypress (Cupressus sempervirens L.). *BMC Complement Altern Med*. Retrieved from http://www.ncbi.nlm.nih.gov/pmc/articles/PMC4052795/

[45] Mori, HM., Kawanami, H., Kawahata, H., Aoki, M. (2016, May 26). Wound healing potential of lavender oil by acceleration of granulation and wound contraction through induction of TGF-ß in a rat model. *BMC Complement Altern Med*. Retrieved from http://www.ncbi.nlm.nih.gov/pubmed/27229681

[46] Pattanayak, P., Behera, P., Das, D., Panda, S.K. (2010, June). Ocimum sanctum Linn. A reservoir plant for therapeutic applications: An overview. *Pharmacogn Rev*. Retrieved from http://www.ncbi.nlm.nih.gov/pmc/articles/PMC3249909/

[47] Misni, N., Nor, ZM., Ahmad, R. (2016, June). New Candidates for Plant-Based Repellents Against Aedes aegypti. *J Am Mosq Control Assoc*. Retrieved from http://www.ncbi.nlm.nih.gov/pubmed/27280349

[48] Cox, E. (2009, July 13). HEALTH: Treating burns with essential oils. *The Mayo News*. Retrieved from http://www.mayonews.ie/component/content/article?id=7130:health-treating-burns-with-essential-oils

[49] Zhou, J., Ma, XM., Qiu, BH., Chen, JX., Bian, L., Pan, LM. (2013, January). Parameters optimization of supercritical fluid-CO_2 extracts of frankincense using response surface methodology and its pharmacodynamics effects. *J Sep Sci*. Retrieved from http://www.ncbi.nlm.nih.gov/pubmed/23255314

50 Flores, FC., De Lima, JA., Da Silva, CR., Benvegnú, D., Ferreira, J., Burger, ME., Beck, RC., Rolim, CM., Rocha, MI., Da Veiga, ML., Da Silva, B. (2015, January). Hydrogels Containing Nanocapsules and Nanoemulsions of Tea Tree Oil Provide Antiedematogenic Effect and Improved Skin Wound Healing. *J Nanosci Nanotechnol.* Retrieved from http://www.ncbi.nlm.nih.gov/pubmed/26328444

51 Ni, X., Suhail, MM., Yang, Q., Cao, A., Fung, KM., Postier, RG., Woolley, C., Young, G., Zhang, J., Lin, HK. (2012, December 13). Frankincense essential oil prepared from hydrodistillation of Boswellia sacra gum resins induces human pancreatic cancer cell death in cultures and in a xenograft murine model. *BMC Complement Altern Med.* Retrieved from http://www.ncbi.nlm.nih.gov/pubmed/23237355

52 Yeo, SK., Ali, AY., Hayward, OA., Turnham, D., Jackson, T., Bowen, ID., Clarkson, R. (2016, March). ß-Bisabolene, a Sesquiterpene from the Essential Oil Extract of Opoponax (Commiphora guidottii), Exhibits Cytotoxicity in Breast Cancer Cell Lines. *Phytother Res.* Retrieved from http://www.ncbi.nlm.nih.gov/pubmed/26666387

53 Miller, JA., Pappan, K., Thompson, PA., Want, EJ., Siskos, AP., Keun, HC., Wulff, J., Hu, C., Lang, JE., Chow, HH. (2015, January). Plasma metabolomic profiles of breast cancer patients after short-term limonene intervention. Cancer Prev Res (Phila). Retrieved from http://www.ncbi.nlm.nih.gov/pubmed/25388013

54 Park, SY., Kim, YH., Kim, Y., Lee, SJ. (2012, December). Aromatic-turmerone attenuates invasion and expression of MMP-9 and COX-2 through inhibition of NF-κB activation in TPA-induced breast cancer cells. *J Cell Biochem.* Retrieved from http://www.ncbi.nlm.nih.gov/pubmed/22740037

55 Aratanechemuge, Y., Komiya, T., Moteki, H., Katsuzaki, H., Imai, K., Hibasami, H. (2002, May). Selective induction of apoptosis by ar-turmerone isolated from turmeric (Curcuma longa L) in two human leukemia cell lines, but not in human stomach cancer cell line. *Int J Mol Med.* Retrieved from http://www.ncbi.nlm.nih.gov/pubmed/11956652

56 Murakami, A., Furukawa, I., Miyamoto, S., Tanaka, T., Ohigashi, H. (2013, April). Curcumin combined with turmerones, essential oil components of turmeric, abolishes inflammation-associated mouse colon carcinogenesis. *Biofactors.* Retrieved from http://www.ncbi.nlm.nih.gov/pubmed/23233214

57 Mansourian, A., Boojarpour, N., Ashnagar, S., Momen Beitollahi, J., Shamshiri, AR. (2014, December). The comparative study of antifungal activity of Syzygium aromaticum, Punica granatum and nystatin on Candida albicans; an in vitro study. *J Mycol Med.* Retrieved from http://www.ncbi.nlm.nih.gov/pubmed/25442923

58 Mitropoulou, G., Fitsiou, E., Stavropoulou, E., Papavassilopoulou, E., Vamvakias, M., Pappa, A., Oreopoulou, A., Kourkoutas, Y. (2015, May 6). Composition, antimicrobial, antioxidant, and antiproliferative activity of Origanum dictamnus (dittany) essential oil. *Microb Ecol Health Dis.* Retrieved from http://www.ncbi.nlm.nih.gov/pubmed/?term=Mitropoulou%20G%5BAuthor%5D&cauthor=true&cauthor_uid=25952773

59 Al-Mariri, A., Safi, M. (2014, January). In Vitro Antibacterial Activity of Several Plant Extracts and Oils against Some Gram-Negative Bacteria. *Iran J Med Sci.* Retrieved from http://www.ncbi.nlm.nih.gov/pubmed/24453392

60 Chami, N., Bennis, S., Chami, F., Aboussekhra, A., Remmal, A. (2005, April). Study of anticandidal activity of carvacrol and eugenol in vitro and in vivo. *Oral Microbiol Immunol.* Retrieved from http://www.ncbi.nlm.nih.gov/pubmed/?term=Oral+Microbiology+%26+Immunology+nystatin+clove

61 Li, XJ., Yang, YJ., Li, YS., Zhang, WK., Tang, HB. (2016, February 17). a-Pinene, linalool, and 1-octanol contribute to the topical anti-inflammatory and analgesic activities of frankincense by inhibiting COX-2. *J Ethnopharmacol.* Retrieved from http://www.ncbi.nlm.nih.gov/pubmed/26721216

62 Majumder, J., Yedoti, P., Dastidar, P. (2015, February 28). A supramolecular topical gel derived from a non-steroidal anti-inflammatory drug, fenoprofen, is capable of treating skin inflammation in mice. *Org Biomol Chem.* Retrieved from http://www.ncbi.nlm.nih.gov/pubmed/25554116

63 Kazemian, H., Ghafourian, S., Heidari, H., Amiri, P., Yamchi, JK., Shavalipour, A., Houri, H., Maleki, A., Sadeghifard, N. (2015, August). Antibacterial, anti-swarming and anti-biofilm formation activities of Chamaemelum nobile against Pseudomonas aeruginosa. *Rev Soc Bras Med Trop.* Retrieved from http://www.ncbi.nlm.nih.gov/pubmed/26312934

64 Mori, HM., Kawanami, H., Kawahata, H., Aoki, M. (2016, May 26). Wound healing potential of lavender oil by acceleration of granulation and wound contraction through induction of TGF-ß in a rat model. *BMC Complement Altern Med.* Retrieved from http://www.ncbi.nlm.nih.gov/pubmed/27229681

65 Shah, G., Shri, R., Panchal, V., Sharma, N., Singh, B., Mann, A.S. (2011, March). Scientific basis for the

therapeutic use of Cymbopogon citratus, stapf (Lemon grass). *J Adv Pharm Technol Res.* Retrieved from http://www.ncbi.nlm.nih.gov/pmc/articles/PMC3217679/

66 Rabiei, Z., Rafieian-Kopaei, M., Mokhtari, S., Shahrani, M. (2014). Effect of Dietary Ethanolic Extract of Lavandula officinalis on Serum Lipids Profile in Rats. *Iran J Pharm Res.* Retrieved from http://www.ncbi.nlm.nih.gov/pmc/articles/PMC4232795/

67 Lee, IS., Lee, GJ. (2006, February). Effects of lavender aromatherapy on insomnia and depression in women college students. *Taehan Kanho Hakhoe Chi.* Retrieved from http://www.ncbi.nlm.nih.gov/pubmed/?term=college+students+sleep+insomnia+lavender

68 Cox, IM., Campbell, MJ., Dowson, D. (1991, March 30). Red blood cell magnesium and chronic fatigue syndrome. *Lancet.* Retrieved from http://www.ncbi.nlm.nih.gov/pubmed/1672392

69 Wang, X., Yin, J. (2015, May 3). Complementary and Alternative Therapies for Chronic Constipation. *Evid Based Complement Alternat Med.* Retrieved from http://www.ncbi.nlm.nih.gov/pmc/articles/PMC4433664/

70 Roberts, RE., Allen, S., Chang, AP., Henderson, H., Hobson, GC., Karania, B., Morgan, KN., Pek, AS., Raghvani, K., Shee, CY., Shikotra, J., Street, E., Abbas, Z., Ellis, K., Heer, JK., Alexander,SP. (2013, November 1). Distinct mechanisms of relaxation to bioactive components from chamomile species in porcine isolated blood vessels. *Toxicol Appl Pharmacol.* Retrieved from http://www.ncbi.nlm.nih.gov/pubmed/23845591

71 Alexandrovich, I., Rakovitskaya, O., Kolmo, E., Sidorova, T., Shushunov, S. (2003, August). The effect of fennel (Foeniculum Vulgare) seed oil emulsion in infantile colic: a randomized, placebo-controlled study. *Altern Ther Health Med.* Retrieved from http://www.ncbi.nlm.nih.gov/pubmed/?term=fennel+seed+oil+motility

72 (2016). Upper Respiratory Infection (URI or Common Cold). *Hopkins Medicine.* Retrieved from http://www.hopkinsmedicine.org/healthlibrary/conditions/pediatrics/upper_respiratory_infection_uri_or_common_cold_90,P02966/

73 Gill, TA., Li, J., Saenger, M., Scofield, SR. (2016, June 2). Thymol-based submicron emulsions exhibit antifungal activity against Fusarium graminearum and inhibit Fusarium head blight in wheat. *J Appl Microbiol.* Retrieved from http://www.ncbi.nlm.nih.gov/pubmed/27253757

74 Hamada, M., Uezu, K., Matsushita, J., Yamamoto, S., Kishino, Y. (2002, April). Distribution and immune responses resulting from oral administration of D-limonene in rats. *J Nutr Sci Vitaminol (Tokyo).* Retrieved from http://www.ncbi.nlm.nih.gov/pubmed/12171437

75 Lissiman, E., Bhasale, AL., Cohen, M. (2014, November 11). Garlic for the common cold. *Cochrane Database Syst Rev.* Retrieved from http://www.ncbi.nlm.nih.gov/pubmed/25386977

76 Pallarito, K. (2009, June 28). Constipation May Lead to Other Problems. *U.S. News.* Retrieved from http://health.usnews.com/health-news/family-health/brain-and-behavior/articles/2009/06/28/constipation-may-lead-to-other-problems

77 Hu, M.L., Rayner, C., Wu, K.L., Chuah, S.K., Tai, W.C., Chou, Y.P., Chiu, Y.C., Chiu, K.W., Hu, T.H. (2011, January 7). Effect of ginger on gastric motility and symptoms of functional dyspepsia. *World J Gastroenterol.* Retrieved from http://www.ncbi.nlm.nih.gov/pmc/articles/PMC3016669/

78 Cappello, G., Spezzaferro, M., Grossi, L., Manzoli, L., Marzio, L. (2007, June). Peppermint oil (Mintoil) in the treatment of irritable bowel syndrome: a prospective double blind placebo-controlled randomized trial. *Dig Liver Dis.* Retrieved from http://www.ncbi.nlm.nih.gov/pubmed/17420159

79 hMulyaningsih, S., Sporer, F., Reichling, J., Wink, M. (2011, September). Antibacterial activity of essential oils from Eucalyptus and of selected components against multidrug-resistant bacterial pathogens. *Pharm Biol.* Retrieved from http://www.ncbi.nlm.nih.gov/pubmed/21591991

80 Plevkova, J., Kollarik, M., Poliacek, I., Brozmanova, M., Surdenikova, L., Tatar, M., Mori, N., Canning, BJ. (2013, July 15). The role of trigeminal nasal TRPM8-expressing afferent neurons in the antitussive effects of menthol. *J Appl Physiol (1985).* Retrieved from http://www.ncbi.nlm.nih.gov/pubmed/23640596

81 Béjaoui, A., Chaabane, H., Jemli, M., Boulila, A., Boussaid, M. (2013, December 1). Essential Oil Composition and Antibacterial Activity of Origanum vulgare subsp. glandulosum Desf. at Different Phenological Stages. *J Med Food.* Retrieved from http://www.ncbi.nlm.nih.gov/pmc/articles/PMC3868303/

82 Bento, A.F., Marcon, R., Dutra, R.C., Claudino, R.F., Cola, M., Pereira Leite, D.F., Calixto, J.B. (2011, March). ß-Caryophyllene Inhibits Dextran Sulfate Sodium-Induced Colitis in Mice through CB2 Receptor Activation and PPARy Pathway. *Am J Pathol.* Retrieved from http://www.ncbi.nlm.nih.gov/pmc/articles/PMC3070571/

[83] Vyas, K.S., Vasconez, H.C. (2014, September). Wound Healing: Biologics, Skin Substitutes, Biomembranes and Scaffolds. *Healthcare (Basel)*. Retrieved from http://www.ncbi.nlm.nih.gov/pmc/articles/PMC4934597/

[84] Rasooli, I., Shayegh, S., Taghizadeh, M., Alipoor Astaneh, S.D. (2008, September). Peppermint and rosemary extract are superior to the chemical chlorhexidine in preventing dental biofilm formation. *Phytother Res*. Retrieved from http://www.greenmedinfo.com/article/peppermint-and-rosemary-extract-are-superior-chemical-chlorhexidine-preventing-dental

[85] Alqareer, A., Alyahya, A., Andersson, L. (2006, November). The effect of clove and benzocaine versus placebo as topical anesthetics. *J Dent*. Retrieved from http://www.ncbi.nlm.nih.gov/pubmed/16530911

[86] Hongratanaworakit, T. (2011, August). Aroma-therapeutic effects of massage blended essential oils on humans. *Nat Prod Commun*. Retrieved from http://www.ncbi.nlm.nih.gov/pubmed/21922934

[87] Conrad, P., Adams, C. (2012, August). The effects of clinical aromatherapy for anxiety and depression in the high risk postpartum woman - a pilot study. *Complement Ther Clin Pract*. Retrieved from http://www.ncbi.nlm.nih.gov/pubmed/22789792

[88] Kirkham, S., Akilen, R., Sharma, S., Tsiami, A. (2009, December). The potential of cinnamon to reduce blood glucose levels in patients with type 2 diabetes and insulin resistance. *Diabetes Obes Metab*. Retrieved from http://www.ncbi.nlm.nih.gov/pubmed/19930003

[89] Anderson, R.A., Cheng, N., Bryden, N.A., Polansky, M.M., Cheng, N., Chi, J., Feng, J. (1997, November). Elevated intakes of supplemental chromium improve glucose and insulin variables in individuals with type 2 diabetes. *Diabetes*. Retrieved from http://www.ncbi.nlm.nih.gov/pubmed/9356027

[90] Ehrlich, S. (2015, August 5). Omega-3 fatty acids. A.D.A.M., Inc. Retrieved from http://umm.edu/health/medical/altmed/supplement/omega3-fatty-acids#ixzz3n4Eutf00

[91] Liju, VB., Jeena, K., Kuttan, R. (2015, January). Gastroprotective activity of essential oils from turmeric and ginger. *J Basic Clin Physiol Pharmacol*. Retrieved from http://www.ncbi.nlm.nih.gov/pubmed/24756059

[92] Cappello, G., Spezzaferro, M., Grossi, L., Manzoli, L., Marzio, L. (2007, June). Peppermint oil (Mintoil) in the treatment of irritable bowel syndrome: a prospective double blind placebo-controlled randomized trial. *Dig Liver Dis*. Retrieved from http://www.ncbi.nlm.nih.gov/pubmed/17420159

[93] Li, XJ., Yang, YJ., Li, YS., Zhang, WK., Tang, HB. (2016, February 17). a-Pinene, linalool, and 1-octanol contribute to the topical anti-inflammatory and analgesic activities of frankincense by inhibiting COX-2. *J Ethnopharmacol*. Retrieved from http://www.ncbi.nlm.nih.gov/pubmed/26721216

[94] Kristinsson, KG., Magnusdottir, AB., Petersen, H., Hermansson, A. (2005, June 1). Effective treatment of experimental acute otitis media by application of volatile fluids into the ear canal. *J Infect Dis*. Retrieved from http://www.ncbi.nlm.nih.gov/pubmed/15871121

[95] Hanifin, JM., Reed, ML., Eczema Prevalence and Impact Working Group. (2007, June). A population-based survey of eczema prevalence in the United States. *Dermatitis*. Retrieved from http://www.ncbi.nlm.nih.gov/pubmed/17498413

[96] Kobayashi, Y., Sato, H., Yorita, M., Nakayama, H., Miyazato, H., Sugimoto, K., Jippo, T. (2016, June). Inhibitory effects of geranium essential oil and its major component, citronellol, on degranulation and cytokine production by mast cells. *Biosci Biotechnol Biochem*. Retrieved from http://www.ncbi.nlm.nih.gov/pubmed/26927807

[97] Haffor, AS. (2010, March). Effect of myrrh (Commiphora molmol) on leukocyte levels before and during healing from gastric ulcer or skin injury. *J Immunotoxicol*. Retrieved from http://www.ncbi.nlm.nih.gov/pubmed/19995243

[98] Whitney, TR., Lee, AE., Klein, DR., Scott, CB., Craig, TM., Muir, JP. (2011, March 10). A modified in vitro larvae migration inhibition assay using rumen fluid to evaluate Haemonchus contortus viability. *Vet Parasitol*. Retrieved from http://www.ncbi.nlm.nih.gov/pubmed/21109354

[99] Silva, GL., Luft, C., Lunardelli, A., Amaral, RH., Melo, DA., Donadio, MV., Nunes, FB., de Azambuja, MS., Santana, JC., Moraes, CM., Mello, RO., Cassel, E., Pereira, MA., de Oliveira, JR. (2015, August). Antioxidant, analgesic and anti-inflammatory effects of lavender essential oil. *An Acad Bras Cienc*. Retrieved from http://www.ncbi.nlm.nih.gov/pubmed/26247152

[100] (2011). Health Benefits of Patchouli Essential Oil. *Organic Facts*. Retrieved from https://www.organicfacts.net/health-benefits/essential-oils/health-benefits-of-patchouli-essential-oil.html

[101] Hongratanaworakit, T. (2010, January). Stimulating effect of aromatherapy massage with jasmine oil. *Nat Prod Commun*. Retrieved from http://www.ncbi.nlm.nih.

gov/pubmed/?term=Hongratanaworakit%20 T%5BAuthor%5D&cauthor=true&cauthor_ uid=20184043

[102] Al-Harrasi, A., Ali, L., Hussain, J., Rehman, NU., Mehjabeen, Ahmed, M., Al-Rawahi, A. (2014, September). Analgesic effects of crude extracts and fractions of Omani frankincense obtained from traditional medicinal plant Boswellia sacra on animal models. *Asian Pac J Trop Med*. Retrieved from http://www.ncbi.nlm.nih.gov/pubmed/?term=frankincense+essential+oil+pain+muscle

[103] Chandola, HC., Chakraborty, A. (2009, October). Fibromyalgia and myofascial pain syndrome-a dilemma. *Indian J Anaesth*. Retrieved from http://www.ncbi.nlm.nih.gov/pmc/articles/ PMC2900090/#CIT21

[104] Schnitzler, P., Schön, K., Reichling, J. (2001, April). Antiviral activity of Australian tea tree oil and eucalyptus oil against herpes simplex virus in cell culture. *Pharmazie*. Retrieved from http://www.ncbi.nlm.nih.gov/pubmed/11338678

[105] (2012). Health Benefits of Thyme Essential Oil. *Organic Facts*. Retrieved from https://www.organicfacts.net/health-benefits/essential-oils/thyme-essential-oil.html

[106] Garozzo, A., Timpanaro, R., Bisignano, B., Furneri, PM., Bisignano, G., Castro A. (2009, December). In vitro antiviral activity of Melaleuca alternifolia essential oil. *Lett Appl Microbiol*. Retrieved from http://www.ncbi.nlm.nih.gov/pubmed/19843207

[107] Zamani-Zadeh, M., Soleimanian-Zad, S., Sheikh-Zeinoddin, M. (2013, October). Biocontrol of gray mold disease on strawberry fruit by integration of Lactobacillus plantarum A7 with ajwain and cinnamon essential oils. *J Food Sci*. Retrieved from http://www.ncbi.nlm.nih.gov/pubmed/24024787

[108] Marya, C., Satija, G., Avinash, J., Nagpal, R., Kapoor, R., Ahmad, A. (2011, December 4). In Vitro Inhibitory Effect of Clove Essential Oil and Its Two Active Principles on Tooth Decalcification by Apple Juice. *Charu M. Marya et al*. Retrieved from http://www.hindawi.com/journals/ijd/2012/759618/

[109] (2012). Health Benefits of Clary Sage Essential Oil. *Organic Facts*. Retrieved from https://www.organicfacts.net/health-benefits/essential-oils/health-benefits-of-clary-sage-essential-oil.html

[110] Ehrlich, S. (2015, January 2). Lavender. *A.D.A.M., Inc*. Retrieved from http://umm.edu/health/medical/altmed/herb/lavender

[111] Göbel, H., Fresenius, J., Heinze, A., Dworschak, M., Soyka, D. (1996, August). Effectiveness of Oleum menthae piperitae and paracetamol in therapy of headache of the tension type. *Nervenarzt*. Retrieved from http://www.ncbi.nlm.nih.gov/pubmed/8805113

[112] Sasannejad, P., Saeedi, M., Shoeibi, A., Gorji, A., Abbasi, M., Foroughipour, M. (2012). Lavender essential oil in the treatment of migraine headache: a placebo-controlled clinical trial. *Eur Neurol*. Retrieved from http://www.ncbi.nlm.nih.gov/pubmed/22517298

[113] Assarzadegan, F., Asgarzadeh, S., Hatamabadi, HR., Shahrami, A., Tabatabaey, A., Asgarzadeh, M. (2016, September). Serum concentration of magnesium as an independent risk factor in migraine attacks: a matched case-control study and review of the literature. *Int Clin Psychopharmacol*. Retrieved from http://www.ncbi.nlm.nih.gov/pubmed/27140442

[114] Ernst, E., Pittler, MH. (2000, December). The efficacy and safety of feverfew (Tanacetum parthenium L.): an update of a systematic review. *Public Health Nutr*. Retrieved from http://www.ncbi.nlm.nih.gov/pubmed/11276299

[115] Ehrlich, S. (2014, July 6). Peppermint. *A.D.A.M., Inc*. Retrieved from http://umm.edu/health/medical/altmed/herb/peppermint

[116] Liju, VB., Jeena, K., Kuttan, R. (2015). Gatroprotective Activity of Essential Oils from Turmeric and Ginger. J Basic Clin Physiol *Pharmacol*. Retrieved from http://www.ncbi.nlm.nih.gov/pubmed/24756059

[117] (2011). Health Benefits of Helichrysum Essential Oil. Organic Facts. Retrieved from https://www.organicfacts.net/health-benefits/essential-oils/health-benefits-of-helichrysum-essential-oil.html

[118] Carson, C.F., Hammer, K.A., Riley, T.V. (2006, January). Melaleuca alternifolia (Tea Tree) Oil: a Review of Antimicrobial and Other Medicinal Properties. *Clin Microbiol Rev*. Retrieved from http://www.ncbi.nlm.nih.gov/pmc/articles/ PMC1360273/

[119] Schnitzler, P., Koch, C., Reichling, J. (2007, March 12). Susceptibility of Drug-Resistant Clinical Herpes Simplex Virus Type 1 Strains to Essential Oils of Ginger, Thyme, Hyssop, and Sandalwood. *Antimicrob Agents Chemother*. Retrieved from http://www.ncbi.nlm.nih.gov/pmc/articles/ PMC1855548/

[120] Lindeman, Z., Waggoner, M., Batdorff, A., Humphreys, T.L. (2014, May 27). Assessing the antibiotic potential of essential oils against Haemophilus ducreyi. *BMC Complement Altern Med*. Retrieved from http://www.ncbi.nlm.nih.gov/pubmed/24885682

[121] (2014). Health Benefits of Frankincense Essential Oil. *Organic Facts*. Retrieved from https://www.organicfacts.net/health-benefits/essential-oils/health-benefits-of-frankincense-essential-oil.html

[122] Seol, G.H., Lee, Y.H., Kang, P., You, J.H., Park, M., Min, S.S. (2013, July). Randomized Controlled Trial for Salvia sclarea or Lavandula angustifolia: Differential Effects on Blood Pressure in Female Patients with Urinary Incontinence Undergoing Urodynamic Examination. *J Altern Complement Med*. Retrieved from http://www.ncbi.nlm.nih.gov/pmc/articles/PMC3700459/

[123] Shah, G., Shri, R., Panchal, V., Sharma, N., Singh, B., Mann, A.S. (2011, March). Scientific basis for the therapeutic use of Cymbopogon citratus, stapf (Lemon grass). *J Adv Pharm Technol Res*. Retrieved from http://www.ncbi.nlm.nih.gov/pmc/articles/PMC3217679/

[124] Nangia-Makker, P., Tait, L., Hogan, V., Shekhar, M.P.V., Funasaka, T., Raz, A. (2007, August 15). Inhibition of breast tumor growth and angiogenesis by a medicinal herb: Ocimum sanctum. *Int J Cancer*. Retrieved from http://www.ncbi.nlm.nih.gov/pmc/articles/PMC3613994/

[125] Gannon, J.M., Forrest, P.E., Roy Chengappa, K.N. (2014, October). Subtle changes in thyroid indices during a placebo-controlled study of an extract of Withania somnifera in persons with bipolar disorder. *J Ayurveda Integr Med*. Retrieved from http://www.ncbi.nlm.nih.gov/pubmed/25624699

[126] Jaber, R. (2002, June). Respiratory and allergic diseases: from upper respiratory tract infections to asthma. *Prim Care*. Retrieved from http://www.ncbi.nlm.nih.gov/pubmed/?term=frankincense+essential+oil+blood+cell

[127] Faramarzi, S., Bozorgmehrifard, M.H., Khaki, A., Moomivand, H., Saeid Ezati, M., Rasoulinezhad, S., Bahnamiri, A.J., Dizaji, B.R. (2013). *Annals of Biological Research*. Retrieved from http://scholarsresearchlibrary.com/ABR-vol4-iss6/ABR-2013-4-6-290-294.pdf

[128] Béjaoui, A., Chaabane, H., Jemli, M., Boulila, A., Boussaid, M. (2013, December 1). Essential Oil Composition and Antibacterial Activity of Origanum vulgare subsp. glandulosum Desf. at Different Phenological Stages. *J Med Food*. Retrieved from http://www.ncbi.nlm.nih.gov/pmc/articles/PMC3868303/

[129] Bento, A.F., Marcon, R., Dutra, R.C., Claudino, R.F., Cola, M., Pereira Leite, D.F., Calixto, J.B. (2011, March). ß-Caryophyllene Inhibits Dextran Sulfate Sodium-Induced Colitis in Mice through CB2 Receptor Activation and PPARγ Pathway. *Am J Pathol*. Retrieved from http://www.ncbi.nlm.nih.gov/pmc/articles/PMC3070571/

[130] Chaudhari, L.K., Jawale, B.A., Sharma, S., Sharma, H., Kumar, C.D., Kulkarni, P.A. (2012, January 1). Antimicrobial activity of commercially available essential oils against Streptococcus mutans. *J Contemp Dent Pract*. Retrieved from http://www.ncbi.nlm.nih.gov/pubmed/22430697

[131] Miller, S.C. (2005, September). Echinacea: a Miracle Herb against Aging and Cancer? Evidence In vivo in Mice. *Evid Based Complement Alternat Med*. Retrieved from http://www.ncbi.nlm.nih.gov/pmc/articles/PMC1193558/

[132] Basch, E., Ulbricht, C., Hammerness, P., Bevins, A., Sollars, D. (2004, February). Thyme (Thymus vulgaris L.), Thymol. *Journal of Herbal Pharmacotherapy*. Retrieved from https://www.researchgate.net/publication/8436790_Thyme_Thymus_vulgaris_L_Thymol

[133] Zava, D.T., Dollbaum, C.M., Blen, M. (1998, March). Estrogen and progestin bioactivity of foods, herbs, and spices. *Proc Soc Exp Biol Med*. Retrieved from http://www.ncbi.nlm.nih.gov/pubmed/9492350

[134] Jalili, C., Salahshoor, M.R., Naseri, A. (2014, June). Protective effect of Urtica dioica L against nicotine-induced damage on sperm parameters, testosterone and testis tissue in mice. *Iran J Reprod Med*. Retrieved from http://www.ncbi.nlm.nih.gov/pubmed/?term=Stinging+Nettles+infertility

[135] Edwards, T. (2005, November). Inflammation, pain, and chronic disease: an integrative approach to treatment and prevention. *Altern Ther Health Med*. Retrieved from http://www.ncbi.nlm.nih.gov/pubmed/16320856

[136] Siddiqui, M.Z. (2011, May). Boswellia serrata, a potential antiinflammatory agent: an overview. Indian J Pharm Sci. Retrieved from http://www.ncbi.nlm.nih.gov/pubmed/22457547

[137] Amsterdam, J.D., Shults, J., Soeller, I., Mao, J.J., Rockwell, K., Newberg, A.B. (2012, September). Chamomile (Matricaria recutita) may provide antidepressant activity in anxious, depressed humans: an exploratory study. *Altern Ther Health Med*. Retrieved from http://www.ncbi.nlm.nih.gov/pubmed/22894890

[138] Kuźma, Ł., Kalemba, D., Różalski, M., Różalska, B., Więckowska-Szakiel, M., Krajewska, U., Wysokińska, H. (2009, February 29). Chemical Composition and Biological Activities of Essential Oil from Salvia sclarea Plants Regenerated in vitro. *Molecules*. Retrieved from http://www.mdpi.com/1420-3049/14/4/1438

[139] Srivastava, J.K., Shankar, E., Gupta, S. (2010,

November 1). Chamomile: A herbal medicine of the past with bright future. *Mol Med Report*. Retrieved from http://www.ncbi.nlm.nih.gov/pmc/articles/PMC2995283/

[140] Liju, VB., Jeena, K., Kuttan, R. (2015, January). Gastroprotective activity of essential oils from turmeric and ginger. *J Basic Clin Physiol Pharmacol*. Retrieved from http://www.ncbi.nlm.nih.gov/pubmed/24756059

[141] Cappello, G., Spezzaferro, M., Grossi, L., Manzoli, L., Marzio, L. (2007, June). Peppermint oil (Mintoil) in the treatment of irritable bowel syndrome: a prospective double blind placebo-controlled randomized trial. *Dig Liver Dis*. Retrieved from http://www.ncbi.nlm.nih.gov/pubmed/17420159

[142] Doheny, K. (2016, July 15). Gut Bacteria May Hold Clues to Chronic Fatigue, Intestinal colonies differ in CFS patients, study finds, bolstering notion the disorder isn't a psychological problem. *HealthDay Reporter*. Retrieved from http://www.webmd.com/chronic-fatigue-syndrome/news/20160715/gut-bacteria-may-hold-clues-to-chronic-fatigue-syndrome

[143] Bartolozzi, E. (2015, May). The natural approach to osteoporosis. *Clin Cases Miner Bone Metab*. Retrieved from http://www.ncbi.nlm.nih.gov/pmc/articles/PMC4625766/

[144] Csoti, I., Jost, W.H., Reichmann, H. (2015, August 23). Parkinson's disease between internal medicine and neurology. *J Neural Transm (Vienna)*. Retrieved from http://www.ncbi.nlm.nih.gov/pmc/articles/PMC4713462/

[145] Taneja, V. (2014, May 27). Arthritis susceptibility and the Gut Microbiome. *FEBS Lett*. Retrieved from http://www.ncbi.nlm.nih.gov/pmc/articles/PMC4246018/

[146] Liu, JH., Chen, G.H., Yeh, H.Z., Huang, C.K., Poon, S.K. (1997, December). Enteric-coated peppermint-oil capsules in the treatment of irritable bowel syndrome: a prospective, randomized trial. *J Gastroenterol*. Retrieved from http://www.ncbi.nlm.nih.gov/pubmed/9430014

[147] Thapa, D., Louis, P., Losa, R., Zweifel, B., Wallace, R.J. (2015, February). Essential oils have different effects on human pathogenic and commensal bacteria in mixed faecal fermentations compared with pure cultures. *Microbiology*. Retrieved from http://www.ncbi.nlm.nih.gov/pubmed/25500493

[148] Kothavade, P.S., Nagmoti, D.M., Bulani, V.D., Juvekar, A.R. (2013, October 1). Arzanol, a potent mPGES-1 inhibitor: novel anti-inflammatory agent. *ScientificWorldJournal*. Retrieved from http://www.ncbi.nlm.nih.gov/pubmed/?term=Helichrysum+autoimmune

[149] Siddiqui, M.Z. (2011, May). Boswellia serrata, a potential antiinflammatory agent: an overview. *Indian J Pharm Sci*. Retrieved from http://www.ncbi.nlm.nih.gov/pubmed/22457547

[150] (2013, August 19). CDC provides estimate of Americans diagnosed with Lyme disease each year. *Centers for Disease Control and Prevention*. Retrieved from http://www.cdc.gov/media/releases/2013/p0819-lyme-disease.html

[151] De Mello, V., Prata, M.C., Da Silva, M.R., Daemon, E., Da Silva, L.S., Guimarães Fdel, G., De Mendonça, A.E., Folly, E., Vilela, F.M., Do Amaral, L.H., Cabral, L.M., Do Amaral Mda, P. (2014, December). Acaricidal properties of the formulations based on essential oils from Cymbopogon winterianus and Syzygium aromaticum plants. *Parasitol Res*. Retrieved from http://www.ncbi.nlm.nih.gov/pubmed/25199555

[152] Zava, D.T., Dollbaum, C.M., Blen, M. (1998, March). Estrogen and progestin bioactivity of foods, herbs, and spices. *Proc Soc Exp Biol Med*. Retrieved from http://www.ncbi.nlm.nih.gov/pubmed/9492350

[153] Lee, K.B., Cho, E., Kang, Y.S. (2014, November). Changes in 5-hydroxytryptamine and cortisol plasma levels in menopausal women after inhalation of clary sage oil. *Phytother Res*. Retrieved from http://www.ncbi.nlm.nih.gov/pubmed/24802524

[154] Shams, T., Setia, M.S., Hemmings, R., McCusker, J., Sewitch, M., Ciampi, A. (2010, January). Efficacy of black cohosh-containing preparations on menopausal symptoms: a meta-analysis. *Altern Ther Health Med*. Retrieved from http://www.ncbi.nlm.nih.gov/pubmed/20085176

[155] Matić, I.Z., Aljančić, I., Žižak, Ž., Vajs, V., Jadranin, M., Milosavljević, S., Juranić, Z.D. (2013, February 18). In vitro antitumor actions of extracts from endemic plant Helichrysum zivojinii. *BMC Complement Altern Med*. Retrieved from http://www.ncbi.nlm.nih.gov/pubmed/?term=helichrysum+immune

[156] Li, Y., Lv, O., Zhou, F., Li, Q., Wu, Z., Zheng, Y. (2015, July). Linalool Inhibits LPS-Induced Inflammation in BV2 Microglia Cells by Activating Nrf2. *Neurochem Res*. Retrieved from http://www.ncbi.nlm.nih.gov/pubmed/26040565

[157] Sosaa, S., Altiniera, G., Politib, M., Bracab, A., Morellib, I., Della Loggiaa, R. (2004, February 2). Extracts and constituents of Lavandula multifida with topical anti-inflammatory activity. *Phytomedicine*. Retrieved from http://www.sciencedirect.com/science/article/pii/S0944711304001412

[158] Chandola, HC., Chakraborty, A. (2009, October).

Fibromyalgia and myofascial pain syndrome-a dilemma. *Indian J Anaesth.* Retrieved from http://www.ncbi.nlm.nih.gov/pmc/articles/PMC2900090/#CIT21

[159] Pillai, A.K., Sharma, K.K., Gupta, Y.K., Bakhshi, S. (2011, February). Anti-emetic effect of ginger powder versus placebo as an add-on therapy in children and young adults receiving high emetogenic chemotherapy. *Pediatr Blood Cancer.* Retrieved from http://www.ncbi.nlm.nih.gov/pubmed/20842754

[160] Prakash, P., Gupta, N. (2005, April). Therapeutic uses of Ocimum sanctum Linn (Tulsi) with a note on eugenol and its pharmacological actions: a short review. *Indian J Physiol Pharmacol.* Retrieved from http://www.ncbi.nlm.nih.gov/pubmed/16170979

[161] Tayarani-Najaran, Z., Talasaz-Firoozi, E., Nasiri, R., Jalali, N., Hassanzadeh, M.K. (2013). Antiemetic activity of volatile oil from Mentha spicata and Mentha × piperita in chemotherapy-induced nausea and vomiting. *ecancer.* Retrieved from http://ecancer.org/journal/7/290-antiemetic-activity-of-volatile-oil-from-mentha-spicata-and-mentha-piperita-in-chemotherapy-induced-nausea-and-vomiting.php

[162] Barbar, A., Raouf, M., Plakogiannis, FM. (1990). In vitro release studies of methyl salicylate from the ointment bases and the commercial dermatological products. Pharm Acta Helv. Retrieved from http://www.ncbi.nlm.nih.gov/pubmed/2371308

[163] Ou, M.C., Lee, Y.F., Li, C.C., Wu, S.K. (2014, October). The effectiveness of essential oils for patients with neck pain: a randomized controlled study. J Altern Complement Med. Retrieved from http://www.ncbi.nlm.nih.gov/pubmed/25192562

[164] Ibrahim, N.A., El-Seedi, H.R., Mohammed, M.M. (2007, August). Phytochemical investigation and hepatoprotective activity of Cupressus sempervirens L. leaves growing in Egypt. *Nat Prod Res.* Retrieved from http://www.ncbi.nlm.nih.gov/pubmed/17680494

[165] Lee Chung, J., Snajberk, K., Zavarin, E. (1973, April 30). Chemical composition of the cortical essential oil from Abies balsamea. *Phytochemistry.* Retrieved from http://www.sciencedirect.com/science/article/pii/S0031942200912901

[166] Durzan, D.J. (2009, February 2). Arginine, scurvy and Cartier's "tree of life". *J Ethnobiol Ethnomed.* Retrieved from http://www.ncbi.nlm.nih.gov/pmc/articles/PMC2647905/

[167] Nikolova, G., Karamalakova, Y., Kovacheva, N.,

Stanev, S., Zheleva, A., Gadjeva, V. (2016, July 2). Protective effect of two essential oils isolated from Rosa damascena Mill. and Lavandula angustifolia Mill. and two classic antioxidants against L-dopa oxidative toxicity induced in healthy mice. *Regul Toxicol Pharmacol.* Retrieved from http://www.ncbi.nlm.nih.gov/pubmed/27381452

[168] Sala, A., Recio, M., Giner, R.M., Máñez, S., Tournier, H., Schinella, G., Ríos, J.L. (2002, March). Anti-inflammatory and antioxidant properties of Helichrysum italicum. *J Pharm Pharmacol.* Retrieved from http://www.ncbi.nlm.nih.gov/pubmed/11902802

[169] Saiyudthong, S., Pongmayteegul, S., Marsden, C.A., Phansuwan-Pujito, P. (2015). Anxiety-like behaviour and c-fos expression in rats that inhaled vetiver essential oil. *Nat Prod Res.* Retrieved from http://www.ncbi.nlm.nih.gov/pubmed/25553641

[170] Saper, R., Boah, A., Eisenberg, D. (2012, May 15). Scientific Abstracts Presented at the International Research Congress on Integrative Medicine and Health 2012. *Volume 12, Supplement 1. Bio Med Central.* Retrieved from http://bmccomplementalternmed.biomedcentral.com/articles/supplements/volume-12-supplement-1

[171] Atsumi, T., Tonosaki, K. (2007, February 28). Smelling lavender and rosemary increases free radical scavenging activity and decreases cortisol level in saliva. *Psychiatry Res.* Retrieved from http://www.ncbi.nlm.nih.gov/pubmed/17291597

[172] American Society for Biochemistry and Molecular Biology. (2010, January 14). Thyme oil can inhibit COX2 and suppress inflammation. *ScienceDaily.* Retrieved from https://www.sciencedaily.com/releases/2010/01/100113122306.htm

[173] Aprahamian, M., Dentinger, A., Stock-Damgé, C., Kouassi, J.C., Grenier, J.F. (1985, March). Effects of supplemental pantothenic acid on wound healing: experimental study in rabbit. *Am J Clin Nutr.* Retrieved from http://www.ncbi.nlm.nih.gov/pubmed/3976557

[174] Society for General Microbiology. (2010, April 4). Essential oils to fight superbugs. *ScienceDaily.* Retrieved from https://www.sciencedaily.com/releases/2010/03/100330210942.htm

[175] Krishnan, T., Yin, W.F., Chan, K.G. (2012, March 27). Inhibition of Quorum Sensing-Controlled Virulence Factor Production in Pseudomonas aeruginosa PAO1 by Ayurveda Spice Clove (Syzygium Aromaticum) Bud Extract. *Sensors (Basel).* Retrieved from http://www.ncbi.nlm.nih.gov/pmc/articles/PMC3355396/

[176] (2012). Health Benefits of Clary Sage Essential Oil. *Organic Facts*. Retrieved from https://www.organicfacts.net/health-benefits/essential-oils/health-benefits-of-clary-sage-essential-oil.html

[177] Lee, K.B., Cho, E., Kang, Y.S. (2014, November). Changes in 5-hydroxytryptamine and cortisol plasma levels in menopausal women after inhalation of clary sage oil. *Phytother Res*. Retrieved from http://www.ncbi.nlm.nih.gov/pubmed/24802524

[178] Pattanayak, P., Behera, P., Das, D., Panda, S.K. (2010, June). Ocimum sanctum Linn. A reservoir plant for therapeutic applications: An overview. *Pharmacogn Rev*. Retrieved from http://www.ncbi.nlm.nih.gov/pmc/articles/PMC3249909/

[179] Hur, M.H., Lee, M.S., Seong, K.Y., Lee, M.K. (2012). Aromatherapy massage on the abdomen for alleviating menstrual pain in high school girls: a preliminary controlled clinical study. *Evid Based Complement Alternat Med*. Retrieved from http://www.ncbi.nlm.nih.gov/pubmed/21949670

[180] Türk, G., Çeribaşı, A.O., Şimşek. Ü.G., Çeribaşı,S., Güvenç, M., Özer Kaya, Ş., Çiftçi, M., Sönmez, M., Yüce, A., Bayrakdar, A., Yaman, M., Tonbak, F. (2016, January). Dietary rosemary oil alleviates heat stress-induced structural and functional damage through lipid peroxidation in the testes of growing Japanese quail. *Anim Reprod Sci*. Retrieved from http://www.ncbi.nlm.nih.gov/pubmed/26656503

[181] Thosar, N., Basak, S., Bahadure, R.N., Rajurkar, M. (2013, September). Antimicrobial efficacy of five essential oils against oral pathogens: An in vitro study. *Eur J Dent*. Retrieved from http://www.ncbi.nlm.nih.gov/pmc/articles/PMC4054083/

[182] Ali, B., Al-Wabel, N.A., Shams, S., Ahamad, A., Khan, S.A., Anwar, F. (2015, May 15). Essential oils used in aromatherapy: A systemic review. *Asian Pacific Journal of Tropical Biomedicine*. Retrieved from http://www.sciencedirect.com/science/article/pii/S2221169115001033

[183] Jiang, L., Liu, Y., He, P., Chen, J., Liu, S., Tan, N. (2016, August). Geraniin ameliorates cisplatin-induced nephrotoxicity in mice. *Free Radic Res*. Retrieved from http://www.ncbi.nlm.nih.gov/pubmed/27043748

[184] Wedler, J., Rusanov, K., Atanassov, I., Butterweck, V. (2016, July). A Polyphenol-Enriched Fraction of Rose Oil Distillation Wastewater Inhibits Cell Proliferation, Migration and TNF-a-Induced VEGF Secretion in Human Immortalized Keratinocytes. *Planta Med*. Retrieved from http://www.ncbi.nlm.nih.gov/pubmed/27093251

[185] Koca Kutlu, A., Ceçen, D., Gürgen, S.G., Sayın. O., Cetin, F. (2013). A Comparison Study of Growth Factor Expression following Treatment with Transcutaneous Electrical Nerve Stimulation, Saline Solution, Povidone-Iodine, and Lavender Oil in Wounds Healing. *Evid Based Complement Alternat Med*. Retrieved from http://www.ncbi.nlm.nih.gov/pubmed/23861704

[186] Sala, A., Recio, M., Giner, R.M., Máñez, S., Tournier, H., Schinella, G., Ríos, J.L. (2002, March). Anti-inflammatory and antioxidant properties of Helichrysum italicum. *J Pharm Pharmacol*. Retrieved from http://www.ncbi.nlm.nih.gov/pubmed/11902802

[187] Wei, N.N., Lv. H.N., Wu, Y., Yang, S.L., Sun, X.Y., Lai, R., Jiang, Y., Wang, K. (2016, Janurary 8). Selective Activation of Nociceptor TRPV1 Channel and Reversal of Inflammatory Pain in Mice by a Novel Coumarin Derivative Muralatin L from Murraya alata. *J Biol Chem*. Retrieved from http://www.ncbi.nlm.nih.gov/pubmed/26515068

[188] Silva, M.R., Paiva, T. (2016, September). Poor precompetitive sleep habits, nutrients' deficiencies, inappropriate body composition and athletic performance in elite gymnasts. *Eur J Sport Sci*. Retrieved from http://www.ncbi.nlm.nih.gov/pubmed/26505326

[189] Jarmuda, S., O'Reilly, N., Zaba, R., Jakubowicz, O., Szkaradkiewicz, A., Kavanagh, K. (2012, November). Potential role of Demodex mites and bacteria in the induction of rosacea. *J Med Microbiol*. Retrieved from http://www.ncbi.nlm.nih.gov/pubmed/22933353

[190] Kasprowicz, S. (2015, August 11). Tea tree oil: What can it do for your patients? *Dermatology Times*. Retrieved from http://dermatologytimes.modernmedicine.com/dermatology-times/news/tea-tree-oil-what-can-it-do-your-patients

[191] Tighe, S., Gao, Y.Y., Tseng, S.C.G. (2013, November). Terpinen-4-ol is the Most Active Ingredient of Tea Tree Oil to Kill Demodex Mites. *Transl Vis Sci Technol*. Retrieved from http://www.ncbi.nlm.nih.gov/pmc/articles/PMC3860352/

[192] Minaiyan, M., Ghassemi-Dehkordi, N., Mahzouni, P., Ahmadi, N.S. (2014, February 28). Anti-inflammatory effect of Helichrysum oligocephalum DC extract on acetic acid - Induced acute colitis in rats. *Adv Biomed Res*. Retrieved from http://www.ncbi.nlm.nih.gov/pubmed/24761395

[193] Pilau, M.R., Alves, S.H., Weiblen, R., Arenhart, S., Cueto, A.P., Lovato, L.T. (2011, October). Antiviral activity of the Lippia graveolens (Mexican oregano) essential oil and its main compound carvacrol against human and animal viruses. *Braz J*

Microbiol. Retrieved from http://www.ncbi.nlm.nih.gov/pubmed/24031796?log$=activity

194 Williamson, I.G., Rumsby, K., Benge, S., Moore, M., Smith, P.W., Cross, M., Little, P. (2007, Devember 5). Antibiotics and Topical Nasal Steroid for Treatment of Acute Maxillary Sinusitis. *The Journal of the American Medical Association.* Retrieved from http://jama.jamanetwork.com/article.aspx?articleid=209649

195 Hotta, M., Nakata, R., Katsukawa, M., Hori, K., Takahashi, S., Inoue, H. (2010, January). Carvacrol, a component of thyme oil, activates PPARalpha and gamma and suppresses COX-2 expression. *J Lipid Res.* Retrieved from http://www.ncbi.nlm.nih.gov/pubmed/19578162

196 Hosseinkhani, F., Jabalameli, F., Banar, M., Abdellahi, N., Taherikalani, M., Leeuwen, W.B., Emaneini, M. (2016, April). Monoterpene isolated from the essential oil of Trachyspermum ammi is cytotoxic to multidrug-resistant Pseudomonas aeruginosa and Staphylococcus aureus strains. *Rev Soc Bras Med Trop.* Retrieved from http://www.ncbi.nlm.nih.gov/pubmed/27192585

197 Badet, C., Furiga, A., Thébaud, N. (2008). Effect of xylitol on an in vitro model of oral biofilm. *Oral Health Prev Dent.* Retrieved from http://www.ncbi.nlm.nih.gov/pubmed/19178100

198 Ben-Arye, E., Dudai, N., Eini, A., Torem, M., Schiff, E., Rakover, Y. (2010, November 1). Treatment of Upper Respiratory Tract Infections in Primary Care: A Randomized Study Using Aromatic Herbs. *Evid Based Complement Alternat Med.* Retrieved from http://www.ncbi.nlm.nih.gov/pmc/articles/PMC2967840/

199 Scandorieiro, S., De Camargo, L.C., Lancheros, C.A.C., Yamada-Ogatta, S.F., Nakamura, C.V., De Oliveira, A.G., Andrade, C.G.T.J., Duran, N., Nakazato, G., Kobayashi, R.K.T. (2016, May 23). Synergistic and Additive Effect of Oregano Essential Oil and Biological Silver Nanoparticles against Multidrug-Resistant Bacterial Strains. *Front Microbiol.* Retrieved from http://www.ncbi.nlm.nih.gov/pmc/articles/PMC4876125/

200 Dagli, N., Dagli, R., Mahmoud, R.S., Baroudi, K. (2015, September). Essential oils, their therapeutic properties, and implication in dentistry: A review. *J Int Soc Prev Community Dent.* Retrieved from http://www.ncbi.nlm.nih.gov/pubmed/26539382

201 Alqareer, A., Alyahya, A., Andersson, L. (2006, November). The effect of clove and benzocaine versus placebo as topical anesthetics. *J Dent.* Retrieved from http://www.ncbi.nlm.nih.gov/pubmed/16530911

202 (2014). Health Benefits of Frankincense Essential Oil. *Organic Facts.* Retrieved from https://www.organicfacts.net/health-benefits/essential-oils/health-benefits-of-frankincense-essential-oil.html

203 Kamatou, G.P., Vermaak, I., Viljoen, A.M., Lawrence, B.M. (2013, December). Menthol: a simple monoterpene with remarkable biological properties. *Phytochemistry.* Retrieved from http://www.ncbi.nlm.nih.gov/pubmed/24054028

204 Selimoğlu Şen, H., Şen, V., Bozkurt, M., Türkçü, G., Güzel, A., Sezgi, C., Abakay, O., Kaplan, I. (2014, October 19). Carvacrol and Pomegranate Extract in Treating Methotrexate-Induced Lung Oxidative Injury in Rats. *Med Sci Monit.* Retrieved from http://www.ncbi.nlm.nih.gov/pmc/articles/PMC4211419/

205 Li, WR., Li, HL., Shi, QS., Sun, TL., Xie, XB., Song, B., Huang, XM. (2016, July 7). The dynamics and mechanism of the antimicrobial activity of tea tree oil against bacteria and fungi. *Appl Microbiol Biotechnol.* Retrieved by http://www.ncbi.nlm.nih.gov/pubmed/27388769

206 Thompson, A., Meah, D., Ahmed, N., Conniff-Jenkins, R., Chileshe, E., O Phillips, C., Claypole, T.C., Forman, D.W., Row, P.E. (2013, November 28). Comparison of the antibacterial activity of essential oils and extracts of medicinal and culinary herbs to investigate potential new treatments for irritable bowel syndrome. *BMC Complement Altern Med.* Retrieved from http://www.ncbi.nlm.nih.gov/pmc/articles/PMC4220539/

207 Ribeiro, A.R., Diniz, P.B., Pinheiro, M.S., Albuquerque-Júnior, R.L., Thomazzi, S.M. (2016, January 25). Gastroprotective effects of thymol on acute and chronic ulcers in rats: The role of prostaglandins, ATP-sensitive K(+) channels, and gastric mucus secretion. *Chem Biol Interact.* Retrieved from http://www.ncbi.nlm.nih.gov/pubmed/26689173

208 Pesavento, G., Maggini, V., Maida, I., Lo Nostro, A., Calonico, C., Sassoli, C., Perrin, E., Fondi, M., Mengoni, A., Chiellini, C., Vannacci, A., Gallo, E., Gori, L., Bogani, P., Bilia, A.R., Campana, S., Ravenni, N., Dolce, D., Firenzuoli, F., Fani, R. (2016, June). Essential Oil from Origanum vulgare Completely Inhibits the Growth of Multidrug-Resistant Cystic Fibrosis Pathogens. *Nat Prod Commun.* Retrieved from http://www.ncbi.nlm.nih.gov/pubmed/27534136

209 Su, S., Wang, T., Duan, J.A., Zhou, W., Hua, Y.Q., Tang, Y.P., Yu, L., Qian, D.W. (2011, March 24). Anti-inflammatory and analgesic activity of different extracts of Commiphora myrrha. *J Ethnopharmacol.* Retrieved from http://www.ncbi.nlm.nih.gov/pubmed/21167270

210 Cronin, H., Draelos, Z.D. (2010, September). Top 10 botanical ingredients in 2010 anti-aging creams. *J Cosmet Dermatol*. Retrieved from http://www.ncbi.nlm.nih.gov/pubmed/?term=citronel-lol+skin+health

211 Youdim, K.A., Deans, S.G. (2000, January). Effect of thyme oil and thymol dietary supplementation on the antioxidant status and fatty acid composition of the aging rat brain. *Br J Nutr*. Retrieved from http://www.ncbi.nlm.nih.gov/pubmed/10703468

212 Sakkas, H., Gousia, P., Economou, V., Sakkas, V., Petsios, S., Papadopoulou, C. (2016, May 30). In vitro antimicrobial activity of five essential oils on multidrug resistant Gram-negative clinical isolates. *J Intercult Ethnopharmacol*. Retrieved from http://www.ncbi.nlm.nih.gov/pubmed/27366345

213 Minami, M., Kita, M., Nakaya, T., Yamamoto, T., Kuriyama, H., Imanishi, J. (2003). The inhibitory effect of essential oils on herpes simplex virus type-1 replication in vitro. *Microbiol Immunol*. Retrieved from http://www.ncbi.nlm.nih.gov/pubmed/14584615

214 Ogden, C.L., Carroll, M.D., Kit, B.K., Flegal, K.M. (2012). How many people are affected by/at risk for obesity and overweight? *Centers for Disease Control and Prevention*. Retrieved from https://www.nichd.nih.gov/health/topics/obesity/conditioninfo/Pages/risk.aspx

215 (2011). Health Benefits of Black Pepper Essential Oil. *Organic Facts*. Retrieved from https://www.organicfacts.net/health-benefits/essential-oils/health-benefits-of-black-pepper-essential-oil.html

216 Shen, J., Niijima, A., Tanida, M., Horii, Y., Maeda, K., Nagai, K. (2005, June 3). Olfactory stimulation with scent of grapefruit oil affects autonomic nerves, lipolysis and appetite in rats. *Neurosci Lett*. Retrieved from http://www.ncbi.nlm.nih.gov/pubmed/15862904

PART IV

Chapter 6

1 Mohd. Razali Salleh. Life Event, Stress and Illness. *Malays J Med Sci. 2008 Oct; 15(4): 9–18*. Retrieved from http://www.ncbi.nlm.nih.gov/pmc/articles/PMC3341916/.

2 Kunz, B. & Kunz, K. (2008). *Evidence-Based Reflexology for Health Professionals and Researchers: The Reflexology Research Series.*

3 Hodgson H. April, 2000. Does reflexology impact on cancer patients' quality of life? Nursing Standard. *Pubmed*, 11973949. Retrieved from http://www.ncbi.nlm.nih.gov/pubmed/11973949

4 Nurul Haswani Embong, Yee Chang Soh, Long Chiau Ming, and Tin Wui Wong. Revisiting reflexology: Concept, evidence, current practice, and practitioner training. *Journal of Traditional and Complementary Medicine. 2015 Oct; 5(4): 197–206*. Retrieved from http://www.ncbi.nlm.nih.gov/pmc/articles/PMC4624523/.

5 Launsø L, Brendstrup E, Arnberg S. May, 1999. An exploratory study of reflexological treatment for headache. Altern Ther Health Med. *Pubmed*, 10234869. Retrieved from http://www.ncbi.nlm.nih.gov/pubmed/10234869

6 Frankel, B.S.M. June, 1997. The effect of reflexology on baroreceptor reflex sensitivity, blood pressure and sinus arrhythmia. *Complementary Therapies in Medicine. Volume 5, Issue 2, pages 80 – 84*. Retrieved from http://www.complementarytherapiesinmedicine.com/article/S0965-2299(97)80003-9/abstract?cc=y

7 Hou WH, Chiang PT, Hsu TY, Chiu SY, Yen YC. July, 2010. Treatment effects of massage therapy in depressed people: a meta-analysis. J Clin Psychiatry. *Pubmed*, 20361919. Retrieved from http://www.ncbi.nlm.nih.gov/pubmed/20361919

8 Weerapong P, Hume PA, Kolt GS. The mechanisms of massage and effects on performance, muscle recovery and injury prevention. *Sports Medicine, 2005;35(3):235-56*. Retrieved from http://www.ncbi.nlm.nih.gov/pubmed/15730338.

9 Li, Y., Wang, F., Feng, C., Yang, X., & Sun, Y. (2014). Massage Therapy for Fibromyalgia: A Systematic Review and Meta-Analysis of Randomized Controlled Trials. *PLoS ONE, 9(2), e89304*. http://doi.org/10.1371/journal.pone.0089304

10 Morhenn V, Beavin LE, Zak PJ. November-December, 2012. Massage increases oxytocin and reduces adrenocorticotropin hormone in humans. Altern Ther Health Med. *Pubmed*, 23251939. Retrieved from http://www.ncbi.nlm.nih.gov/pubmed/23251939

11 Crane JD, Ogborn DI, Cupido C, Melov S, Hubbard A, Bourgeois JM, Tarnopolsky MA. February, 2012. Massage therapy attenuates inflammatory signaling after exercise-induced muscle damage. *Sci Transl Med. Pubmed*, 22301554. Retrieved from http://www.ncbi.nlm.nih.gov/pubmed/22301554

INDEX

Page numbers in bold
indicate main articles.